STRESS DOPPLER ECHOCARDIOGRAPHY

Developments in Cardiovascular Medicine

VOLUME 105

STRESS DOPPLER ECHOCARDIOGRAPHY

Edited by

STEVE M. TEAGUE

Department of Medicine, University of Oklahoma,
Oklahoma City, Oklahoma, U.S.A.

KLUWER ACADEMIC PUBLISHERS
DORDRECHT / BOSTON / LONDON

Library of Congress Cataloging-in-Publication Data

```
Stress Doppler echocardiography / edited by Steve M. Teague.
       p.   cm. -- (Developments in cardiovascular medicine ; v. 105)

     1. Doppler echocardiography.   2. Treadmill exercise tests.
   3. Heart--Diseases--Diagnosis.    I. Teauge, Steve M., 1949-   .
   II. Series.
     [DNLM: 1. Coronary Disease--physiopathology.   2. Echocardiography,
   Doppler--methods.   3. Heart Ventricle--physiopathology.   4. Stress.
   W1 DE007VMe v. 105 / WG 141.5.S915]
   RC683.5.U5S77   1990
   616.1'207543--dc20
   DNLM/DLC
   for Library of Congress                                   89-24433
                                                                 CIP
```

ISBN-13: 978-94-010-6700-3   e-ISBN-13: 978-94-009-0477-4
DOI: 10.1007/978-94-009-0477-4

Published by Kluwer Academic Publishers,
P.O. Box 17, 3300 AA Dordrecht, The Netherlands.

Kluwer Academic Publishers incorporates
the publishing programmes of
D. Reidel, Martinus Nijhoff, Dr W. Junk and MTP Press.

Sold and distributed in the U.S.A. and Canada
by Kluwer Academic Publishers,
101 Philip Drive, Norwell, MA 02061, U.S.A.

In all other countries, sold and distributed
by Kluwer Academic Publishers Group,
P.O. Box 322, 3300 AH Dordrecht, The Netherlands.

Printed on acid-free paper

Contents

Preface

For almost 40 years, a small but intense group of cardiovascular investigators have evaluated cardiac performance by measuring the mass, velocity, and acceleration of blood ejected from the left ventricle. These studies reveal that energy is transferred from ventricle to blood very early in systole, and that the left ventricle is characterized as an impulse generator. Recent explosive developments in Doppler echocardiography have allowed study of the energetics of ventricular contraction through noninvasive acceleration, velocity, and volumetric flow measurements. Compared against reference standards of ejection fraction, dP/dt, and instantaneous pressure gradient across the aortic valve, Doppler acceleration and velocity measurements are highly sensitive to changes in ventricular performance.

Most patients seeking cardiovascular care present with coronary artery disease as a chief concern. This book focuses upon identification of coronary disease presence and severity through the evaluation of left ventricular Doppler ejection responses to stress loading. Chapters 1 through 4 detail basic research on the dynamics of left ventricular ejection in ischemic and nonischemic animal models. Chapters 5 through 13 present clinical correlates of changes in the Doppler systolic ejection pulse during exercise and under pharmacologic stress loading. Angiographic anatomy, thallium perfusion defects, and radionuclear ejection fraction responses serve as reference standards. Chapters 14, 15 and 16 address applications of Doppler echocardiography during the stresses of brief coronary occlusion, myocardial infarction and post infarction recovery, while chapters 17 and 20 illustrate applications of stress Doppler techniques in valvular heart disease. Chapters 18 and 19 explore theoretical analysis of the ejection pulse from Newtonian and Fourier perspectives.

In this day of medical cost containment, cost-effectiveness of new noninvasive tests must receive highest consideration. Stress Doppler echocardiography affords inexpensive, portable, accurate evaluation of ventricular performance under the demanding conditions present in the treadmill laboratory and the coronary care unit. This book summarizes the basic, clinical, and theoretical research supporting these important applications of Doppler ultrasound in the evaluation of patients with coronary artery disease.

Steve M. Teague, MD

Contributing authors

David Bennett, MD, FRCP, Department of Medicine 1, St. George's Medical School, London, SW 17 ORE England

James F. Brymer, MD, Henry Ford Hospital, 2799 West Grand Boulevard, Detroit, Michigan 48202

Robert J. Bryg, MD, Associate Professor, University of Nevada, 1000 Locust St., Reno, Nevada 89520

John W. Cooper, Assistant Technical Director, Echocardiography Laboratory, University of Alabama, Birmingham, Alabama 35294

Jorge Constantino, MD, Fellow in Cardiology, Bay State Medical Center, Springfield, Massachusetts 01199

Carolyn R Corn, MD, Assistant Professor, University of Oklahoma Health Sciences Center, P.O. Box 26901, Oklahoma City, Oklahoma 73190

Anthony D. DeMaria, MD, Professor of Medicine, University of Kentucky, College of Medicine, Lexington, Kentucky 40536–0084

Julius M. Gardin, MD, Professor of Medicine, Director, Noninvasive Laboratory, University of California, 101 City Drive South, Irvine, California 92668–3297

Robert S. Gibson, MD, Professor of Medicine, Director, Cardiac Noninvasive Laboratory, University of Virginia Health Sciences Center, Charlottesville, Virginia 22908

Michael R. Harrison, MD, Assistant Professor, University of Kentucky, College of Medicine, Lexington, Kentucky 40536–0084

Karl Isaaz, MD, Service the Cardiologie A, CHU de Nancy-Brabois, Université de Nancy, 54511 Vandoeuvre-les-Nancy, France

Fareed Khaja, MD, Director, Cardiac Catheterization Laboratory, Henry Ford Hospital, 2799 West Grand Boulevard, Detroit, Michigan 48202

Arthur J. Labovitz, MD, Associate Professor of Medicine, St. Louis University Medical Center, P.O. Box 15250, St. Louis, Missouri 63110–0250

Navin C. Nanda, MD, Professor of Medicine, University of Alabama, Birmingham, Alabama 35294

Farshad J. Nosratian, MD, Fellow in Cardiology, Department of Medicine, University of California, 101 City Drive South, Irvine, California 92668–3297

Nawzer Mehta, Ph.D., Department of Medicine 1, St. George's Medical School, London, SW 17 ORE England

George D. Mitchell, MD, Assistant Professor of Medicine, University of Connecticut, School of Medicine, Saint Francis Hospital and Medical Center, 114, Woodland Street, Hartford, Connecticut 06105

Robert Rothbart, MD, Assistant Professor, Division of Cardiology, Box B 130, 4200 East Ninth Avenue, Denver, Colorado 80262

Robert F. Rushmer, MD, Professor of Bioengineering (Emeritus), University of Washington, Seattle, Washington 98115

Hani N. Sabbah, Ph.D., Associate Director, Cardiovascular Institute, Henry Ford Heart and Vascular Institute, 2799 W. Grand Blvd., Detroit, Michigan 48202–2689

Kiran B. Sagar, MD, Assistant Professor, Medical College of Wisconsin, Cardiology Division, 8700 W. Wisconsin Ave. Milwaukee Wisconsin 53226

Abdul-Majeed Salmasi MD, Ph.D., FACA, Irvine Laboratory for Cardiovascular Investigation and Research, St. Mary's Hospital, London, W2 1NY England

Ronald Smalling, MD, Fellow in Cardiology, University of California, Los Angeles, California

Paul D. Stein, MD, Director of Cardiovascular Research, Henry Ford Heart and Vascular Institute, 2799 W. Grand Boulevard, Detroit, Michigan 48202–2689

Steve M. Teague, MD, Director, Noninvasive Laboratory, MetroHealth Medical Center, 3395 Scranton Road, Cleveland, Ohio 44109

Udho Thadani, MD, Professor of Medicine, University of Oklahoma Health Sciences Center, P.O. Box 26901, Oklahoma City, Oklahoma 73190

Wyatt F. Voyles, MD, Assistant Professor of Medicine, University of Oklahoma Health Sciences Center, P.O. Box 26901, Oklahoma City, Oklahoma 73190

L. Samuel Wann, MD, Professor of Medicine, Division of Cardiology, Milwaukee County Medical Complex, 8700 W. Wisconsin Ave., Milwaukee, Wisconsin 53226

1. The left ventricular impulse

ROBERT F. RUSHMER

University of Washington, Seattle, WA 98115, U.S.A.

1.1 Introduction

Assessment of cardiac performance and reserve capacity is a crucial element in evaluating health status and prognosis in patients with evidence of heart disease. In the past few decades, a technical revolution has provided cardiologists with an expanding array of methods for dynamic, clinical evaluation of the heart in terms of changes in pressures, dimensions, flow rates and related variables. Widespread application of these advanced technologies have converted cardiology from a highly subjective clinical discipline into a more comprehensive and quantitative analysis of the human circulation as a hydraulic system. The significance of this profound change is more readily appreciated by comparing current concepts with the generally accepted tenets of the recent past.

1.2 Historical perspective

Prior to mid-century, cardiology was more of an art than science, relying very largely on history, auscultation, and percussion supplemented by some objective indicators from vascular pressures, electrocardiography and roentgenographic evidence of changes in size and configuration of the heart. Clinical emphasis on heart size stemmed rather directly from generally accepted concepts of cardiac function embodied in Starling's law of the heart: namely that the energy released by contracting myocardium was directly related to their initial length (diastolic volume).

This generally accepted dogma was based on experiments on dog hearts that had been isolated or exposed by thoracotomy. Under these conditions, hearts beat rapidly and without change for long period unless the investigator induces responses (i.e. by adjusting inflow or outflow pressures.) There was an implied assumption that the artificially induced responses were equivalent to corresponding changes under normal control mechanisms and environmental conditions and were therefore applicable to intact animals and man.

It was an intuitively appealing concept that cardiac control was embodied in an intrinsic property of myocardium fibers, such that it would respond to either an increased volume or pressure load by distending to larger diastolic dimensions.

Steve M. Teague (ed.) Stress Doppler Echocardiography, 1–13.
© 1990 *Kluwer Academic Publishers.*

It was recognized that such innate reactions could be modulated by neurohumeral control mechanisms affecting the 'contractility' or the 'vigor' of contraction. However, these vague terms were poorly defined and lacking in recognizeable units.

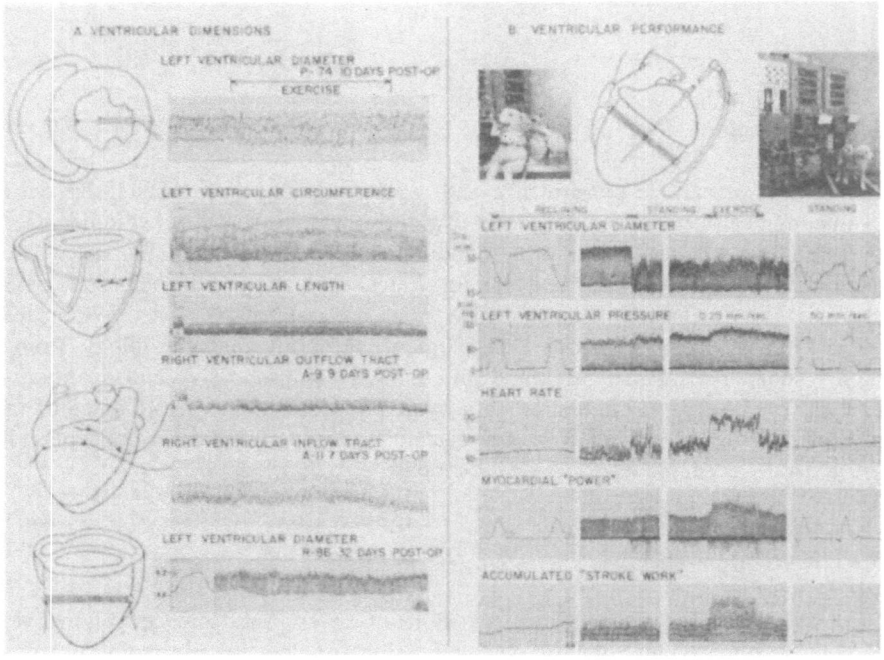

Figure 1. A) Changes in ventricular dimensions were recorded continuously during exercise and other conditions by means of recording devices surgically installed in side and on the surface of the ventricles. B) Left ventricular diameter, recorded by sonocardiometer, was at nor near maximum while reclining and diminished abruptly on standing. This unpredicted change was accompanied by changes in left ventricular pressure, heart rate and derived variables.

When samples of myocardium were stretched beyond some critical length, further elongation resulted in progressive decline in contractile energy output. This was accepted as the rationale for the dilation of cardiac chambers typically associated with heart failure. The combination of elevated venous pressure and enlargement of the affected chambers were generally associated with impaired cardiac performance at advanced stage of disease. Assessment of cardiac performance in normal subjects or at early stages of disease was dependent primarily on signs and symptoms appearing during exercise.

During the first half of this century, these attractive concepts so dominated physiological and cardiological thought that alternative views were not seriously considered. They led to widespread preoccupation with changes in the venous and

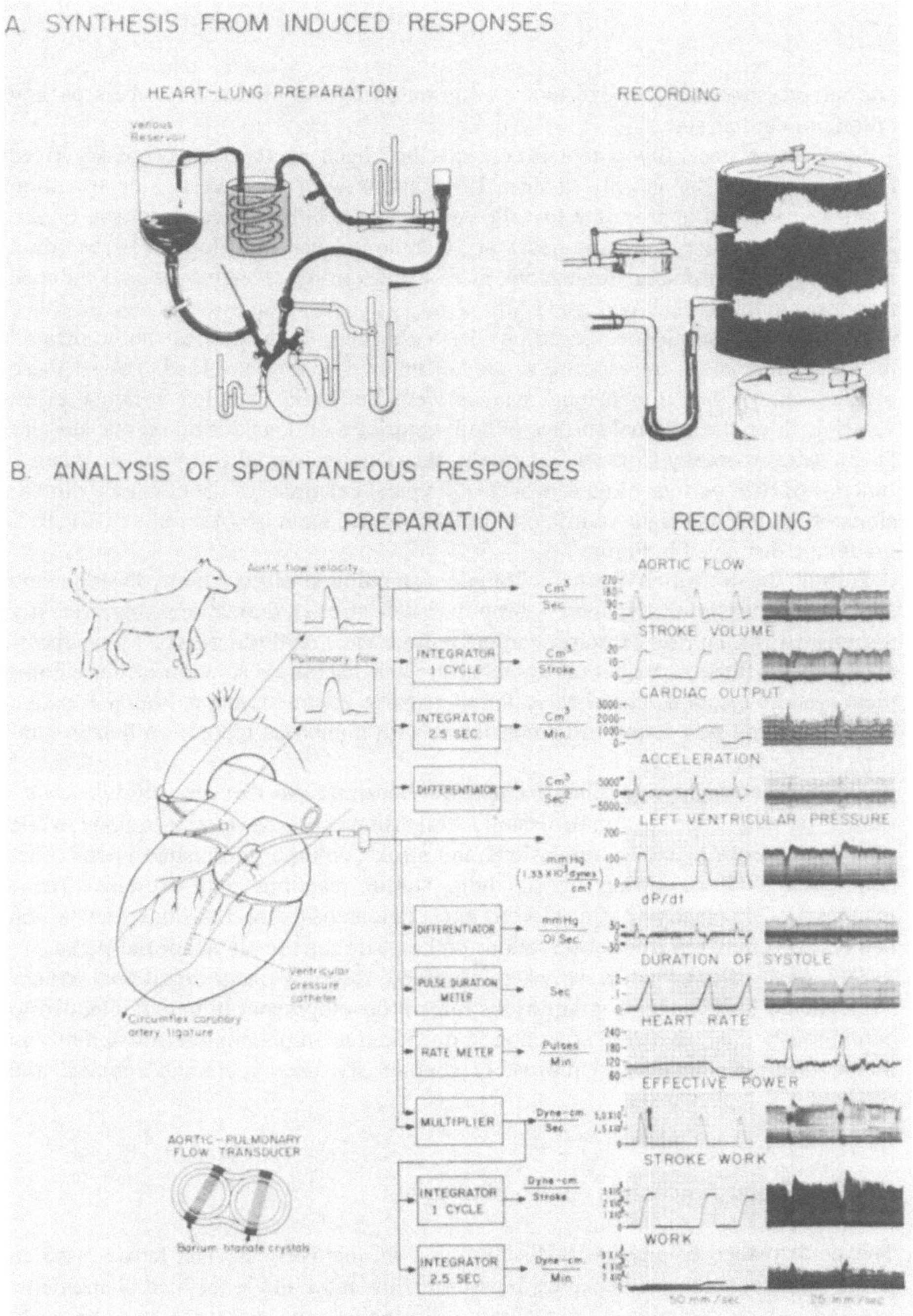

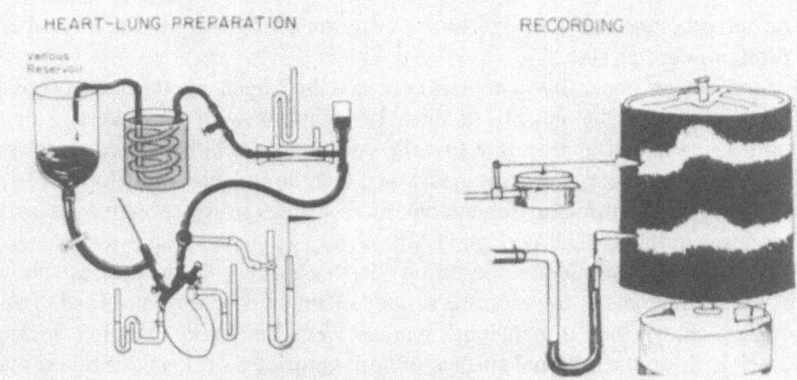

A. SYNTHESIS FROM INDUCED RESPONSES

HEART–LUNG PREPARATION

RECORDING

B. ANALYSIS OF SPONTANEOUS RESPONSES

PREPARATION

RECORDING

Figure 2. A) The traditional concepts of cardiac function and control were synthesized from studies on isolated or exposed hearts, responding to changes imposed by the investigator. B) To study cardiac function under more normal conditions, devices were developed to record and continuously analyze ventricular function quantitatively in engineering terms.

arterial pressure and the size and configuration of the cardiac chambers as key criteria of cardiac status.

Since these generally accepted concepts had been synthesized originally from hearts studied under grossly abnormal conditions with the investigator assuming control, it seemed appropriate to validate them in healthy active dogs (see Figure 2). For this purpose, new and necessary techniques were developed for recording the changing ventricular dimensions at rest and during spontaneous and induced responses in intact healthy dogs [1, 2].

According to predictions based on Starling's Law, the ventricles should distend to larger dimensions in response to greater volume or pressure load. To test these predictions, various dimensional gauges were built and installed within the left ventricle or on the external surface of both ventricles of dogs during aseptic surgery [1–3]. After recovery from the operation, the dogs recovered fully and the gauges functioned over periods of days or weeks. Typical examples of the changing dimensions of the left and right ventricles during treadmill exercise (4.5 m.p.h. on a 10% grade) are displayed in Figure 1A.

During the transition from reclining to standing postures, both diastolic and systolic dimensions declined abruptly and stroke deflections significantly diminished [4]. During exercise, cardiac output was greatly increased by tachycardia with very little contribution by either greater diastolic distention or more complete systolic ejection. The observation that stroke volume remained fairly constant during exertion was found to be consistent with numerous reports on human subjects during exercise [5].

From these and myriad other examples, it became clear that the ventricles function at or near their maximal diastolic dimensions in dogs resting quietly while recumbant. Both diastolic dimensions and stroke volume diminished under other conditions such as sitting or standing, startle reactions and exercise. These responses were clearly contrary to our expectations based on Starlings Law which had been synthesized from observations on hearts in manifestly abnormal states.

The gross discrepancies between observed responses and traditional theory stimulated a long range program of instrument development ultimately intended to continuously analyze cardiac function in quantitative engineering terms, initially in intact, healthy animals and ultimately adapted for use on human subjects and patients.

1.3 Ventricular function in engineering terms

The performance of any hydraulic pumping mechanism can best be assessed in terms of the changing dimensions, pressures, flow rates and associated phenomena. We had in hand techniques for recording dimensions and pressures, but obviously required means of continuously monitoring blood flow, specifically, ejection of blood from the ventricles.

To measure instantaneous flow velocities, pulsed ultrasonic flowmeters were developed expressly for application to the aorta, pulmonary artery and other major vessels [6]. This device was a natural outgrowth of the ultrasonic diameter gauge (sonocardiometer in Figure 1B) since it depends upon measuring extremely small differences in the transit time of brief bursts of ultrasound alternately traveling upstream and downstream diagonally across a blood vessel enclosed in a lucite cylinder (Figure 2B). An indwelling plastic tube extended from the left atrium through the posterior thoracic wall to provide access to the left ventricle for high fidelity pressure records. These devices were installed under aseptic surgical conditions for recording after the animals had fully recovered.

Additional information was obtained by means of dedicated analog computers to provide a unique, continuous, comprehensive hydraulic analysis of left ventricular function [7] as illustrated in Figure 2B. Instantaneous aortic flow velocities were recorded directly. In addition, stroke volume was indicated by steps representing the area under the flow velocity curve using integrating circuits. Successive stroke volumes were added over constant periods of 2.5 seconds to indicate changes in cardiac output.

The rate of change of velocity (acceleration) was derived from the flow signal using a differentiating circuit to register the steepness of the upslope and downslope of the flow velocity waveform. Similarly the upslope and downslope of left ventricular pressure was recorded by a differentiator to indicate the rate of change of pressure (dP/dt). The heart rate and the duration of systole were registered by interval timers triggered by the ventricular pressure signal. Effective power (the rate of performing work) was derived by a multiplier circuit giving the instantaneous product of flow and pressure. Work per stroke and work per unit time (i.e. 2.5 seconds) were also derived by means of appropriate integrating circuits.

1.4 Left ventricular dynamics

The characteristics of left ventricular function can be derived in considerable detail from the waveforms of records of aortic flow velocity and ventricular pressure and diameter (Figure 3). At the onset of systole, left ventricular pressure rises abruptly to exceed the pressure in the root of the aorta. The resultant pressure gradient rapidly accelerates blood into the aorta producing a steeply rising ejection velocity, reaching a peak in early systole. The sudden acceleration of blood is represented by the steep upslope on the velocity record which represents the rate of change of velocity or acceleration. Aortic flow acceleration is derived from the flow velocity record and displays a very steep spike in early systole, dipping below baseline as the aortic velocity slows progressively during the latter part of systole. The area under the ejection velocity waveform represents stroke volume. Cardiac output is represented by summing the successive stroke volume over a specified period of time (in this instance 2.5 seconds).

The ventricular pressure record has very steep upslopes and downslopes which can be registered as the rate of change of pressure (dP/dt): recognized for many years as an important indicator of ventricular performance. Using a multiplier circuit, the continuous product of outflow rate and ventricular pressure represents

6

the power (rate of performing work) generated by the ventricle.

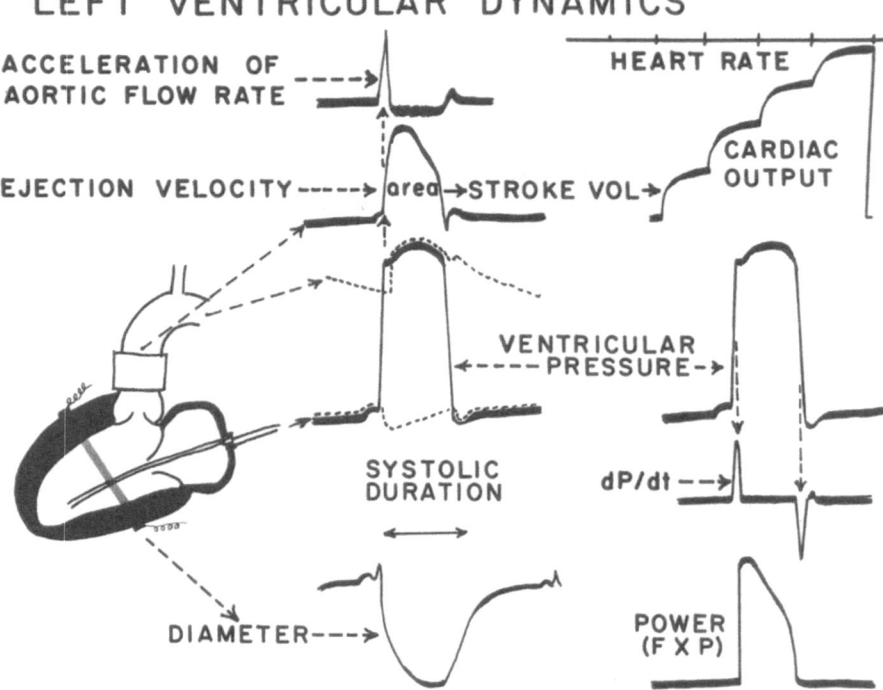

Figure 3. The dynamics of left ventricular function are indicated by the changes in ejection velocity, ventricular pressure, and derived variables such as ejection acceleration, stroke volume, heart rate, cardiac output, rate of change of pressure and power (flow X pressure).

These recordings represent a comprehensive quantitative analysis utilizing physical characteristics which can be defined and calibrated in precise engineering terms. Such variables help clarify the underlying meaning of vague terms like 'contractility' or 'vigor' of contraction as they change during exercise, startle reactions, sympathetic stimulation, administration of catecholamines and simulated pathological conditions. Examination of extensive records obtained under these conditions disclosed some characteristic changes in the various wave forms illustrated in Figure 3.

1.5 Characteristics of increased 'contractility'

Changes in 'contractility' of the ventricles are generally recognized as occurring in response to stimulation of cardiac sympathetic nerves, administration of certain catechol amines and exercise. Comprehensive analysis of left ventricular performance was recorded continuously under these and many other conditions which are generally accepted as increasing 'contractility' (Figure 4).

COMPONENTS OF INCREASED VENTRICULAR CONTRACTILITY

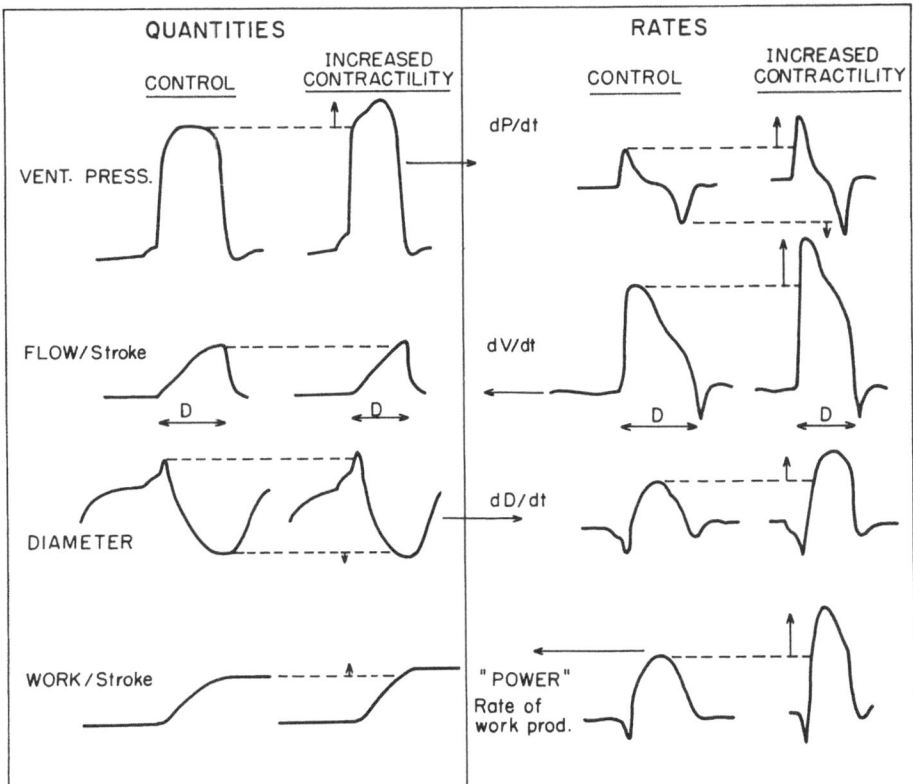

Figure 4. The most significant physical characteristics implied by the vague term 'contractility' are rate-related variables such as rate of change of pressure (dP/dt), peak velocity (rate of movement), rate of change of diameter and Power (rate of doing work). Changes in the 'quantities' displayed are less prominent or consistent.

In response to these perturbations, all of the recorded variables were affected to some degree. For example ventricular pressure, stroke volume, change in diameter during systole and work per stroke were increased somewhat. In contrast to these quantities, the rate-related variables consistently increased much more markedly. For example, heart rate, rate of change of pressure (dP/dt), flow rates (velocity) and rate of change of diameter (dD/dt) were more obviously and consistently elevated. Similarly, ventricular power (the rate of performing work) varied more than work/stroke.

8

1.6 Functional effects of increased 'contractility'

Increased contractility (i.e. during exercise) was characterized by greatly increased heart rate and slightly increased stroke volumes. Tachycardia is associated with shortened systolic intervals. Thus, increased contractility maintains stroke volume by ejecting similar volumes in shorter times. This means that the ejection velocity must increase by an amount sufficient to compensate for the shorter ejection times. By the same token, the initial acceleration of blood out of the ventricle is also enhanced. Clearly the status of ventricular function could be most readily assessed by observing the rate-related variables that best describes their dynamic properties.

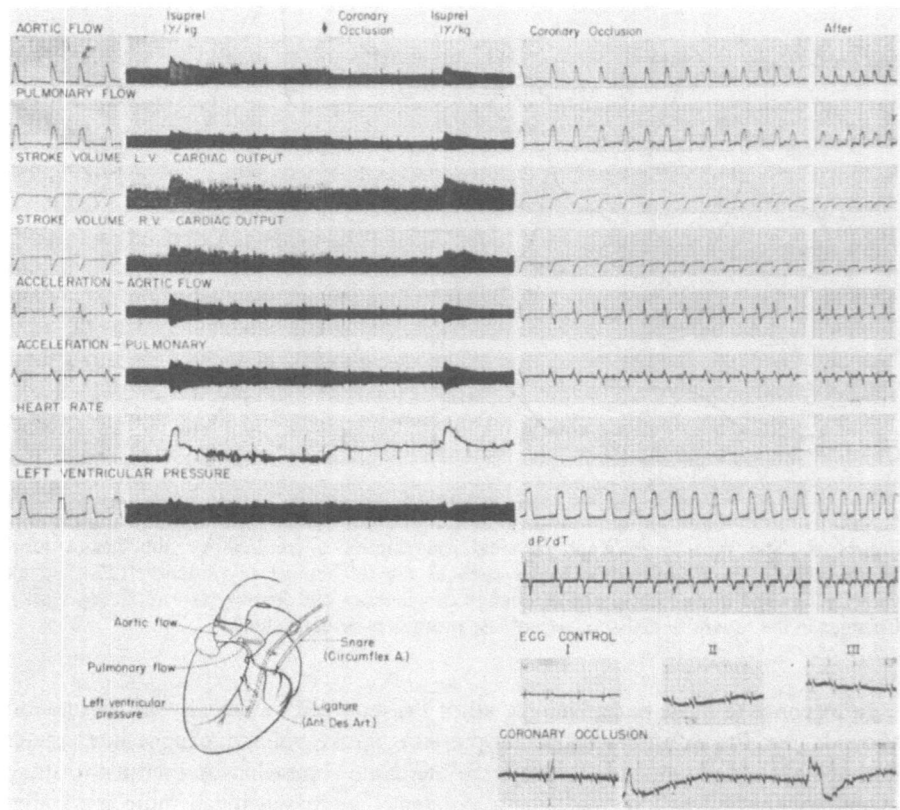

Figure 5. Acute occlusion of the circumflex coronary artery (with anterior descending coronary artery previously ligated) produced prompt reduction in pulmonary and aortic flow velocity and ejection acceleration along with depression of virtually all derived variables except for heart rate which accelerated.

LEFT VENTRICULAR IMPULSE

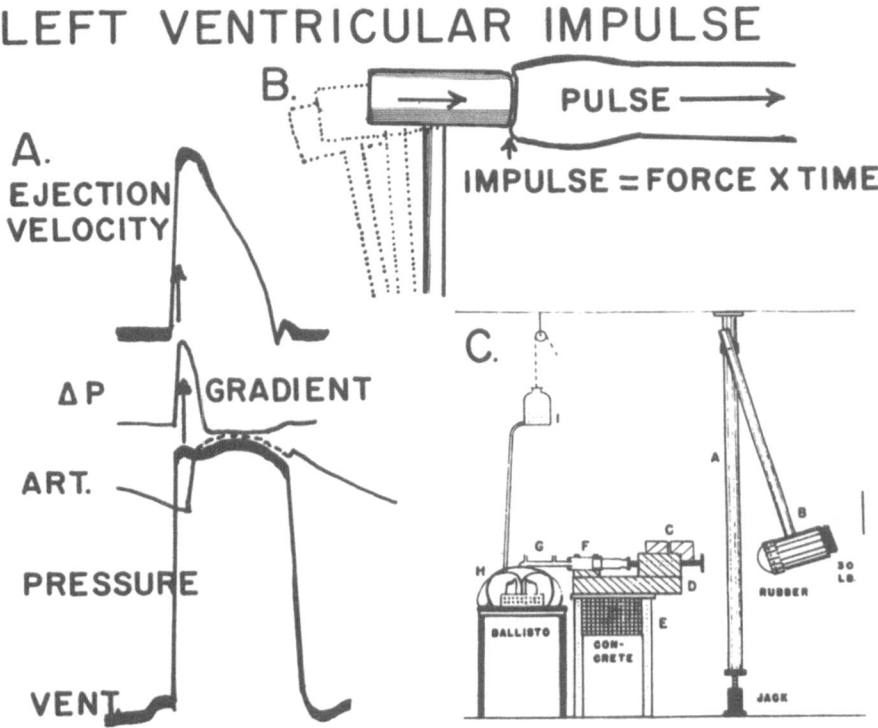

Figure 6. A) The left ventricle abruptly impels blood into the aorta by a steep pressure gradient at the onset of systole when steeply rising ventricular pressure overshoots aortic pressure. B) Left ventricular contraction resembles the impact of a heavy mallet striking the end of a column of fluid as evidenced by the experience of Isaac Starr *et al.* attempting to simulate the normal ballistocardiogram in a cadaver [10].

1.7 Acute coronary occlusion

Obstruction of a single coronary artery in dogs has little effect because collaterals from a large septal artery protect the myocardium. For this reason, we ligated the anterior descending coronary artery at the time of surgery and installed a snare around the circumflex artery in a series of experiments (Figure 5). After recovery, with the animal reclining but alert, the circumflex artery was abruptly occluded while the ventricular function was being recorded [8]. The most prominent changes in this and similar experiments were the depression of virtually all of the recorded variables of both right and left ventricles except for heart rate (Figure 5). The rate-related variables (see Figure 4) were the most severely depressed.

These observations consistently confirmed that those features of ventricular performance that were most noticeably enhanced by exercise and autonomic stimulation were also most obviously depressed by acute coronary occlusion, severe hypotension from exsanguination or administration of anesthetics (e.g. sodium pentobarbital or halothane). Indeed, the myocardial depression accompanying such anesthesia appeared to be about as severe as occurred with acute coronary occlusion.

The dominance of the rate-related characteristics of ventricular contraction under conditions specifically designed to impair function led a critical examination of these variables as potential criteria of overall ventricular performance.

1.8 The left ventricle as an impulse generator

The velocity of blood pumped by the left ventricle into the aorta has a very characteristic wave form illustrated in Figure 6A. At the onset of systole, the ejection velocity ascends abruptly to a peak after which the velocity declines to the baseline where aortic valve closure produces brief oscillations. One way to visualize such a wave form is to consider the effects of a heavy mallet forcefully striking a column of fluid contained within a distensible hose (Figure 6B). The kinetic energy in the moving mallet is delivered to the liquid at the point of impact and induces abrupt increase in velocity or acceleration of flow [9]. At the initial impact, the liquid in the proximal end of the tube accelerates rapidly to a peak velocity and then slows down as momentum carries it forward. The long column of fluid cannot accelerate instantly along its length because of its inertia. Instead, the proximal part of the column is distended and this localized region of distention proceeds at high velocity along the tube in the form of a pulse.

The impetus for the sudden acceleration of ejection velocity was clarified by a timely report by Spencer and Greiss [10] who measured simultaneously the pressures in the left ventricle and in the aorta just above the valve. Their high fidelity records clearly disclosed that ventricular pressure rises abruptly at the onset of systole and overshoots the pressure in the root of the aorta. A brief but powerful pressure difference or gradient occurs at the onset of systole, precisely when the sudden acceleration occurs. During the remainder of the systolic interval, the aortic pressure slightly exceeds ventricular pressure as the ejected bolus of blood slows down.

This series of hydraulic events indicates that the contracting ventricle generates a sudden impulse. In the case of ventricular systole, the force is extremely powerful acting over a very brief period. Confirmation of this perception stemmed from a completely unexpected source; namely the experience of Isaac Starr and his colleagues [11] in attempting to simulate the ballistocardiographic deflections of normal human subjects by driving blood into the aorta of a cadaver lying on a ballistocardiographic table. They had difficulty impelling blood into the aorta with sufficient force to approach the amplitude of deflections that occur with human heart beats. They finally found it necessary to utilize the force of a 30 pound mass swinging downward on an 8 foot arm to impact a large syringe and drive blood into the aorta of the cadaver, as illustrated in Figure 6C. To match the impact of a heavy mallet, the contracting myocardium must shorten convulsively to accelerate blood into the aorta so quickly to its peak velocity.

The most striking and useful criteria for assessing the performance of the left ventricle in dogs are illustrated in Figure 7. Striking differences between normal controls, sympathetic stimulation and impaired function (i.e. acute coronary occlusion) are manifest in acceleration, peak ejection velocity and rate of change of ventricular pressure (dP/dt) as shown schematically in Figure 7.

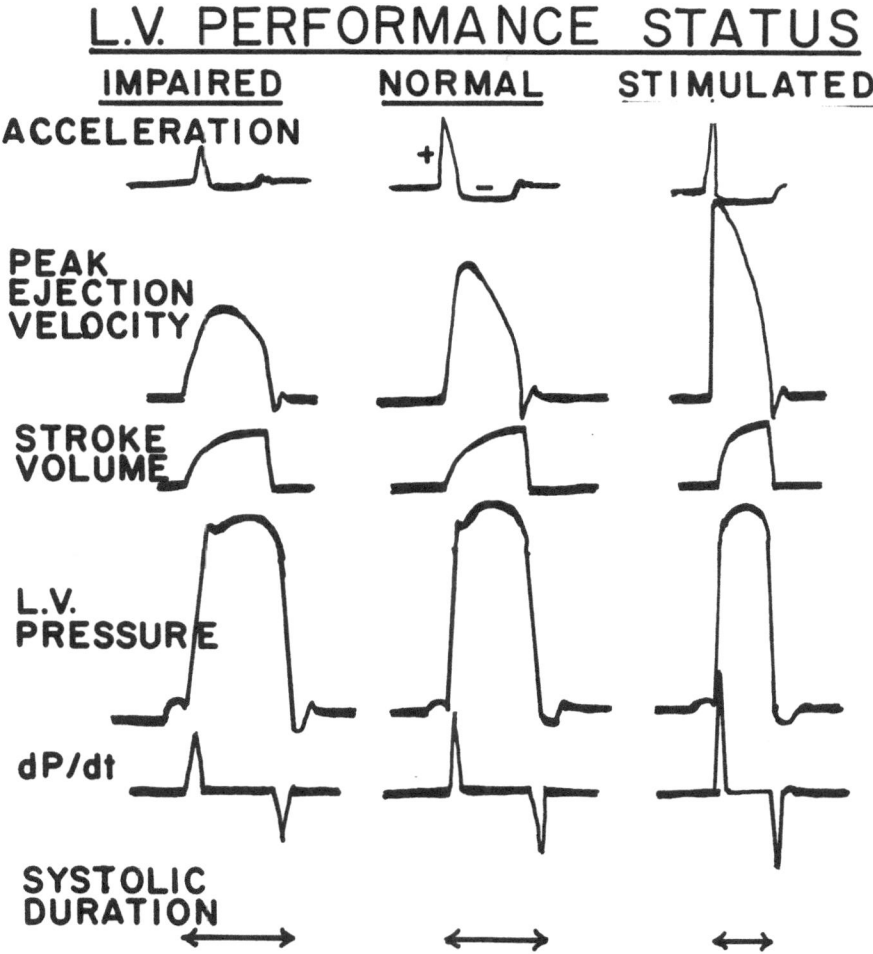

Figure 7. Left ventricular performance can best be assessed in terms of the changes in peak ejection velocity, acceleration and rate of change of ventricular pressure (dP/dt) under conditions which either enhance or depress its function.

1.9 Evaluating ventricular performance in humans

Decrements in performance of such an impulse generator should logically be manifest in reduction in both the peak acceleration and the peak velocity attained during systolic contraction. Fortunately both of these crucial variables can be readily registered in human subjects and patients using ultrasonic Doppler flow sensors positioned at the suprasternal notch.

The ultrasonic Doppler flowmeter [12] was designed to replace the transit-time flowmeter because it was more stable and reliable. Since it was based on the change in frequency of continuous waves of ultrasound, backscattered from moving red blood cells, it was readily adaptable to recording of blood flow velocity in blood vessels deep within the body when the transducers were applied to the skin at appropriate locations on the body surface. Thus, the ultrasonic Doppler flowmeter was adapted for use in human subjects and patients as a non-invasive method of measurement. By positioning the transducer in the supersternal notch, the flow velocity (and acceleration) of blood ejected into the root of the aorta could be recorded continuously [13,14]. Being painless and risk-free, this method could be used routinely for screening or monitoring the status of ventricular performance at rest or even during certain types of exercise (i.e. recumbant or on a stationary bicycle). Dimensional measurements indicating the position and movement of the walls of the heart can be recorded by means of echocardiography in one or two dimensions.

Left ventricular pressure is not yet accessible by non-invasive techniques. For this reason, it is not now possible to achieve such as comprehensive an analysis of left ventricular function routinely in man as can be achieved in dogs with implanted gauges. However, the combination of peak flow velocity, ejection acceleration and the movements of ventricular walls by means of ultrasonic echocardiography represent rational approaches to assessment of performance and status of the heart by totally non-invasive methods. Their application to basic and clinical investigations will be fully covered in other chapters of this publication.

Acknowledgements

This report is based largely on a series of studies conducted as a team effort in research and development involving invaluable contributions by Don Baker, Dick Ellis, Dean Franklin, Don Harding, John Ofstad, Wayne Quinton, Jack Reid, Bill Schlegel, Dennis Watkins, and Robert Van Citters.

References

1. Rushmer RF, Crystal DK, and Wagner C. The functional anatomy of ventricular contraction. Circ Res 1953; 4:684–688.
2. Rushmer RF. Initial phase of ventricular contraction; asynchronous contraction. Am J

Physiol 1956; 184:188–194.

3. Rushmer RF, Franklin DL, and Ellis RM. Left ventricular dimensions recorded by sonocardiometry. Circ Res 1956; 4:684–688.

4. Rushmer RF. Postural effects on the baselines of ventricular performance. Circulation 1959; 20:897–905.

5. Rushmer RF. Constancy of stroke volume in ventricular responses to exertion. Am J Physiol 1959; 196:745–750.

6. Franklin DL, Baker DW, Ellis RM, and Rushmer RF. A pulsed ultrasonic flowmeter. IEEE Trans on Med Electronics 1959; ME. 6:204–206.

7. Franklin DL, Van Citters RL, and Rushmer RF. Left ventricular function described in physical terms. Circ Res 1962; 11:702–711.

8. Rushmer FR, Watson N, Harding C and Baker. Effects of acute coronary occlusion on performance of right and left ventricles in intact, unanesthetized dogs. Am Heart J 1963; 66:522–531.

9. Rushmer RF. Initial ventricular impulse; a potential key to cardiac evaluation. Circulation 1964; 24:268–283.

10. Spencer MP, and Greiss FS. Dynamics of ventricular ejection. Circ Res 1962; 10:274–279.

11. Starr I, Schnabel TG, Jr. and Maycock RL. Studies made by simulating systole at necropsy, II. Experiments on the relation of cardiac and peripheral factors to the generation of the pulse wave and ballistocardiogram. Circulation 1953; 8:44–61.

12. Franklin DL, Schlegel W, and Rushmer RF. Blood flow measured by Doppler frequency shift of back-scattered ultrasound. Science 1961; 134:564.

13. Light H. Noninjurious ultrasonic technique for observing flow in the human aorta. Nature 1969; 224–119.

14. Huntsman LL, Gams C, Johnson CC, and Fairbanks E. Transcutaneous determination of aortic blood flow velocities in man. Am Heart J 1975; 89:605–612.

2. Effect of preload, afterload, and inotropic state on Doppler ejection dynamics

L. SAMUEL WANN and KIRAN B. SAGAR

Cardiology Division, Medical College of Wisconsin, 8700 W. Wisconsin Avenue, Milwaukee, Wisconsin 53226, U.S.A.

2.1 Introduction

Early studies on isolated papillary muscle [1] emphasized the importance of the initial velocity of ventricular muscle shortening as an index of muscular function and contractility. Rushmer [2] popularized the concept of the 'initial ventricular impulse' as a manifestation of left ventricular function over 20 years ago. Using electromagnetic flowmeters, the velocity and acceleration of blood flow in the ascending aorta have been shown to be closely related to left ventricular function [3–5] to be effected in a characteristic fashion by myocardial ischemia and infarction [6, 7] and by interventions such as the administration of catecholamines [8] and propranolol [9].

Light [10] reported the non-invasive use of Doppler ultrasound to study flow in the ascending aorta in 1969. This technique has subsequently been shown to be an

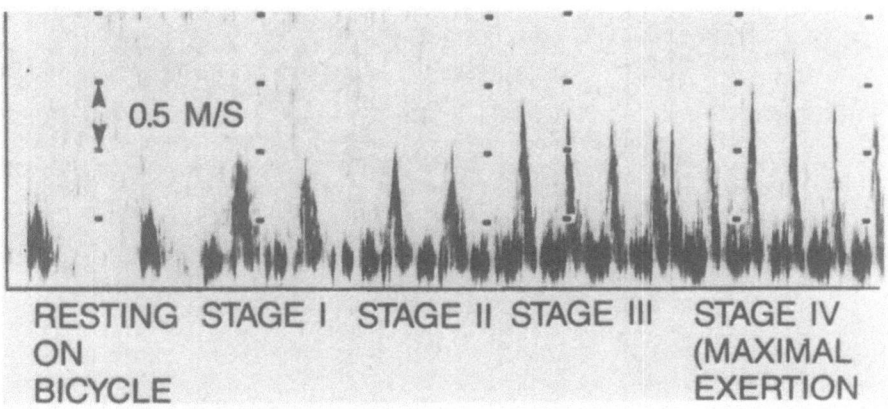

Figure 1. Suprasternal Doppler velocity profiles in a single subject at rest and during each stage of exercise. Recordings were made with a Pedof transducer in the continuous wave mode at a paper speed of 50 mm/sec.

Steve M. Teague (ed.) Stress Doppler Echocardiography, 15–23.
© 1990 *Kluwer Academic Publishers.*

16

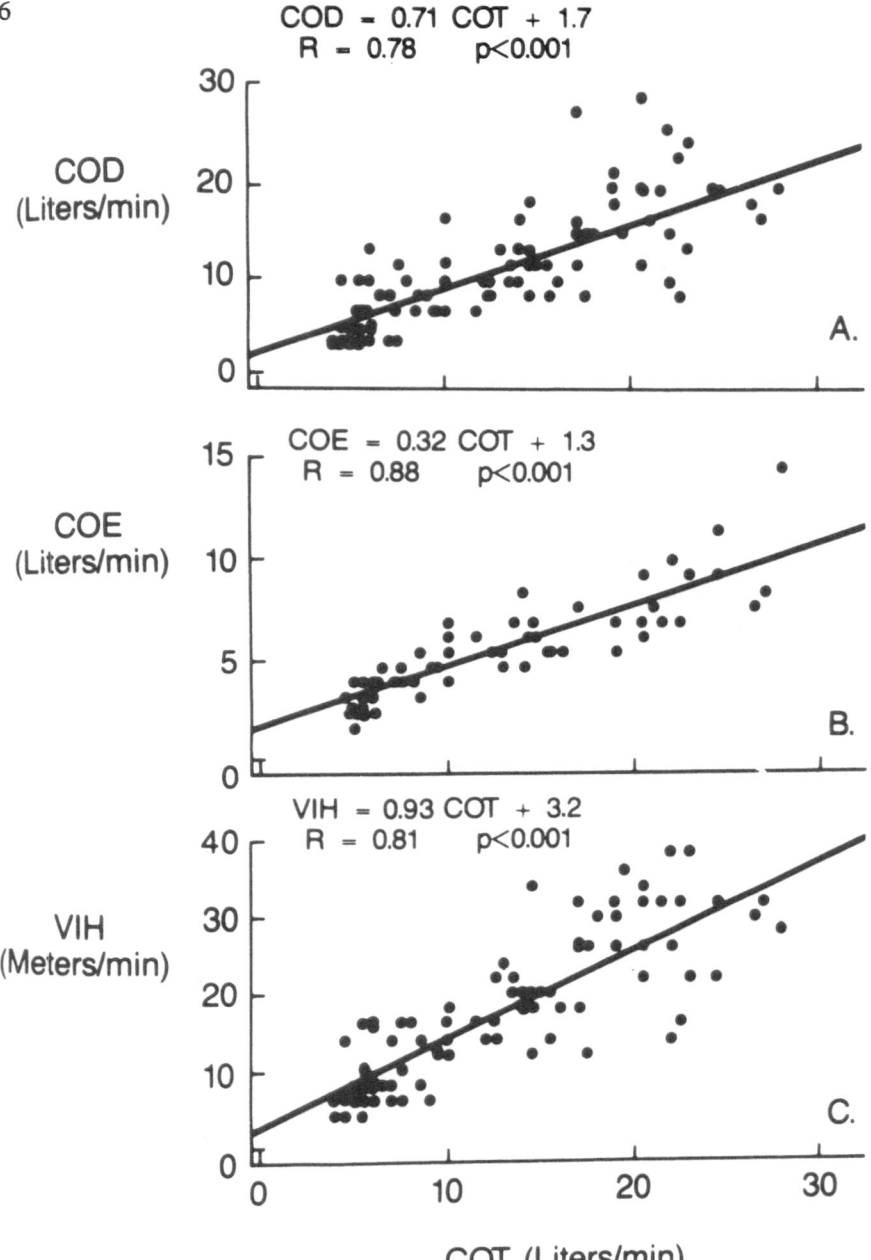

Figure 2. Regression plots comparing exercise Doppler-derived cardiac output estimates (COD), cross-sectional echocardiographic cardiac output estimates (COE), and the product of velocity integral and heart rate (VIH) with thermodilution cardiac output estimates (COT). (Doppler estimates made with aortic areas calculated from resting diameters measured at the aortic annulus with the leading edge-to-leading edge method.)

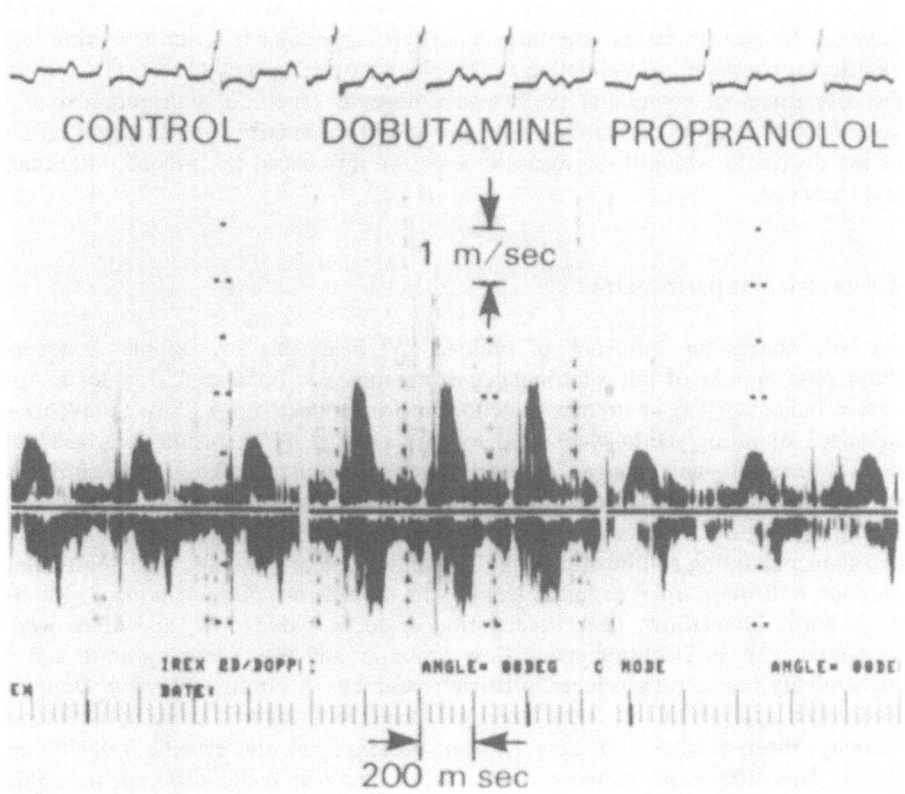

CONTROL   DOBUTAMINE PROPRANOLOL

1 m/sec

200 m sec

Figure 3. Doppler recordings and simultaneous electrocardiogram taken from a representative animal in the control state, during the infusion of dobutamine (10 ug/kg/min iv), and after administration of propranolol (1 mg/kg iv).

accurate means of detecting beat-to-beat changes in stroke volume both in experimental animals [11–13] and in man [14–17] Doppler ultrasound can be used to determine stroke volume not only at rest but also during exercise [18–20].

Unlike conventional use of ultrasound to image cardiac structures [21] little deterioration of signal due to chest wall motion and hyperventilation is seen in Doppler recordings, which we usually performed from the suprasternal notch. Shown in Figure 1 is an example of Doppler velocity profiles recorded from the suprasternal notch in a normal subject at rest and during upright bicycle exercise. Note a progressive increase in the peak velocity of flow with exercise and little deterioration of signal. Figure 2 compares regression plots of exercise cardiac output measured by Doppler and cross-sectional echocardiography to those made with thermodilution. The accuracy of Doppler cardiac output measurements during exercise appears reasonable enough to be clinically relevant.

In addition to using the Doppler derived stroke velocity integral to calculate stroke volume, Doppler ultrasonic measurements of the velocity and acceleration of flow can be used to assess other aspects of left ventricular function including left ventricular contractility. Validation of Doppler echocardiography as a useful tool in the assessment of ventricular performance depends on the demonstration of the sensitivity of Doppler measurements to changes in contractility and an appreciation of the degree to which these measurements are influenced by preload, afterload, and heart rate.

2.2 Ventricular performance

To help clarify the influence of preload and heart rate on Doppler echocardiographic indices of left ventricular performance, we compared Doppler to invasive indices of left ventricular function in 6 open-chest dogs [2,3]. Intravenous infusions of nitroglycerin were used to vary preload, atrial pacing was used to control heart rate, and changes in inotropic state were induced by 2 different doses of dobutamine (5 and 10 ug/kg/min iv) and by administration of propranolol (1 mg/kg iv). Figure 3 shows a representative Doppler recording obtained in the control state and during administration of dobutamine and propranolol. Left ventricular anterior wall myocardial segment length was used as an index of preload. Maximum aortic blood flow, peak acceleration of aortic blood flow, and dP/dt were measured with an electromagnetic flow probe around the ascending aorta and a high-fidelity pressure transducer in the left ventricle. A continuous wave Doppler transducer applied to the aortic arch was used to measured peak aortic blood velocity, mean acceleration, time to peak velocity, and the systolic velocity integral. The differences between mean values obtained under different inotropic conditions were significant at the $p < 0.01$ level for peak velocity and at the $p < 0.05$ level for mean acceleration. Within a given animal, Doppler measurements of peak velocity correlated very closely with maximum aortic flow ($r = 0.96$), maximum acceleration of aortic flow ($r = 0.95$) and with maximum dP/dt ($r = 0.92$). Mean acceleration measured by Doppler echocardiography also correlated very closely with conventional indexes, but was subject to greater interobserver variability. Doppler measurements of time to peak and the systolic velocity integral correlated less well with conventional hemodynamic indexes. Doppler measurements of peak aortic blood velocity and mean acceleration appeared to offer an effective means to noninvasively assess short-term changes in left ventricular performance under conditions of varying preload, heart rate, and inotropic state.

2.3 Afterload effects

We also investigated the influence of afterload on Doppler indices of left ventricular performance in an animal model [24]. Eight dogs with their chests opened were studied in 4 inotropic states at varying levels of heart rate and mean aortic blood pressure. Data were collected in the control state, at 2 different levels of dobutamine administration (5 and 10 ug/kg/min iv), and after administration of propranolol (0.5 mg/kg iv). In each inotropic state, phenylephrine was infused intravenously to produce at least 2 successive steady state increased of 10 mm Hg or more in mean aortic blood pressure. Within a given animal, peak velocity emerged as the Doppler index most closely correlated with changes in Q_{max}, dQ/dt, and dP/dt ($r = 0.94$, 0.91, and 0.89, respectively). Mean acceleration also correlated closely with the invasive indexes ($r = 0.87$, 0.89, and 0.89). The effect of changes in mean aortic blood pressure on Doppler index measurements was not statistically significant in any of the inotropic states and did not affect the closeness of their correlation with the invasive indexes. Doppler echocardiographic measurements of aortic blood peak velocity and mean acceleration remained as sensitive to changes

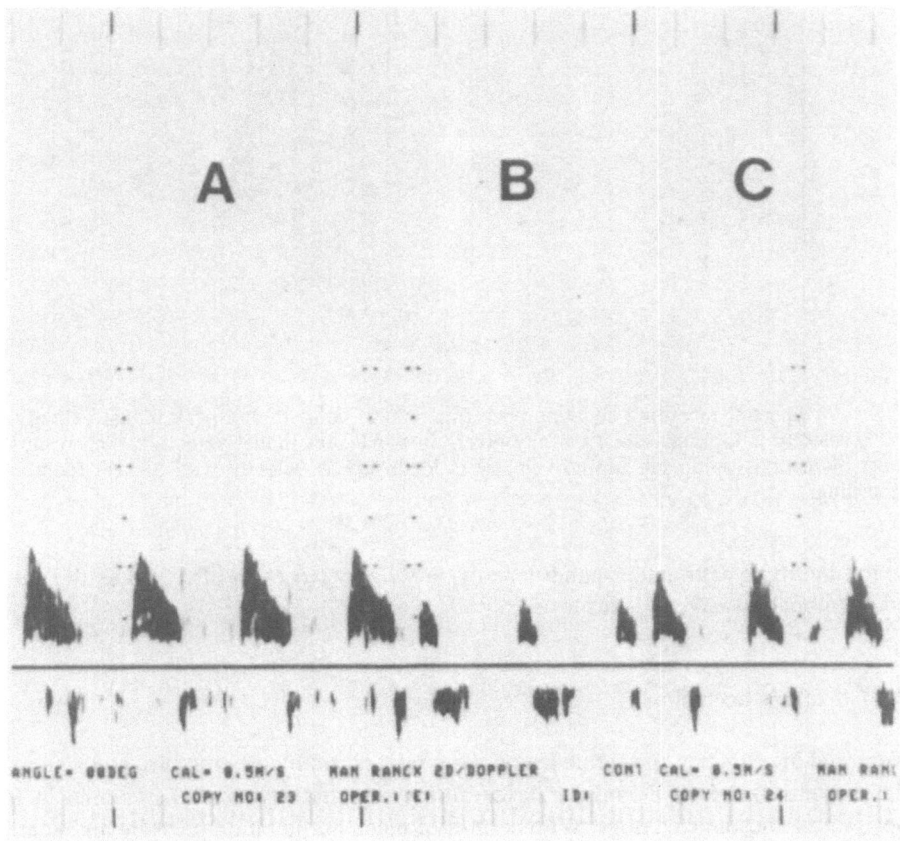

Figure 4. Effect of changes in mean aortic blood pressure on the Doppler indexes. Baseline recording (A). Proximal cx plus LAD occlusion with heart rate and blood pressure controlled by aortic compression (B). Descending aortic compression released with pacing continued (C). Note the increase in aortic blood flow velocity when aortic blood pressure was no longer controlled.

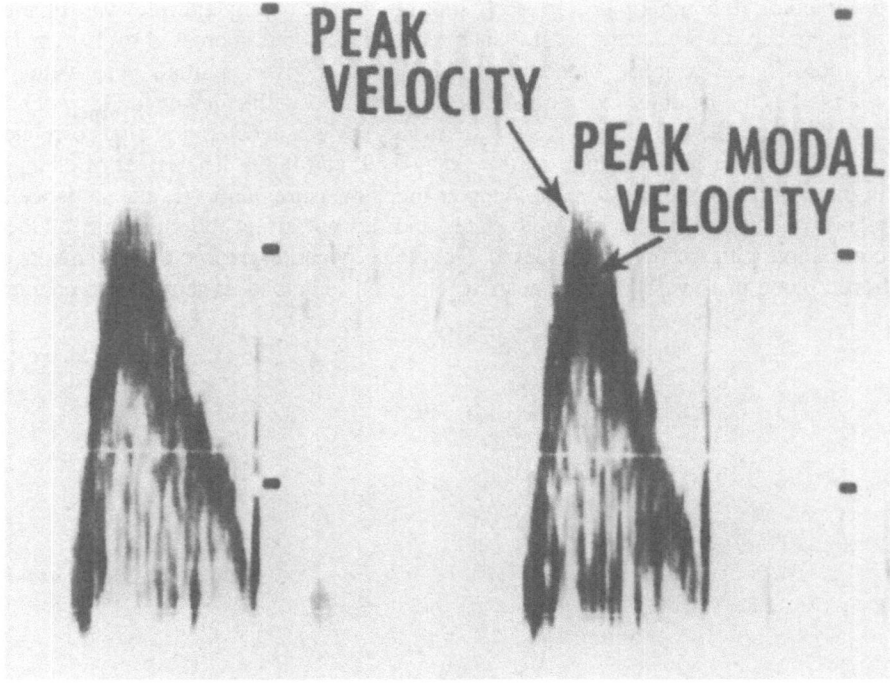

Figure 5. Spectral recording showing peak (maximum) velocity and peak modal velocity. Peak velocity is highest velocity at any given time, whereas modal velocity which occurs most often or is dominant. Modal velocity is identified as velocity with darkest spectral recording.

in the inotropic state under conditions of varying increases in afterload as did the conventional invasive indexes tested.

2.4 Coronary occlusion

Next, we investigated the influence of heart rate, aortic blood pressure, and size of the ischemic zone on Doppler indexes during regional myocardial ischemia in 8 open-chest anesthetized dogs. With control of mean aortic blood pressure and heart rate, transient coronary artery occlusion resulted in a statistically significant decline in peak velocity and mean velocity when as little as 24% of left ventricular myocardium was rendered ischemic. However, when heart rate and mean aortic blood pressure were not controlled, significant declines in peak velocity and mean velocity occurred only with simultaneous two-vessel occlusions involving > 47% of left ventricular myocardium. Although transient coronary artery occlusions generally produced no significant change in heart rate in the absence of atrial pacing, significant declines in aortic blood pressure were observed. Figure 4 shows typical changes seen in the Doppler recordings at baseline and during LAD occlusion with and without control of heart rate and blood pressure. Doppler indexes of left ventricular performance obtained during myocardial ischemia appear to be influenced not only by the extent of myocardium rendered ischemic, but also by changes in mean aortic blood pressure.

The previous studies were performed with a non-imaging continuous wave Doppler instrument which gave hard copy output of the Doppler spectral envelope using a strip chart recorder. A new type of Doppler instrument has recently become available (Exerdop-Quinton Instruments) which automatically gives an alphanumeric printout of modal velocity, peak acceleration and stroke velocity integral (Figure 5).

2.5 Accuracy assessment

To determine the accuracy of Doppler-derived modal and maximum velocity and peak and mean acceleration of ascending aortic blood for the assessment of left ventricular systolic function, we studied 6 anesthetized open-chest dogs [26]. Doppler-derived modal velocity, maximum velocity, and peak and mean acceleration were compared with left ventricular dP/dt, maximum aortic blood flow (Q_{max}), and rate of blood flow measured with an electromagnetic flow probe under varying inotropic states. Maximum Doppler velocity showed better correlation ($r = 0.94$, $y = 0.34 + 3.95$) with maximum aortic blood flow than the modal velocity ($r = 0.85$, $y = 1.49 + 3.85x$). Peak acceleration also correlated better with the rate of blood flow ($r = 0.92$, $y = 1.23 + 4.92x$) than the mean acceleration ($r = 0.83$, $y = 12.2 + 4.27x$). Modal and maximum velocity and mean and peak acceleration correlated with left ventricular dP/dt. Peak modal and peak maximum velocity and peak and mean acceleration appeared to be accurate measurements of left ventricular function. Maximum velocity and peak acceleration are more accurate than modal velocity and mean acceleration. Thus automated digital signals and conventional Doppler among signals both appear to be reliable indicators of left ventricular function.

2.6 Conclusion

We conclude from these results that Doppler echocardiographic recording of the velocity of blood flow in the ascending aorta is a useful means of assessing left ventricular function. Measurements derived from Doppler recordings closely track other independent measures of left ventricular function and are altered by clinically significant intervention such as exercise and myocardial ischemia. Doppler recordings of ascending aortic flow velocity are easy to record and the equipment used is relatively inexpensive. While the Doppler parameters are not load independent and certainly are not pure measurements of left ventricular contractility, they do appear to be clinically relevant and should achieve widespread utility.

References

1. Sonnenblick EH. Force velocity relations in mammalian heart muscle. Am J Physiol 1962; 202:931.
2. Rushmer RF. Initial ventricular impulse – a potential key to cardiac evaluation. Circulation 1964; 39:268.
3. Nobel MIM, Trenchard D, Guz A. Left ventricular ejection in conscious dogs – measurement and significance of the maximum acceleration of blood from the left ventricle. Circ Res 1966; 19:139.
4. Gabe IT, Gault JH, Ross J, Mason DT, Mills C, Schillingford JP, Braunwald E. Measurement of instantaneous blood flow velocity and pressure in conscious man with a catheter-tip velocity probe. Circulation 1969; 40:603.
5. Kolettis M, Jenkins BS, Webb-Peploe MM. Assessment of left ventricular function by indices derived from aortic flow velocity. Br Heart J 1976; 38:18.
6. Bennett ED, Else W, Miller GAH, Sutton GC, Miller HC, Nobel MIM. Maximum acceleration of blood from the left ventricle in patients with ischemic heart disease. Clin Sci and Molecular Med 1974; 46:49.
7. Kezdi P, Stanley EL, Marshall WJ, Kordenat RK. Aortic flow velocity and acceleration as an index of ventricular performance during myocardial infarction. Am J Med Sci 1969; 257:61.
8. Immiuk WEGA, Beijer HJM, Brouwer FAS, Charbon GA. Norepinephrine and isoprenaline induced changes of peripheral blood flow acceleration caused by changes of cardiac inotropy. Pflugers Arch 1976; 365:119.
9. Klinke WP, Christie LG, Nichols WW, Ray ME, Curry RC, Pepine CJ, Conti CG. Use of catheter-tip velocity-pressure transducer to evaluate left ventricular function in man. Effects of intravenous propranolol. Circulation 1980; 61:94.
10. Light LH. Non-injurious ultrasonic technique for observing flow in the human aorta. Nature 1969; 224:119.
11. Colocousis JS, Huntsman LL, Curreri PW. Estimation of stroke volume changes of ultrasound Doppler. Circulation 1977; 56:914.
12. Steingart RM, Meller J, Barovick J, Patterson R, Herman MV, Teichholz LE. Pulsed Doppler echocardiographic measurements of beat-to-beat changes in stroke volume in dogs. Circulation 1980; 62:542.
13. Fisher DC, Sahn DJ, Friedman MJ, Larson D, Valdez-Cruz LM, Horowitz S, Goldberg SJ, Allen HD. The effect of variations on pulsed Doppler sampling site on calculation of cardiac output: An experimental study in open-chest dogs. Circulation 1983; 67:370.
14. Buchtal A, Hanson GC, Pealsach AR. Transcutaneous aortovelography: Potentially useful technique in management of critically ill patients. Br Heart J 1976; 38:451.
15. Sequeira RF, Light LH, Cross G, Raftery EB. Transcutaneous aortovelography: A quantitative evaluation. Br Heart J 1976; 38:443.
16. Magnin PA, Stewart JA, Myers S, von Ramm O, Kisslo JA. Combined Doppler and phased-array echocardiographic estimation of cardiac output. Circulation 1981; 63:388.
17. Huntsman LL, Stewart DK, Barnes SR, Franklin SB, Colocousis JS, Hessel EA: Noninvasive Doppler termination of cardiac output in man. Clinical validation. Circulation 1983; 67:593.
18. Daley PJ, Sagar KB, Wann LS. Supine versus upright exercise: Doppler echocardiographic measurement of ascending aortic flow velocity. Br Heart J 1985; 54:562.
19. Loeppky JA, Greene ER, Hockanga DE, Caprihan A, Luft UC. Beat-by-beat stroke

volume assessment by pulsed Doppler in upright and supine exercise. J Appl Physiol 1981; 50:1173.

20. Christie J, Sheldahl L, Tristani F, Sagar K, Ptacin M, Wann LS. Determination of stroke volume and cardiac output during exercise: comparison of two-dimensional and Doppler echocardiography, Fick oximetry and thermodilution. Circulation 1987; 76:539–547.

21. Wann LS, Faris JV, Childress RH, Dillon JC, Weyman AE, Feigenbaum H. Exercise cross-sectional echocardiography in ischemic heart disease. Circulation 1979; 60:1300.

22. Czanski P, Sagar KB, Wann LS. Two-dimensional echocardiographic measurement of the diameter and area of the aortic annulus and ascending thoracic aorta. Am J Card Imag 1988; 2(2):142–147.

23. Wallmeyer K, Wann LS, Sagar KB, Kalbfleisch J, Klopfenstein HS. The influence of preload and heart rate on Doppler echocardiographic indexes of left ventricular performance: Comparison with invasive indexes in an experimental preparation. Circulation 1986; 74:181–186.

24. Wallmeyer K, Wann LS, Sagar KB, Czanski P, Kalbfleisch J, Klopfenstein HS. The effect of changes in afterload on Doppler echocardiographic indexes of left ventricular performance. J Am Soc Echo 1988; 1:135–140.

25. Mathias DW, Wann LS, Sagar KB, Klopfenstein HS. The effect of regional myocardial ischemia on Doppler echocardiographic indexes of left ventricular performance: influence of heart rate, aortic blood pressure, and the size of the ischemic zone. Am Heart J 1988; 116:953.

26. Sagar KB, Wann LS, Boerboom LE, Kalbfleisch J, Rhyne TL, Olinger GN. Comparison of peak and modal aortic blood flow velocities with invasive measures of left ventricular performance. J Am Soc Echo 1988; 1:194–200.

3. Effects of beta blockade, beta stimulation, and afterload upon Doppler ejection dynamics

WYATT F. VOYLES, RONALD SMALLING, UDHO THADANI, and STEVE M. TEAGUE

University of Oklahoma Health Sciences Center, P.O. Box 26901, Oklahoma City, OK 73190, U.S.A.

3.1 Introduction

Studies of the early phase of ventricular ejection and aortic blood flow primarily have involved pressure and flow measurements in the left ventricle and the ascending aorta [1–3]. Early studies in dogs used electromagnetic flowmetry and fluid-filled catheter systems with adequate frequency responses (> 50 Hz) to demonstrate that peak acceleration occurred at the time of the peak transvalvular pressure gradient [1]. Peak velocity of flow was thought to coincide with the time of transvalvular pressure crossover. Murgo *et al.* [2] studied pressure and flow relationships in humans using high fidelity pressure and velocity catheter tip transducers. Their data confirmed that peak acceleration and the peak transvalvular pressure gradient were temporally related at rest, but that peak velocity occurs prior to the time of left ventricular-aortic pressure crossover.

These observations reflect the importance of the effects of blood mass (inertia), vessel distensibility (compliance), and peripheral resistance on the pressure and flow characteristics of the central cardiovascular system. The simultaneous occurrence of peak acceleration and peak transvalvular pressure gradient suggests that during early systole, inertia is the major component governing pressure and flow relationships across the aortic valve. However, if inertia were to continue to dominate throughout systole, then peak velocity (zero acceleration) would occur at the time of zero pressure gradient.

As noted above, peak velocity occurs prior to the time of pressure crossover. This observation implies that other factors such as compliance and peripheral resistance become important influences on the pattern of ventricular ejection during the middle third of ejection.

The characteristics of early ventricular ejection prompted Rushmer [3] to describe the left ventricular performance in terms of force and time. He proposed that indices of early left ventricular ejection, such as peak blood velocities and acceleration, could be useful as measures of ventricular performance. His experiments in dogs were designed to examine the effects of exsanguination, hypotension, general anesthesia, and acute coronary occlusion on the initial ventricular

Steve M. Teague (ed.) Stress Doppler Echocardiography, 25–34.

impulse determined from measurements of left ventricular pressures and aortic flows. Each of these experimental stressors reduced the initial ventricular impulse as measured by acceleration of blood flow and peak flow velocity in the ascending aorta. These experiments were some of the first to specifically apply peak acceleration and velocity in studies of abnormal ventricular performance.

The present study examined the effects of beta blockade, beta stimulation and afterload on simultaneous measurements of isometric and isotonic ventricular ejection indices. Changes in acceleration and velocity of blood flow were correlated with rate of ventricular pressure change, transvalvular pressure gradient, and velocity of ventricular circumferential shortening during periods of pharmacologic stress. The results show that acceleration of blood in the ascending aorta is strongly associated with changes in the rate of ventricular pressure development, transvalvular pressure gradient, and velocity of circumferential shortening. Both acceleration and peak velocity are sensitive to beta stimulation. Beta blockade and afterload result in contrasting effects on these indices. Acceleration is relatively sensitive to beta blockade and insensitive to afterload when compared to peak velocity.

3.2 Methods

Instrumentation

Eight male mongrel dogs were anesthetized (30 mg/kg of sodium pentobarbital given i.v.) for instrumentation. All observations were made in closed chest animals (mean weight = 21.8 kg and range = 20 to 24 kg). Active ventilator support (tidal volume = 10 to 12 ml/kg; rate = 12 cycles/min; end expiratory pressure = 5 to 7 cm of water; room air) using a volume ventilator (Harvard Apparatus Company, Millis, MA) and cuffed endotracheal tube provided periods of stable gas exchange. Additional doses of intravenous pentobarbital (1 to 2 mg/kg) were used as needed to prevent resistance to ventilatory support and/or limb extensor responses. No observations were recorded within 5 minutes of an intravenous dose of pentobarbital.

Both carotid arteries were exposed for cannulation with pressure and velocity sensor catheter systems. A 6F dual pressure sensor (3cm spacing) catheter (Millar Instruments, Inc., Houston, TX) was inserted after balancing and calibration. This catheter was advanced using fluoroscopy so that both sensors were positioned just above the sinotubular junction of the ascending aorta. Pressure amplifiers were balanced such that electronic subtraction of analog signals (Textronix 546B 2 channel oscilloscope; Tektronix, Inc., Portland, OR) resulted in an analog output representing a pressure difference equal to 0 mmHg (10 mV = 10 mmHg). The catheter was then advanced using fluoroscopy such that the distal sensor was in the LV outflow tract and transvalvular pressure gradients could be recorded.

A 20 mHz microvascular Doppler system (MF20, Eden Medizinische Electronik and Carolina Medical Electronics, King, NC) was used with an introducer catheter to record intraaortic velocities. An 8F pigtail catheter was cut so that the catheter tip formed approximately a thirty degree angle to the catheter body. The ultrasound transducer (1.0 mm diameter) was inserted through a Y shaped swivel hub connector into this catheter such that the ultrasound transducer could be easily advanced through the catheter tip. Forward and reverse audio signals from the velocimeter (pulse repetition frequency = 100 kHz) were recorded on tape (Teac XR-310 multichannel cassette data recorder; Teac Corp, Japan; tape speed = 38.1 cm/s and band width = 75 kHz) for offline spectral analysis. This velocimeter-catheter system was fluoroscopically positioned in the ascending aorta such that the catheter tip (and ultrasound transducer) was at the level of the proximal sensor of the pressure catheter system. Range gating (up to 7 mm) was done to optimize Doppler audio frequencies.

Catheter positions were fixed using silk ligatures for ties at the carotid insertion sites. The right thorax was shaved and the dogs positioned right side down such that the shaved portion of the thorax was over a cut out portion (wooden insert) of the fluoroscopy/surgical table. A 5 mHz real time imaging transducer (Mark III Echo Imager; Advanced Technology Laboratories; Belluve, WA) was positioned from beneath the dog. Transducer orientation was adjusted to image the left ventricular cavity in the short axis plane at the midpapillary level. This transducer position was fixed using a mechanical transducer holder so that the left ventricular scan plane was maintained constant throughout each experiment.

Echocardiographic video images (including text generator output) and the electrocardiogram (lead II) were recorded (Panasonic NV8200 video cassette recorder) for off-line digitization and data processing. Doppler audio signals and all analog signals (pressures and electrocardiogram) were recorded (TEAC SR-310 multichannel cassette data recorder) for off-line data processing. A common synchronization signal was used for beat-by-beat matching of pressure, velocities and ventricular endocardial circumferences.

Experimental protocols

After instrumentation and a 15–30 minute equilibration period (less than 10% variation in heart rate and peak systolic pressure), control measurements of pressures, velocities and ventricular endocardial circumferences were recorded for at least 10 consecutive beats. An intravenous infusion of phenylephrine (0.2 mg/min) was started and titrated to produce approximately a 50% increase (±10%) in peak systolic pressure. Pressures, velocities, and ventricular endocardial circumferences were then recorded for at least 10 consecutive beats and the phenylephrine infusion was discontinued. After heart rate and peak systolic pressures returned to control levels (±10%), an intravenous bolus of isoproterenol (4 mg) was administered. At or just following the peak heart rate response, pressures, velocities and ventricular endocardial circumferences were recorded for at least 10 consecutive beats. Heart rate and peak systolic pressure were allowed to return to control values (±10%). Following return to control status, an intravenous bolus of propranolol (1 mg/kg) was administered. Pressures, velocities and ventricular endocardial circumferences were recorded for at least 10 consecutive beats at one and four minutes post injection. This sequence of administering three pharmacologic stressors was followed in all dogs.

Data compilation

Left ventricular pressures, aortic pressures, transvalvular pressure gradients and electrocardiograms were transcribed to hardcopy (Gould ES 1000 electrostatic recorder, Gould Instrument Division, Cleveland, OH) at a paper speed of 250 mm/sec. Doppler frequency shift spectra were processed by fast Fourier transform spectral analysis (MK 500 real time spectral analyzer; Advanced Technology Laboratories, Bellevue, WA) and transcribed to hardcopy. By reducing the recorder playback speed by 50% (recording speed = 38.1 cm/s), aliased frequencies (if any) could be displayed without spectral wrap-around at a paper speed of 200 mm/s. End systolic and diastolic freeze frame images (frame rate = 30/s) and accompanying electrocardiographic signals were printed on hardcopy (Mitsubishi Video Copy Processor, Mitsubishi America, Inc., Cypress, CA). These hardcopy recordings of images, waveforms, and calibration scales were digitized (Sigma-Scan software; Jandel Scientific electronic tablet, Jandel Corp, Sausalito, CA) for computing linear distances, slopes and circumferences. Five consecutive and simultaneous cycles were averaged for the following response variables:

1) heart rate (calculated from R-R intervals) (bpm);
2) peak systolic blood pressure (mmHg);
3) maximum transvalvular pressure gradient (mmHg);
4) maximum rate of rise of systolic ventricular pressure (mmHg/s);
5) peak systolic velocity (cm/s);
6) peak acceleration (m/s/s); and
7) velocity of endocardial circumferential shortening (1/s).

Statistical methods

Results from all response variables were summarized as mean ± standard deviation. Nonparametric methods (sign test) were used to determine the significance of changes relative to control values. Differences yielding p values < 0.05 were considered statistically significant.

3.3 Results

Average (± SD) hemodynamic responses to the three pharmacologic stressors used in this study are shown in Table 1. Nonparametric methods were used to test for significant responses to stressors because of inter-animal variations in control measurements (coefficients of variation range from 13 to 50%). These results are shown in Table 2. Phenylephrine resulted in: (1) significant increases in peak sys-

Table 1. Average (± SD) responses to pharmacologic stressors (n=8).

	CTRL	PE	ISO	PRO
HR	146	119	180	113
(bpm)	(±19)	(±27)	(±24)	(±12)
PSP	170	245	168	149
(mmHg)	(±28)	(±62)	(±28)	(±39)
Max Press Grad	6	5	20	4
(mmHg)	(±3)	(±3)	(±11)	(±2)
DP/DT	2609	3114	8515	1353
(mmHg/s)	(±1232)	(±1204)	(±3697)	(±668)
VCF	1.8	1.2	6.0	1.2
(1/s)	(±1.1)	(±0.8)	(±2.8)	(±0.6)
Peak Acc	23.3	17.4	85.5	12.7
(m/s/s)	(±3.7)	(±9.2)	(±26)	(±4.4)
Peak Vel	60	47	105	52
(cm/s)	(±12)	(±14)	(±242)	(±14)

Abbreviations: CTRL = control; PE = phenylephrine; ISO = isoproterenol; PRO = propranolol; HR = heart rate; PSP = peak systolic blood pressure; Max Press Grad = maximum systolic pressure gradient; DP/DT = maximum rate of left ventricular pressure rise; VCF = velocity of endocardial circumferential shortening; Peak Acc = peak acceleration; Peak Vel = peak velocity.

Table 2. Summary of significant directional responses to pharmacologic stressors relative to control state (n=8).

	PE	ISO	BB
HR (bpm)	NC	+	−
PSP (mmHg)	+	NC	−
Max Press Grad (mmHg)	NC	+	−
DP/DT (mmHg/s)	+	+	−
VCF (1/s)	−	+	−
Peak Acc (m/s/s)	NC	+	−
Peak Vel (cm/s)	−	+	NC

Abbreviations: + = Increase; − = Decrease; NC = No Change; Otherwise as in Table 1.

tolic pressure (8 of 8 animals) and maximum rate of rise in left ventricular pressure (7 of 8 animals); (2) significant decreases in velocity of endocardial circumferential shortening (8 of 8 animals) and peak velocity (8 of 8 animals); and (3) no significant directional changes in heart rate, maximum systolic pressure gradient, or peak acceleration. Isoproterenol resulted in: (1) significant increases in heart rate, maximum systolic pressure gradient, maximum rate of rise in left ventricular pressure, velocity of endocardial circumferential shortening, peak acceleration, and peak velocity (8 of 8 animals for all response variables); and (2) no significant directional changes in peak systolic pressure. Propranolol (4 minutes post infusion) resulted in: (1) significant decreases in heart rate, peak systolic pressure, maximum systolic pressure gradient, maximum rate of rise in left ventricular pressure, velocity of endocardial circumferential shortening, and peak acceleration (8 of 8 animals for all response variables); and (2) no significant directional change in peak velocity.

Figures 1 through 3 show correlations for absolute changes from control values (stress minus control measurements) between early ventricular ejection indices (peak acceleration and velocity) and three other measures of systolic ventricular performance: (1) maximum rate of rise in left ventricular pressure; (2) maximum systolic pressure gradient; and (3) velocity of endocardial circumferential shortening. Correlation coefficients for the relationships between both peak acceleration and peak velocity and each of these measures of systolic ventricular performance were statistically significant. However, the strongest relationships were between peak acceleration and (1) maximum rate of rise in left ventricular pressure (dP/dt) ($r = 0.90$ vs 0.73 for peak velocity), (2) maximum systolic pressure gradient ($r = 0.94$ vs 0.69); and (3) velocity of endocardial circumferential shortening ($r = 0.83$ vs 0.72).

3.4 Discussion

An association between the timing of peak acceleration and maximum transvalvular pressure gradient (within the first 50 ms of valve opening) has been shown in studies by other investigators [1, 2]. This study demonstrates that maximum transvalvular pressure gradients can be altered by pharmacologic agents (particularly beta stimulation with isoproterenol). Furthermore, peak acceleration is strongly correlated with changes in maximum transvalvular pressure gradient as well as maximum rate of rise in ventricular pressure, and velocities of circumferential shortening. There was complete concordance with respect to directional changes in peak acceleration, maximum transvalvular pressure gradient and heart rate for each pharmacologic stressor. Peak acceleration was not significantly changed by phenylephrine. This response indicates that peak acceleration is insensitive to increases (up to 50%) in peak systolic pressure, and supports the assertion by Murgo et al. [2], that inertia is the major factor governing early pressure and flow relationships across the aortic valve. The increase in the rate of rise of ventricular pressure with phenylephrine infusion probably reflects the presence of intramyocardial alpha receptors in the species, and a resultant positive inotropic effect [4]. This effect was not translated into increases in peak acceleration, but may have played a role in preventing decreases in peak acceleration with phenylephrine induced increases in afterload.

Alternatively, the associations between peak velocity and other measures of ventricular performance were less impressive. In this study, changes in peak velocity were unrelated to changes in heart rate, but concordant with changes in end-systolic circumference. Peak velocity was sensitive to beta stimulation, but not influenced by beta blockade. Clearly, peak blood velocities in the ascending aorta

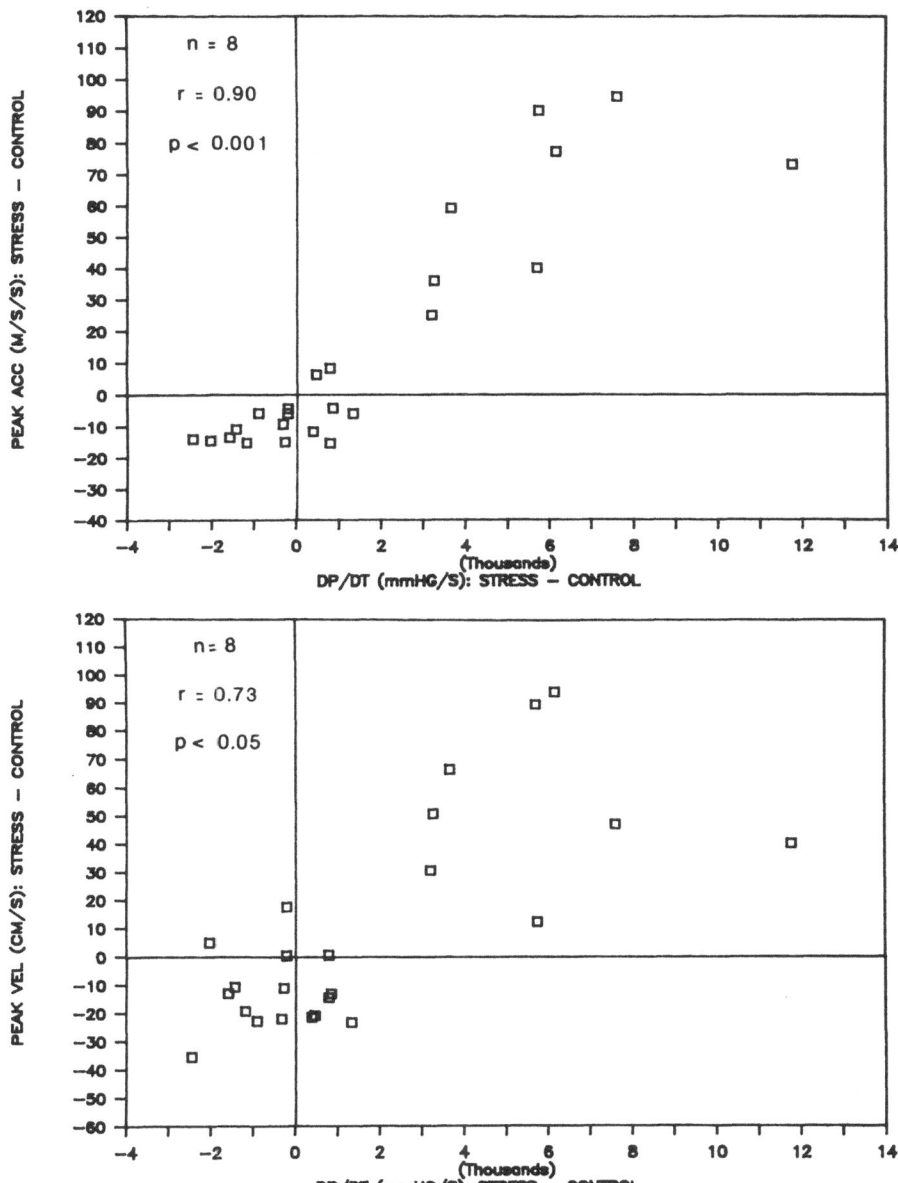

Figure 1. Correlation between absolute changes (stress minus control measurements) in maximum rate of rise in left ventricular pressure and (1) peak acceleration (Panel A) and (2) peak velocity (Panel B). Abbreviations: DP/DT = rate of rise in left ventricular pressure; Peak Acc = peak acceleration; Peak Vel = peak velocity; n = 8 animals (three measurements each); r = correlation coefficient.

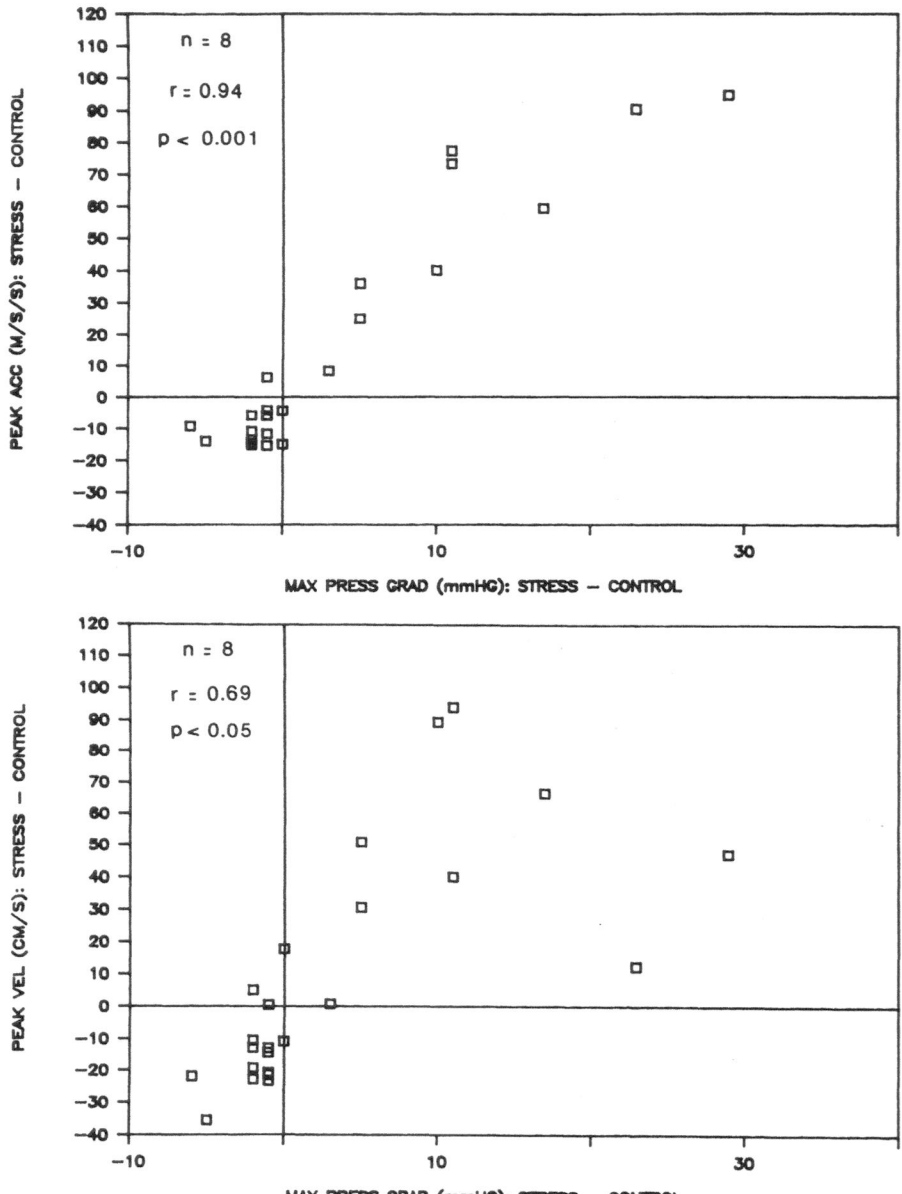

Figure 2. Correlation between absolute changes (stress minus control measurements) in maximum systolic pressure gradient and (1) peak acceleration (Panel A) and (2) peak velocity (Panel B). Abbreviations: Max Press Grad = maximum pressure gradient; otherwise as in Figure 1.

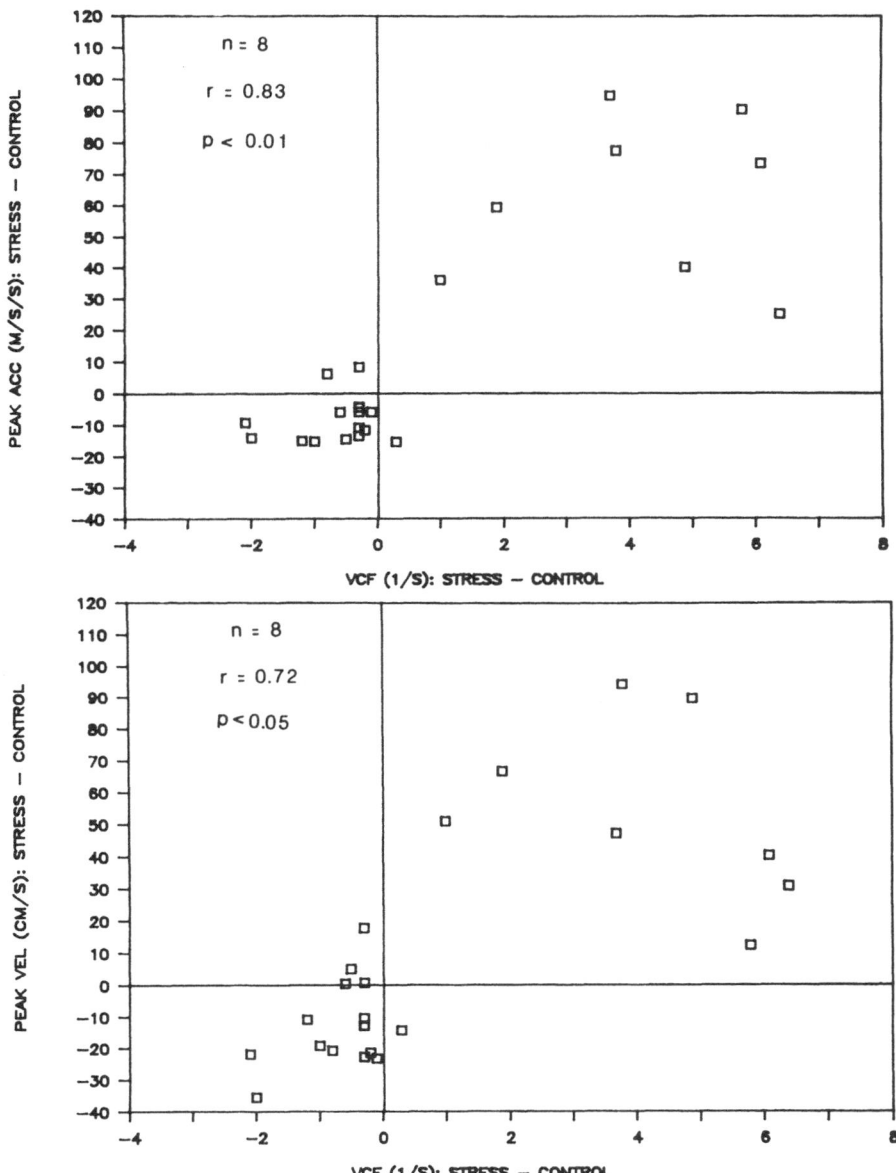

Figure 3. Correlation between absolute changes (stress minus control measurements) in velocity of endocardial circumferential shortening and (1) peak acceleration (Panel A) and (2) peak velocity (Panel B). Abbreviations: VCF = velocity of endocardial circumferential shortening; otherwise as in Figure 1.

34

are influenced by factors other than changes in contractility. As Murgo *et al.* [2] have suggested, peak velocities are probably influenced to some extent by arterial compliance and peripheral resistance. Additionally, peak velocities may also be a function of ventricular size and shape [5].

3.5 Conclusion

In conclusion, experiments using pharmacologic stressors in a closed chest animal model show that acceleration of blood in the ascending aorta is strongly associated with changes in the rate of ventricular pressure development, transvalvular pressure gradient, and velocity of circumferential shortening. Both acceleration and peak velocity are sensitive to beta stimulation. Beta blockade and afterload resulted in contrasting effects on these indices. Acceleration is relatively sensitive to beta blockade and insensitive to afterload when compared to peak velocity.

Acknowledgement

The authors gratefully acknowledge the technical support of Ms. Barbara Cleeney (Oklahoma University Health Sciences Center), and Mr. George O'Shea (VA Hospital) in the preparation of this manuscript.

References

1. Spencer MP, Greiss FC. Dynamics of ventricular ejection. Circ Res 1962; 10:274.
2. Murgo JP, Altobelli SA, Dorethy JF, *et al.* Normal ventricular ejection dynamics in man during rest and exercise. In: Leon DF, Shaver JA (ed.). Physiologic principles of heart sounds and murmurs. American Heart Association Monograph. Dallas, TX 1975. pp 92–101.
3. Rushmer, RF. Initial ventricular impulse – a potential key to cardiac evaluation. *Circulation* 1964; 29:268.
4. Corr PB, Sharma AD. Alpha-adrenergic-mediated effects on myocardial calcium. In: Opie, LH (ed.). *Calcium Antagonists and cardiovascular disease*. Raven, NY. 1984, pp 193–204.
5. Teague SM, Buro R, Voyles WF. A mathematical model that couples Doppler ejection indices to ventricular contraction. *Circulation* 1988; 78:II–549 (abstract).

4. Effects of regional myocardial ischemia on Doppler ejection dynamics

HANI N. SABBAH, and PAUL D. STEIN
Henry Ford Heart and Vascular Institute, 2799 West Grand Boulevard, Detroit, Michigan 48202, U.S.A.

4.1 Introduction

Global left ventricular performance evaluated on the basis of peak acceleration of blood in the ascending aorta and combined with exercise stress testing may potentially offer a noninvasive modality for detecting coronary artery disease in patients. Current clinical noninvasive approaches used in the detection of latent coronary artery disease include real time radionuclide cineangiography [1] and myocardial perfusion scintigraphy with [201]thallium [2] both of which can be performed following isoproterenol infusion [3] has also been used to detect the presence of coronary artery disease, although less frequently. Both exercise stress testing and infusion of inotropic agents are maneuvers which increase myocardial oxygen demands beyond the capabilities of a stenosed coronary artery to supply adequate blood flow and, therefore, lead to regional myocardial ischemia. The presence of a latent coronary artery stenosis, therefore, is identifiable on the basis of a perfusion defect, regional left ventricular wall motion abnormality or electrocardiographic changes compatible with ischemia.

Peak acceleration of blood in the ascending aorta has long been considered a sensitive indicator of global left ventricular performance [4–7]. Its routine use in patients has, over the years, been limited by the need to invasively measure phasic aortic blood velocity. Recent advances in Doppler technology, however, have overcome this hurdle and now allow a noninvasive measurement of phasic aortic blood velocity from which peak acceleration can be derived [8, 9]. In the present chapter, we will discuss the results of two animal studies which support the notion that Doppler derived ejection indices of global left ventricular performance, specifically peak blood acceleration, when combined with exercise stress testing, may potentially offer another approach for the detection of a latent coronary stenosis in patients.

4.2 Effects of regional ischemia

When contemplating the use of an index of global left ventricular function during

Steve M. Teague (ed.) Stress Doppler Echocardiography, 35–44.
© 1990 *Kluwer Academic Publishers.*

exercise stress testing as an adjunct for the detection of latent coronary artery disease one must be certain that the selected index is sensitive to the presence of regional myocardial ischemia. After all, during such testing, the developing ischemia is the identifier of latent coronary artery disease. In the first of the two animal studies to be described in this chapter we will examine the effects of regional left ventricular ischemia on Doppler ejection dynamics by evaluating the relationship between Doppler indices of left ventricular function and the extent of ischemic left ventricular mass at risk of infarction [10].

Ischemic regions of varying sizes were produced in 24 open-chest anesthetized dogs by acute ligation at different levels of the anterior descending coronary artery or circumflex coronary artery. To produce large ischemic zones, the proximal portion of either the left anterior descending or circumflex coronary artery was ligated. For smaller ischemic zones, distal portions or branches of theses vessels were ligated.

Doppler ejection indices of left ventricular function namely, peak velocity, peak acceleration and the systolic velocity integral, were measured using a continuous wave Doppler transmitter and receiver operating at 3.0 MHz (ExerDop, Quinton Instruments Co., Seattle, WA). The Doppler system and its use in laboratory animals and in patients has been described in detail [9, 11]. In all dogs, the Doppler transducer was placed directly on the surface of the aorta pointing in the direction of the aortic valve. Whenever Doppler measurements were made, a minimum of 20 consecutive sinus beats were obtained and the average values are reported. The need for averaging multiple beats is due to beat-to-beat variability often encountered when Doppler techniques are used to measure phasic aortic velocity [9]. Left ventriculograms were obtained in each dog for comparison of the ejection fraction with Doppler indices of left ventricular performance. Measurements of Doppler indices and ventriculograms were obtained at baseline and were repeated within minutes of coronary ligation.

Left ventricular ischemic mass at risk was quantitated at postmortem in each of the 24 dogs. With the appropriate coronary arteries still occluded, the left main coronary artery was cannulated and the myocardium was perfused with Evans blue dye. Accordingly, the normally perfused myocardium was stained blue and the ischemic myocardium was unstained. After removing the right ventricular free wall, large epicardial arteries and valvular structures, the left ventricular myocardium was sliced serially into five to seven slices. Blue stained myocardium was carefully separated from unstained myocardium and both were weighed separately. Ischemic mass at risk of infarction was defined as the anatomic bed of the occluded coronary artery and was calculated as the ratio of ischemic mass to total left ventricular mass $\times$ 100.

In order to examine the sensitivity of the Doppler indices of left ventricular function to varying degrees of ischemia, dogs were divided into three groups according to the extent of the left ventricular ischemic mass at risk. Group I consisted of 8 dogs in which the ischemic mass was $\leq 20\%$ of total left ventricular mass. Group II consited of 8 dogs in which the ischemic mass was 21% to 40% of total left ventricular mass. Group III also consisted of 8 dogs in which the ischemic mass

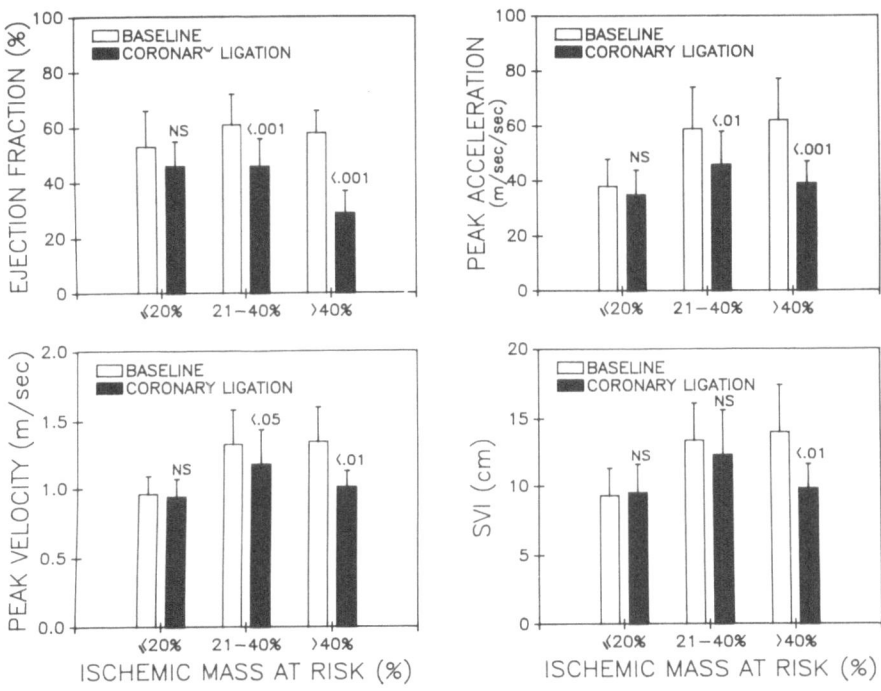

Figure 1. Bar graphs depicting the mean and standard deviation of measured values of ejection fraction (upper left), peak acceleration (upper right), peak velocity (bottom left), and the systolic velocity integral (SVI) (bottom right). Values are shown during baseline conditions (open bars) and during coronary ligation (filled bars) in all three groups of dogs divided according to the extent of left ventricular ischemic mass at risk. Probability values represent paired comparisons between baseline and coronary ligation for each group. NS = not significant.

was > 40% of total left ventricular mass.

The measured values of the various Doppler indices and of left ventricular ejection fraction during baseline conditions and following coronary ligation are shown in Figure 1 for each of the 3 groups. Among dogs with an ischemic mass ≤ 20%, none of the Doppler indices, including peak acceleration, nor left ventricular ejection fraction changed significantly in response to this limited ischemic insult. In dogs with an ischemic mass between 21% and 40% of total left ventricular mass, however, both peak acceleration and ejection fraction decreased significantly. In this group, the reduction of peak velocity, was only borderline significant and there was no significant reduction of the systolic velocity integral. Dogs with an ischemic mass > 40% showed the greatest reduction of peak acceleration, peak velocity and ejection fraction following coronary ligation in comparison to baseline. In this group, the systolic velocity integral also decreased significantly. The percent reduction of peak velocity, peak acceleration, systolic velocity integral and ejection fraction between baseline measurements and measurements obtained during coronary ligation are shown in Figure 2 for all three groups.

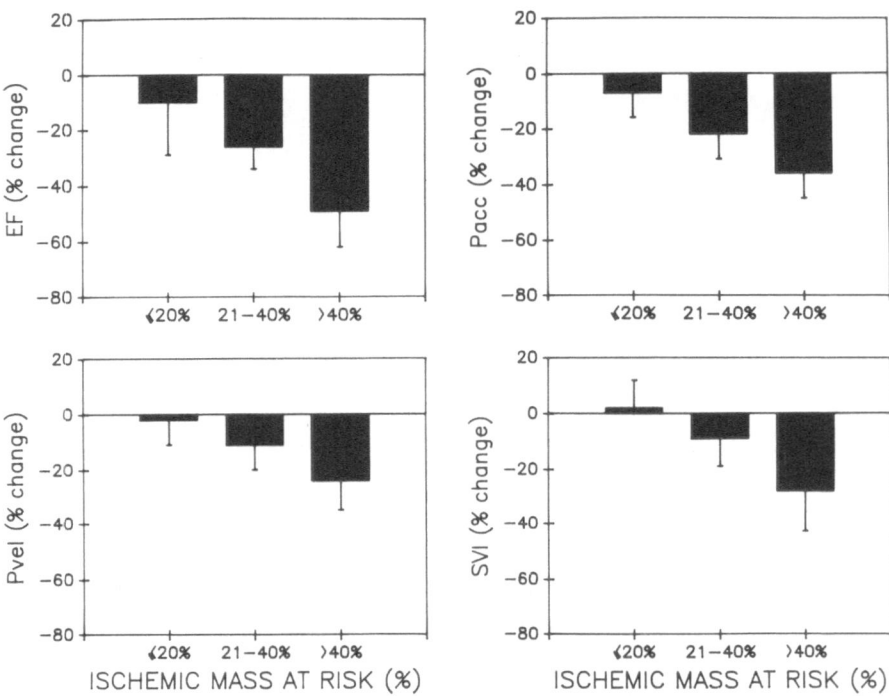

Figure 2. Bar graphs depicting the mean and standard deviation of the percent change between baseline and coronary ligation of ejection fraction (EF) (upper left), peak acceleration (Pacc) (upper right), peak velocity (Pvel) (bottom left) and the systolic velocity integral (SVI) (bottom right). In each panel, bars are shown individually for each of the three groups of dogs divided according to the extent of left ventricular ischemic mass at risk.

Correlation between the percent reduction of the various Doppler indices of left ventricular performance and the percent ischemic mass at risk are shown in Figure 3. The percent change of peak acceleration correlated best with the percent ischemic mass at risk (r = 0.88). It was followed by ejection fraction (r = 0.84), systolic velocity integral (r = 0.80) and peak velocity (r = 0.77).

The above observations suggest that among the Doppler ejection indices of left ventricular performance peak acceleration is the most sensitive to the presence of regional ischemia and can reflect the extent of left ventricular ischemic mass at risk. This, however, is not without a caveat. None of the Doppler indices nor the ejection fraction were capable of detecting ischemic dysfunction associated with a ≤ 20% ischemic mass at risk. This is likely to be due to adequate compensation by the normally perfused myocardium.

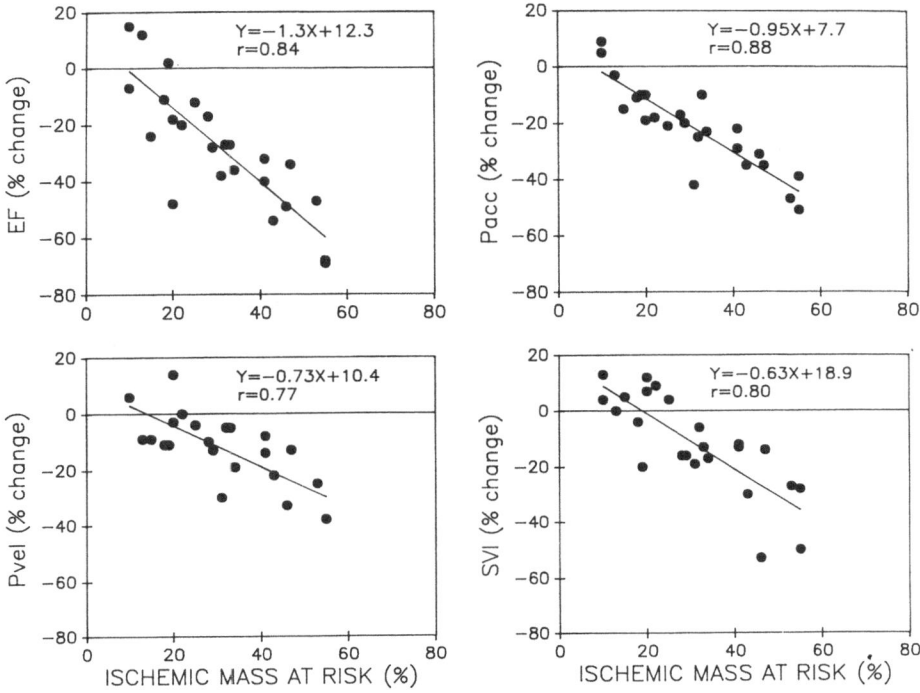

Figure 3. Relationship between the percent change of ejection fraction (EF) (upper left), peak acceleration (Pacc) (upper right), peak Velocity (Pvel) (bottom left) and systolic velocity integral (SVI) (bottom right) and left ventricular ischemic mass at risk. r = correlation coefficient. Reproduced in part from H.N. Sabbah *et al.* [10] with permission.

4.3 Detection of critical coronary stenosis

The sensitivity of peak aortic blood acceleration to the presence of acute regional ischemia and its relation to ischemic mass at risk provided the necessary foundation needed for examining its potential use in detecting ischemic dysfunction caused by the presence of a critical coronary stenosis. Such dysfunction is not present at rest, but occurs under conditions which increase myocardial oxygen demands. Doppler indices of left ventricular function, including peak acceleration, were eveluted in 20 open-chest anesthetized dogs in which a critical coronary artery stenosis was induced in either the left anterior descending or circumflex coronary artery [12]. As with the previous study, Doppler parameters were measured with a continuous wave Doppler velocimeter (ExerDop) with the transducer placed directly over the surface of the ascending aorta in the direction of the aortic valve. Peak rate of change of pressure during isovolumic contraction, dP/dt, was also measured for comparison with Doppler ejection indices.

40

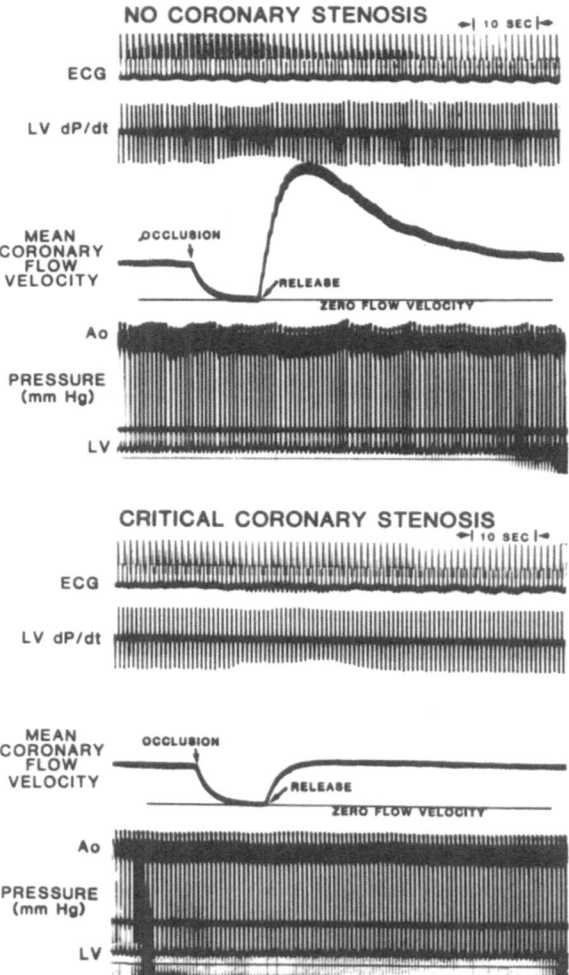

Figure 4. Top: reactive hyperemic response following 10 sec occlusion of the left anterior descending coronary artery in the absence of a stenosis. Bottom: response in the presence of a critical coronary stenosis. ECG = lead II of the electrocardiogram. LV dP/dt = left ventricular isovolumic rate of change of pressure. Ao = aortic pressure and LV = left ventricular pressure. Reproduced from H.N. Sabbah *et al.* [12] with permission.

. In this series of animals, a critical coronary stenosis was defined as the degree of coronary narrowing that eliminates reactive hyperemic flow at rest [13, 14]. To create the stenosis, a snare was placed on the proximal portion of either the left anterior descending (10 dogs) or circumflex coronary artery (10 dogs). The snare was progressively tightened until the reactive hyperemic response, after a 10 second coronary occlusion, was essentially abolished indicating depletion of coronary vasodilatory reserve [13]. Coronary blood flow velocity was measured with a single crystal Doppler flow velocity probe placed proximal to the site of stenosis [12, 15]. A typical record of mean coronary flow velocity during reactive hyperemia in the absence and presence of a critical coronary stenosis is shown in Figure 4.

At the completion of the surgical procedure and prior to inducing a critical coronary stenosis, Doppler indices were evaluated at rest and again following intravenous infusion of isoproterenol. The infusion rate of isoproterenol was adjusted in each dog to achieve approximately a 50% increase of heart rate. Both the baseline measurements and the isoproterenol infusion were repeated in each dog, in an identical fashion, after inducing a critical coronary stenosis. The use of isoproterenol in these animals is not intended to advocate its use in patients. Contraindications for the use of isoproterenol in patients with coronary artery disease have been fully elucidated. Instead, isoproterenol was used only to illustrate the effect on global left ventricular performance of an intervention which increases myocardial oxygen requirements in the presence of a critical coronary artery stenosis.

Table 1. Hemodynamics at rest and during isoproterenol stimulation in the presence and absence of a critical coronary stenosis.

	No stenosis		Critical stenosis	
	Rest	Isop	Rest	Isop
Heart rate (beat/min)	97 ± 28	152 ± 30	101 ± 32	154 ± 31
Systolic pressure (mm Hg)	120 ± 14	110 ± 17	121 ± 14	106 ± 20
Diastolic pressure (mm Hg)	90 ± 15	75 ± 19	94 ± 14	72 ± 22
Peak/dP/dt (mm Hg/sec)	2600 ± 600	4400 ± 1200 $P < 0.01$	2700 ± 700	3500 ± 1200 $P < 0.01$
Peak velocity (m/sec)	1.18 ± 0.19	1.63 ± 0.27 $P < 0.001$	1.17 ± 0.20	1.45 ± 0.30 $P < 0.001$
Peak acceleration (m/sec/sec)	45 ± 11	78 ± 14 $P < 0.001$	46 ± 10	64 ± 12 $P < 0.001$
Systolic velocity integral (cm)	12.3 ± 2.9	11.3 ± 2.7	12.9 ± 2.5	11.4 ± 3.5

Isop = isoproterenol.

The hemodynamics at rest and during stimulation with isoproterenol in the absence of a coronary stenosis are shown in Table 1. Peak acceleration during isoproterenol increased by 33 ± 11 m/sec/sec which was significantly higher than during resting conditions. Both peak velocity and peak left ventricular dP/dt also increased during isoproterenol but the systolic velocity integral remained relatively unchanged. The percent increase of the various Doppler parameters and of dP/dt between rest and isoproterenol are shown in Figure 5.

The hemodynamics at rest and during stimulation with isoproterenol in the presence of a critical coronary stenosis are also shown in Table 1. In the presence of a critical coronary stenosis, peak acceleration during isoproterenol increased only 18 ± 7 m/sec/sec. Even though this increase was significantly higher than resting conditions it was markedly diminished in comparison to the increase observed in the absence of a coronary stenosis. This behavior was also true with respect to peak velocity and left ventricular dP/dt. The percent increase of the various Doppler indices and of dP/dt between rest and isoproterenol in the presence of a critical coronary stenosis are also depicted in Figure 5.

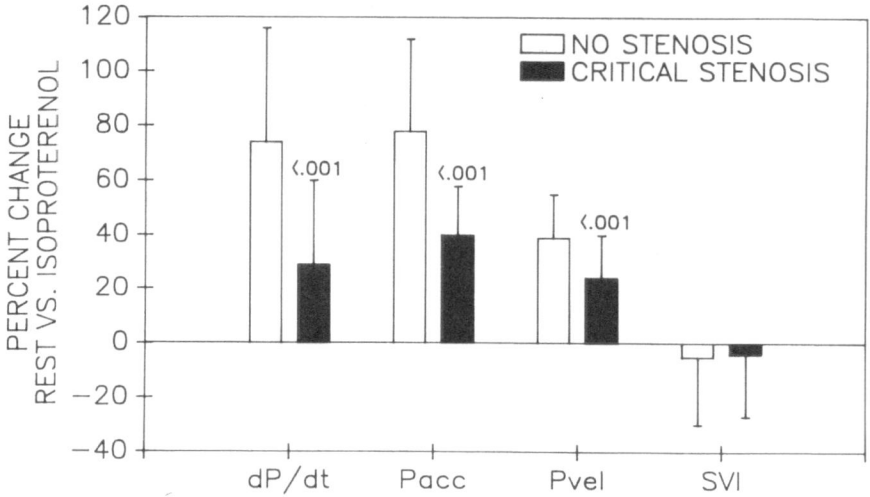

Figure 5. Bar graph depicting the mean and standard deviation of the percent change between rest measurements and isoproterenol measurements of peak dP/dt, peak acceleration (Pacc), peak velocity (Pvel) and systolic velocity integral (SVI). Bars depict changes which occurred in the absence of a coronary stenosis (open bars) and in the presence of a critical coronary stenosis (filled bars). Probabilities are based on paired comparisons between stenosis and no stenosis conditions for each of the functional indices.

The observations made in the two animal studies described in this chapter suggest that among the various Doppler indices of global left ventricular performance, peak acceleration of blood in the ascending aorta is the most sensitive indicator of regional myocardial ischemia. This is true provided the left ventricular ischemic mass is sufficiently large to mask the compensatory response of the residual normally perfused myocardium. With this in mind, the observations also indicate that peak acceleration can be useful in detecting regional ischemia caused by the presence of a critical coronary stenosis during conditions which increase myocardial oxygen requirements. In this setting, peak acceleration of blood in the ascending aorta reflects the presence of a critical coronary stenosis by identifying a relative impairment of global left ventricular performance between rest and simulated exercise rather than an overt reduction of function. Specifically, peak acceleration and other global indices of left ventricular function, in the presence of a critical coronary stenosis, fail to increase to levels reached in the absence of a coronary stenosis. The results overall lend support to the notion that Doppler ejection indices, specially peak acceleration, when measured during graded treadmill exercise testing, can be useful as an adjunct to the diagnosis of latent coronary artery disease in man.

References

1. Borer JS, Bacharach SL, Green MV, Kent KM, Epstein GE, Johnston GS. Real time radionuclide cineangiography in the noninvasive evaluation of global and regional left ventricular function at rest and during exercise in patients with coronary artery disease. N Eng J Med 1977; 296:839–844.
2. Joye JA, Glass EC, Takeda P, Lee G, Hines H, Low RI, Amsterdam EA, DeMaria AN, DeNardo GL, Mason DT. Quatification of the extent of coronary artery disease using noninvasive radionuclide imaging techniques and the evaluation of myocardial revascularization interventions. In: Mason DT, Collins JJ, Jr (eds.). Myocardial Revascularization. New York, Yorke Medical Books, 1981, pp 52–61.
3. Combs DT, Martin CM. Evaluation of isoproterenol as a method of stress testing. Am Heart J 1974; 87:711-715.
4. Rushmer RF. Initial ventricular impulse. A potential key to cardiac evaluation. Circulation 1964; 29:268–283.
5. Noble MIM, Trenchard D, Guz A. Left ventricular ejection in conscious dogs. 1. Measurement and significance of maximum acceleration of blood from the left ventricle. Circ Res 1966; 19:139–147.
6. Bennett ED, Else W, Miller GAH, Sutton GC, Miller HC, Noble MIM. Maximum acceleration of blood from the left ventricle in patients with ischemic heart disease. Clin Sci Mol Med 1974; 46:49–59.
7. Stein PD, Sabbah HN. Rate of change of ventricular power. An indicator of ventricular performance during ejection. Am Heart J 1976; 91:219–226.
8. Bennett ED, Barclay SA, David AL, Mannering D, Mehta N. Ascending aortic blood velocity and acceleration using Doppler ultrasound in the assessment of left ventricular function. Cardiovasc Res 1984; 18:632–638.
9. Sabbah HN, Khaja F, Brymer JF, McFarland TM, Albert DE, Snyder JE, Goldstein S, Stein P.: Noninvasive evaluation of left ventricular performance based on peak aortic blood acceleration measured with a continuous-wave Doppler velocity meter. Circulation 1986; 74:323–329.
10. Sabbah HN, Pryzybylski J, Albert DE, Stein PD. Peak aortic blood acceleration reflects the extent of left ventricular ischemic mass at risk. Am Heart J 1987; 113:885–890.
11. Stein PD, Sabbah HN, Albert DE, Snyder JE. Continuous-wave Doppler for the noninvasive evaluation of aortic blood velocity and rate of change of velocity; Evaluation in dogs. Med Instr 1987; 21:177–182.
12. Sabbah HN, Albert DE, Stein PD. Detection of critical coronary stenosis in dogs: global left ventricular response to isoproterenol. J Appl Cardiol 1987; 2:21–35.
13. Gallagher KP, Osakada G, Matsuzaki M, Kemper WS, Ross J, Jr. Myocardial blood flow and function with critical coronary stenosis in exercising dogs. Am J Physiol 1982; 243:H698–H707.
14. Schwartz JS, Carlyle PF, Cohn JN. Effect of dilation of the distal coronary bed on flow and resistance in severely stenotic coronary arteries in the dog. Am J Cardiol 1979;

44

43:219–223.
15. Vatner SF, Franklin D, VanCitters RL. Simultaneous comparisons and calibration of the Doppler and electromagnetic flowmeters. J Appl Physiol 1970; 29:907–910.

5. Practical considerations in Doppler stress testing

STEVE M. TEAGUE

Noninvasive Laboratory, MetroHealth Medical Center,
3395 Scranton Road, Cleveland, Ohio, 44109, U.S.A.

5.1 Introduction

Although other chapters detail the scientific and clinical basis for Doppler stress testing, this book would be less effective if practical aspects were not discussed. It is the purpose of this chapter to orient the beginner to equipment, stress testing protocols, details of patient study, discrimination of good and bad data, and data analysis. With these issues in mind, it should be possible for novices to confidently approach patients in the stress testing laboratory.

5.2 Equipment considerations for suprasternal examinations

Equipment designed for the echocardiography laboratory is usable for Doppler stress testing, but poorly suited for that task. Probes must be specially angled for fit and position in the suprasternal notch, and the analysis of data so acquired should be automated to relieve the drudgery of data reduction. Many of the features of traditional clinical echocardiographic equipment are not utilized during Doppler stress testing, while many sorely needed features are missing. To fill this niche, Exerdop (Quinton Instruments, Seattle, WA) was developed. This is the instrument employed in most of the studies reported in this book.

As illustrated in Figure 1, sonication of the upper mediastinum from the suprasternal notch returns signals from the ascending aorta, and often the innominate artery [1,2]. This window has the advantage of minimizing the Doppler angle, realized as cosine theta in the Doppler equation. This angle must be as small as possible to reduce errors in velocity assessments from the ascending aorta. In most humans, this solid angle is ± 20% from the suprasternal notch, affording confidence in the measurement (Figure 2) [3]. However, subjects with kyphosis, extensive emphysema, or an uncoiled, aged aorta may present higher angles of approach, resulting in thetas of 30 degrees or greater. Although nothing can be done in these cases to alter the velocity or acceleration measurements thus acquired and scaled by cosine theta, analytical schemes can be devised to diminish or neutralize the effects of angle. Recently, novel Doppler techniques have been introduced to overcome the effects of Doppler angle during cardiac output determinations [4, 5, 6].

Steve M. Teague (ed.) Stress Doppler Echocardiography, 45–59.
© 1990 *Kluwer Academic Publishers.*

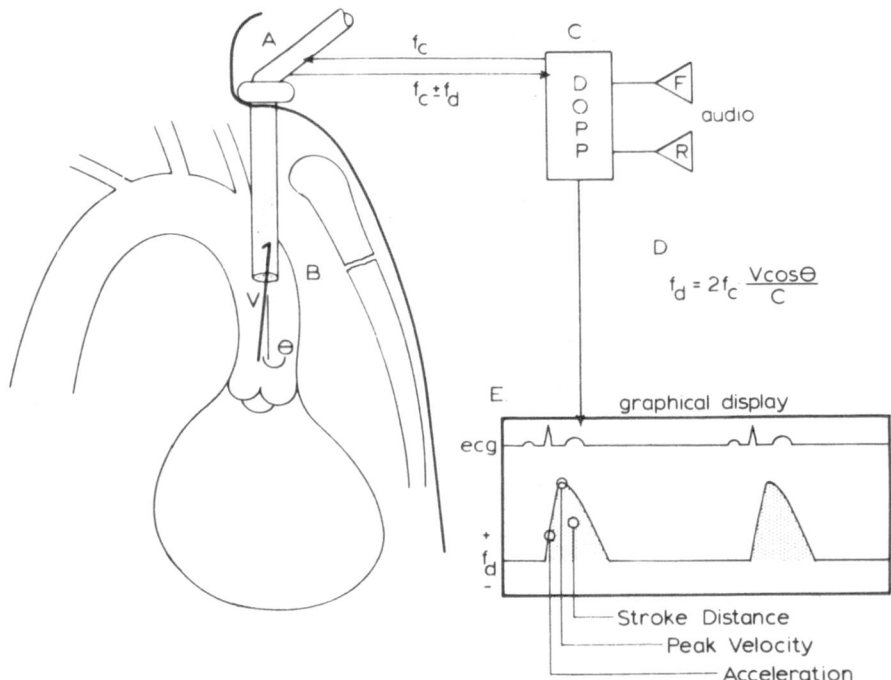

$$f_d = 2f_c \frac{V\cos\Theta}{C}$$

Figure 1. Interaction of Doppler ultrasound from the suprasternal notch with ascending aortic blood flow. A Doppler transducer (A) interrogates blood ejected from the left ventricle (B). The frequency of the reflected ultrasound is determined by the Doppler equation (D). Doppler instrumentation (C) calculates the difference between transmitted and received signals, and displays this information as forward (F) or reverse (R) flow velocity in a video display (E) or stereo speakers. Doppler acceleration, peak velocity, and stroke distance are derived from the systolic ejection pulse.

One can be confident in ascending aortic sonication if aortic valve opening and closure clicks are appreciated in either the acoustical or video graphic display. However, an aortic valve opening click early in systole can easily 'fool' the maximal acceleration detecting circuitry in an exercise Doppler instrument, so the beam should be positioned slightly off axis from the aortic valve.

We should examine whether pulsed wave or continuous wave Doppler would be optimal for Doppler stress testing. Suprasternal pulsed wave Doppler assessments of ascending aortic flow would have the advantage of predictable sample volume depth within the mediastinum, lending reasonable assurance that data were collected from the ascending aorta rather than the innominate artery [7, 8]. On the other hand, sample volumes are difficult to position consistenly during the adverse conditions presented by exercise studies. Most allow that continuous wave Doppler, which reports all velocity information within the sonication path, offers a reasonable trade-off between ease of data acquisition and uncertainty of data sampling site. Data are available suggesting that velocities within proximal thoracic arteries are similar to ascending aortic flow velocity during perturbations of inotropic state, however [9].

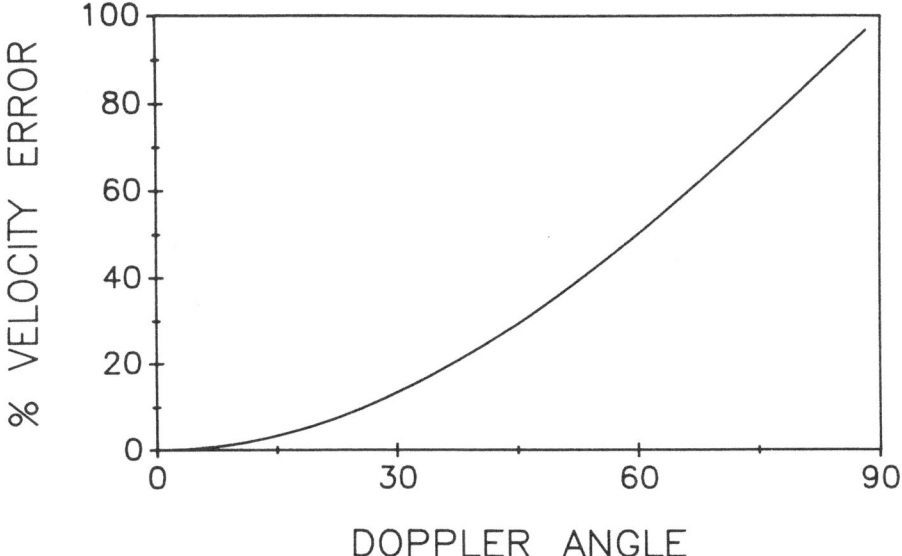

Figure 2. The relationship of velocity estimation errors, plotted as a percentage, against the Doppler angle, theta, as it varies from 0 to 90 degrees. Doppler angles ± 30° result in less than 10% errors.

Most equipment dedicated to stress Doppler echocardiography rely upon 3 to 3.5 mHz transducers. Data display is important. All echocardiographic equipment allow direct appreciation of Doppler shift information in acoustic speakers registering Doppler shifts in forward and reverse directions. Most experienced Doppler echocardiographers come to rely upon the acoustic information primarily, as the ear is exquisitely sensitive to data quality, velocity, and transient events. Certainly most beginners would desire some form of graphical display, affording visual appreciation of data quality and integrity. However, video display adds to the expense of the equipment, and once the beginner is beyond the novice stage aural means will be naturally used to evaluate data quality.

Instruments must have analytical functions automating the analysis of acquired Doppler data, returning parameters such as peak ejection velocity, maximal or average acceleration, and systolic velocity integral as well as the systolic time intervals (Figure 3). Considering the minutes of continuous data acquired during stress testing, and the tachycardias almost always evoked, a stress Doppler study can easily generate 1,000 to 5,000 beats for analysis. If this step is not automated, one quickly looses interest in this method of ventricular performance evaluation.

48

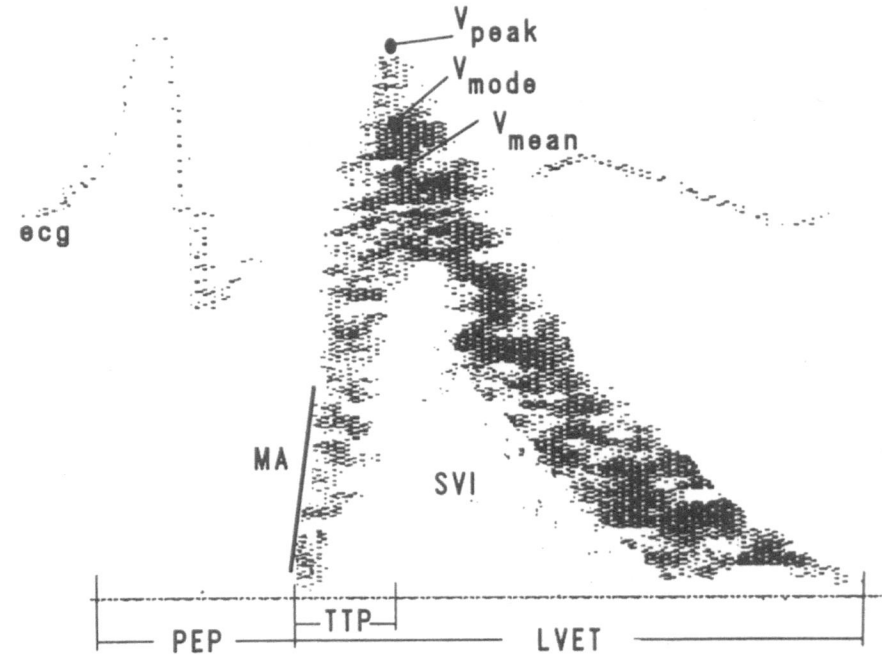

Figure 3. Detail on the systolic Doppler ejection pulse with respect to the electrocardiogram. The preejection period (PEP), the acceleration time (TTP), and the total left ventricular ejection time (LVET), can be measured. From deflection measurements, maximal acceleration (MA) can be estimated as the maximal rate of change of the upstroke, while 'peak velocity' is calculated variously as maximal observable velocity (peak); the modal velocity in the population distribution (mode); or the mean velocity (mean) calculated over the instantaneous spectrum (not shown). The systolic velocity integral (SVI) is the area bounded by the ejection pulse.

5.3 Patient selection

Optimally, patients would not need selection for Doppler echocardiographic studies, as the study should apply to everyone entering the stress testing laboratory. As equipment and approaches improve, we may be able to eliminate the 5 to 8% of studies in which signals can not be acquired from the suprasternal notch. Solutions may include acquisition of ventricular performance data from the common carotid artery, a brachial artery, descending aorta (using esophageal probes), or even (utilizing transcranial Doppler ultrasound) a cerebral artery. However, one must anticipate failure in a finite number of suprasternal examinations, usually attributable to aortic valve disease, obesity, emphysema, unusual body habitus, mediastinal shift, short neck, or previous anterior cervical surgery. It is unusual that patients with adequate data acquisition at rest become impossible to study during exercise if the examiner has prior experience at data acquisition during exercise.

5.4 Stress test protocols

Most cardiac stress testing involves exercise, and these studies represent the bulk of clinical evaluations of stress Doppler echocardiography reported in this book. Studies can be performed during graded treadmill exercise, or during graded bicycle exercise in upright or supine postures. For beginners, probably the easiest studies are performed upon seated bicycling patients, while the most difficult studies are during upright exericse on the treadmill.

Certainly, not all patients suspected of cardiac disease are suitable candidates for exercise stress testing. Orthopedic limitations, pulmonary insufficiency, advance peripheral vascular disease, neuropathy, or neurologic degeneration may make exercise impossible or futile. For these patients, pharmacologic testing protocols must be selected to induce cardiac stresses (Chapter 13). Appropriate stressors would include intervenous isoproterenol, epinephrine, dipyridamole, and dobutamine. Most of these agents reduce peripheral vascular resistance, elevate heart rate, and augment inotropic state, thus mimicking the physiologic effects of exercise [10, 11, 12].

5.5 Probes and positioning

Adequate ultrasonic probes for Doppler stress testing from the suprasternal notch include long handles for easy manipulation, with angulation between the handles and transducer elements for comfortable positioning towards the ascending aorta. In turn, the equipment should incorporate a recording switch for easy data acquisition during the stress testing. A switch may be incorporated in the probe, or reside below the sonographer's foot. Trying to acquire data and reach the recording switch on an ultrasonic machine with a free hand can be a frustrating and fatiguing experience.

For stable and reproducible data acquisition from an exercising subject the probe must be held properly. As seen in Figure 4, we hold the probe like a pencil and rest the palm of the hand on the exercising patient's sternum. This configuration allows easy sonication of the ascending aorta while the subject bobs and weaves during treadmill exercise. Stable positioning of the palm against the patient is particularly important at the higher levels of treadmill exercise. It may be advantageous to apply pressure with the palm of the examining hand against the patient's sternum to help stabilize the probe as the patient approaches jogging on the treadmill.

The Doppler information is optimized by sweeping the probe through multiple arcs and planes in the suprasternal notch. The probe is steered right and left, forward and backward, and in circles to maximize the power or signal size appreciated in the speakers and video displays, or data values appearing on the digital printout. Data should be acquired prestress, at each stage of stress testing, and at least for the

50

first few minutes of the recovery phase. It is necessary to minimize operator fatigue by alternating rest with repeated applications of the transducer during the last 1 to $1^1/_2$ minutes of exercise in each 3 minute stress stage. For data integrity, these repeated applications must result in similar angles of approach to the same flow region. Experience, concentration, and a sharp ear are necessary to correctly orient the transducer during successive applications.

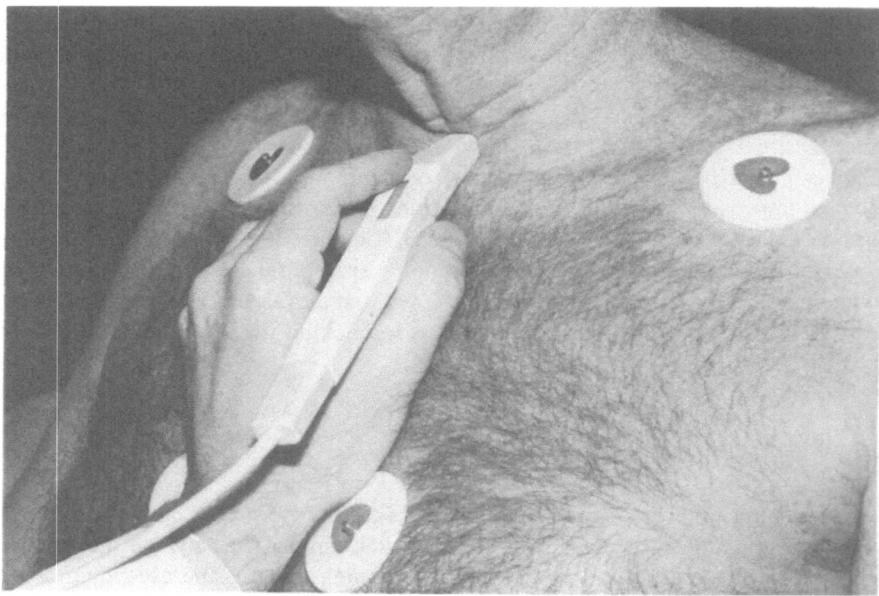

Figure 4. We have found it most practical to hold a suprasternal Doppler probe like a pencil, resting in the palm of the hand on the patient's sternum. This stabilizes the probe during bobbing and weaving induced by treadmill or bicycle exercise.

The sonographer attends the exercising subject very closely, standing beside the treadmill or the bicycle apparatus. As illustrated in Figure 5, we usually find it easiest to approach the patient opposite the electrocardiographic recording apparatus and monitoring technician. This allows the exercise technologist to record blood pressure and stress electrocardiograms unimpeded while exercise Doppler data are acquired. During supine bicycle exercise, we have found it easiest to position the examining sonographer above the patient's head, exerting downward pressure on the transducer with the thumb.

5.6 Performance testing

As previously mentioned, data should be acquired at rest in the exercise posture, during each stage of exercise, at peak exercise, and at successive minutes for at least two minutes into the recovery phase. Collecting data in the last 1 to ½ minutes of each stage assures that the patient has reached physiologic equilibrium at the new stress level, and that data will be representative of that cardiac workload.

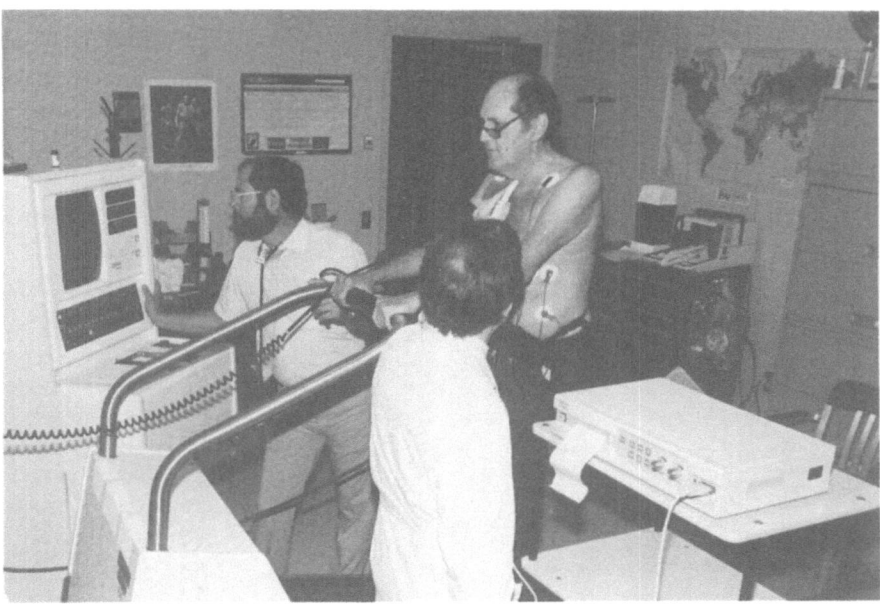

Figure 5. The Stress Testing Laboratory. The sonographer stands on the opposite side of the treadmill so that electrocardiographic, blood pressure, and Doppler data can be acquired in a noncompetitive fashion. Adequate space must be afforded this examination.

To assure an adequate database for subsequent analysis, high quality data must be obtained. We usually insist on 14 to 20 adequate beats during each recording, and optimally these beats will be sequential. Sequential acceptable beats assure that physiologic fluctuations attributable to respiration will be averaged over the recording session. If data are corrupted by noise or difficult conditions, one must persevere to get 14 or 15 adequate beats.

Adequacy, in turn, must be determined by the quality of the individual pulses, interpulse measurement variation, and standard deviation or variance of data acquired during a single recording (Figure 6). Exerdop incorporates a variance algorithm, such that data lying outside ± 20% of the running mean are automatically excluded from subsequent analysis. If calculating data by hand, this mean and variance calculation should be performed for each record to identify acceptable data.

The most important data are acquired at rest, at peak exercise, and in earliest recovery. The data between rest and peak exercise determine the degree of augmentation in Doppler ejection dynamics under the stress load. In turn, data acquired during earliest recovery corroborate those data acquired at peak exercise, as the values should be similar. If marked discrepancies (50% variation) are observed between peak and early recovery, the data obtained at peak exercise must be doubted.

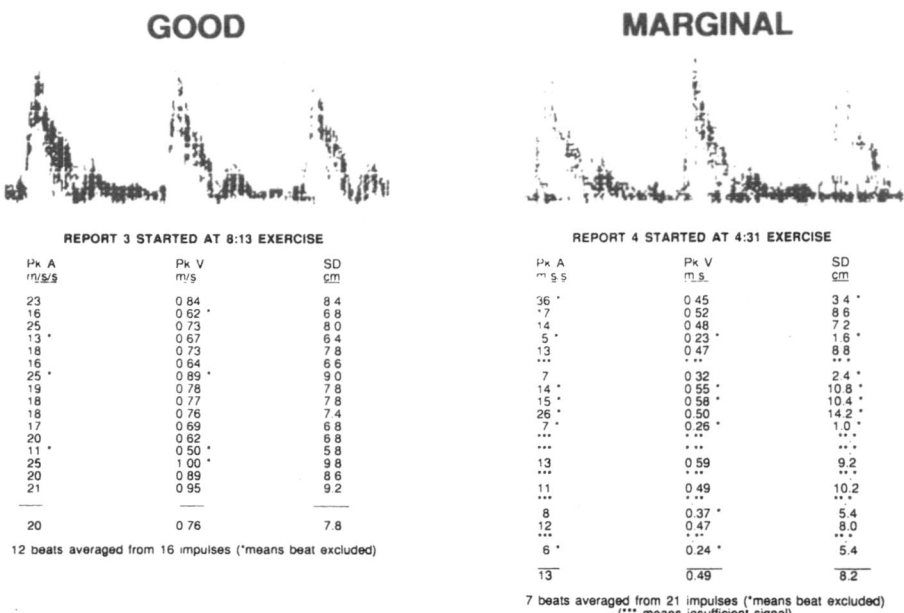

GOOD

REPORT 3 STARTED AT 8:13 EXERCISE

Pk A m/s/s	Pk V m/s	SD cm
23	0 84	8 4
16	0 62 *	6 8
25	0 73	8 0
13 *	0 67	6 4
18	0 73	7 8
16	0 64	6 6
25 *	0 89 *	9 0
19	0 78	7 8
18	0 77	7 8
18	0 76	7 4
17	0 69	6 8
20	0 62	6 8
11 *	0 50 *	5 8
25	1 00 *	9 8
20	0 89	8 6
21	0 95	9.2
20	0 76	7.8

12 beats averaged from 16 impulses (*means beat excluded)

MARGINAL

REPORT 4 STARTED AT 4:31 EXERCISE

Pk A m/s/s	Pk V m/s	SD cm
36 *	0 45	3 4 *
*7	0 52	8 6
14	0 48	7 2
5 *	0 23 *	1.6 *
13	0 47	8 8
***	* **	** *
7	0 32	2.4 *
14 *	0 55 *	10.8 *
15 *	0 58 *	10.4 *
26 *	0.50	14.2 *
7 *	0.26 *	1.0 *
***	* **	** *
***	* **	** *
13	0 59	9.2
***	* **	** *
11	0 49	10.2
***	* **	** *
8	0.37 *	5.4
12	0.47	8.0
***	* **	** *
6 *	0.24 *	5.4
13	0.49	8.2

7 beats averaged from 21 impulses (*means beat excluded)
(*** means insufficient signal)

Figure 6. Illustration of analog and digital estimates of 'Good' and 'Marginal' Doppler data. Good data are consistent, have strong signals, and similar digital measurements from beat-to-beat. Few data are excluded from the running average. Marginal data are inconsistent, variable from beat-to-beat, and have fluctuating signal-to-noise levels. Subsequent digital analysis excludes many beats or rejects many signals with insufficient signal strength.

There are reasons to prefer data obtained during exercise to data obtained during recovery. Exercise physiology includes vasodilation, augmented venous return, increased preload, and increased respiratory excursion. In recovery, muscular pumping activity ceases and venous return is no longer augmented, dropping preload, afterload, and the resultant level of cardiac stress. For diagnostic studies, we have thus relied on data obtained at peak exercise, and have used recovery data only to corroborate and validate the accuracy of peak exercise recordings. We have also observed that Doppler ejection values decrease dramatically during the first $1^1/_2$ minutes following exercise, so that the time of acquisition in recovery is a very important variable.

5.7 Data reduction and analysis

During a stress Doppler test, a host of variables are recorded. From time domain Doppler analysis, principally maximal acceleration, peak velocity, and systolic velocity integral are obtained. Heart rate, blood pressure, and stress electrocardiographic ST segment data are also acquired. Contained in the Doppler record, but of lesser interest are the systolic time intervals (preejection period and left ventricular ejection time) afforded by simultaneous electrocardiographic and Doppler monitoring, and the acceleration time, which is the time from the onset of ejection to the achievement of peak velocity. These measurements are illustrated in Figure 3.

Both velocity and acceleration are variably measured among instruments and investigators. It must be emphasized that Doppler information is a composite of reflections from a population of red cells all moving with slightly different velocities. So ejection velocity, rather than being a single numerical value at any instant in time, is actually a population density function, moving and changing within systole. The bulk of reflecting red cells possess mean velocity, while the fastest moving red cells may be two standard deviations above the mean, and the slowest ones two standard deviations below the mean. Some investigators have reported peak velocity as the highest detectable velocities in the ejection pulse, thus describing ventricular performance on the basis of the velocities of only a small fraction of the red cells in the ejected blood. However, most investigators have realized that mean or modal velocity is more representative of the greatest number of moving red cells (60–70%), and so lower values have been quoted. The reader must be aware of this problem when interpreting published Doppler data.

In turn, acceleration may be measured as a maximal value or an average value. Although the upstroke of the Doppler ejection profile is nonlinear, average acceleration is usually measured linearly between the onset of ejection and achievement of peak velocity. One approach to average acceleration is to merely divide peak velocity by acceleration time, determining the value by triangulation. More sophisticated approaches rely upon electronic derivation to find the maximal first time derivative of the modal velocity curve, thus determining maximal acceleration. In all cases acceleration is derived rather than directly measured.

Recent theoretical analysis has illustrated that the shape of the ejection pulse contains information only partially described by peak velocity, maximal acceleration and systolic velocity integral measurements (Chapter 19). Until clinical validation of shape analysis can be achieved, time domain measurements will be relied upon for diagnostic merit.

Most evaluators of Doppler ultrasound during stress testing have identified maximal acceleration as the index most sensitive to variations in ventricular performance during stress exposure [13–16]. Variably, peak velocity and systolic velocity integral have fallen into second and third place for diagnostic merit. However, the order of second and third place may depend heavily on the disease state being studied and the specific type of stress applied.

54

5.8 Stress variables

Although interest has been shown in defining the most sensitive and diagnostic Doppler ejection variable, opinion remains divided regarding the independent variable that should be chosen to gage the level of cardiac stress. The importance of the independent variable, or quantification of level of stress, is paramount.

The study of cardiac function through Doppler ejection dynamics is an assessment of a physiologic functional element (the heart) through evaluation of output data. To correctly describe the performance of any organ or system, descriptors of input and output variables such as left ventricular filling pressure, inotropic state, and afterload are necessary. In the exercise laboratory most of these parameters are not obtainable easily or nonivasively.

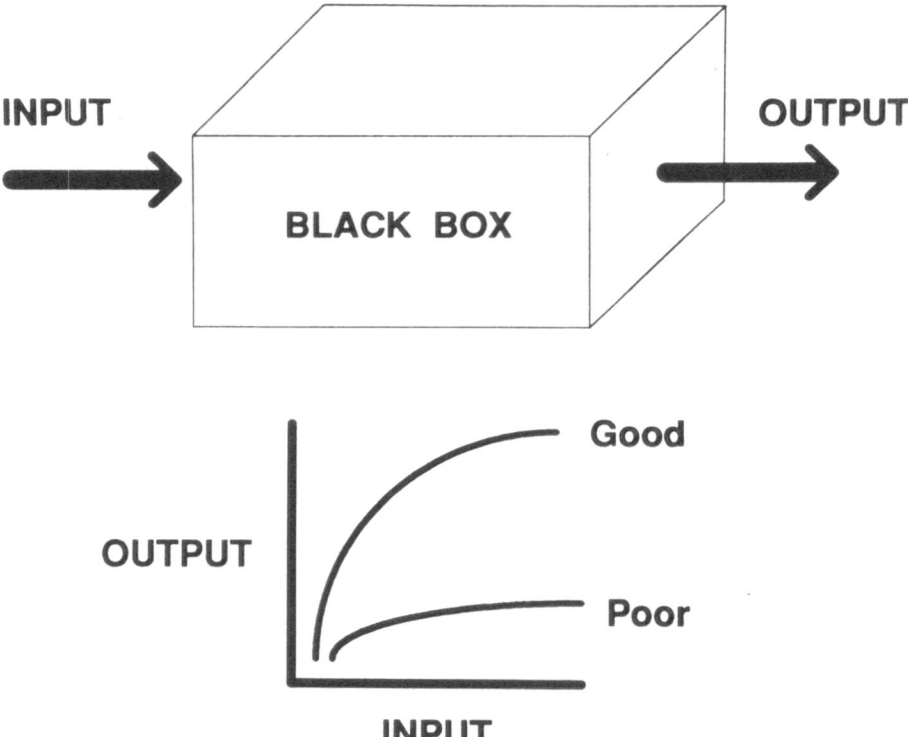

Figure 7. The performance of any physiologic system can be evaluated by comparing the input with the output, even though the functions of the system remain a 'black box'. Good performance results in high output for low input values, while poor system performance has a much flatter relationship between output and increasing input.

We can conceptualize the heart as a 'black box', where we know the output by our Doppler measurements, but only partially know the input (Figure 7). Ultimately, the goal of a Doppler stress test is to compare the changes in the output to the changes in the input, thereby classifying cardiac performance as 'good' or 'bad'. If the input variable can not be quantified, then the stress performance of the 'black box' can not be ascertained. The input variable should define the level of physical stress applied to the left ventricle. Most investigators have simply graded the level of stress as 'rest' and 'peak'; however, this qualitative description does not serve well as an independent variable, which should be quantitative. Other investigators have taken steps toward quantification by grading the applied workload in watts, KPM, or treadmill exercise stage. Due to variation in patient body habitus, age, body surface area, conditioning, and specific exercise protocol chosen, this again remains a rough and only semiqualitative independent variable against which to judge Doppler stress response.

We have evaluated a number of numerical independent variables possessing physiologic rationale as input variables. We have evaluated changes in the heart rate between rest and peak stress, changes in systolic and diastolic blood pressure, and changes in heart rate x systolic blood pressure product. The physiologic bases for these choices owe to the experimentally linear relationship between heart rate and coronary blood flow [17, 18], the linear relationship between myocardial oxygen demand and double product [19, 20], and the linear relationship between myocardial oxygen demand and heart rate [21, 22]. We have contrasted Doppler stress responses in patients with variable coronary disease extent against augmentation of heart rate during various exercise and pharmacologic stresses [12, 14, 23].

5.9 Thresholds and reference standards

It is our consistent observation that in normal individuals (and most coronary patients) peak velocity and maximal acceleration change linearly with increments in stress heart rate. Stress responses may be characterized as slopes by plotting the change in Doppler maximal acceleration or peak velocity against the change in heart rate from rest to peak tolerated exercise [23]. This analysis returns a single number (slope) to characterize the response of myocardial contractile performance to incrementally increasing stress (Figures 8, 9). The responses of patients with coronary disease show slope values in inverse proportion to anatomic disease extent and physiologic functional impairment under stress. In severe coronary disease, slope values may be negative. We have suggested thresholds based upon slope measurements for both maximal acceleration and peak velocity to discriminate patients with coronary disease from those with insignificant or no coronary disease [14, 23]. Other investigators have observed changes in Doppler ejection dynamical variables between rest and peak exertion in patients with and without coronary disease with similar results [13, 16, 24–27].

However, a binary decision threshold must be chosen for calculation of the sensitivity and specificity of the Doppler test profile against the reference standard. In our laboratory, that reference standard has always been the coronary angiogram; however, creditable laboratories have compared Doppler stress responses against

56

stress thallium scintigraphy, or stress radionuclide angiography for the detection of coronary artery disease (Chapters 7, 9). In studies to date, binary decision thresholds for Doppler stress responses have returned specificity and sensitivity superior to that of electrocardiographic testing, but inferior to the results of thallium scintitraphy.

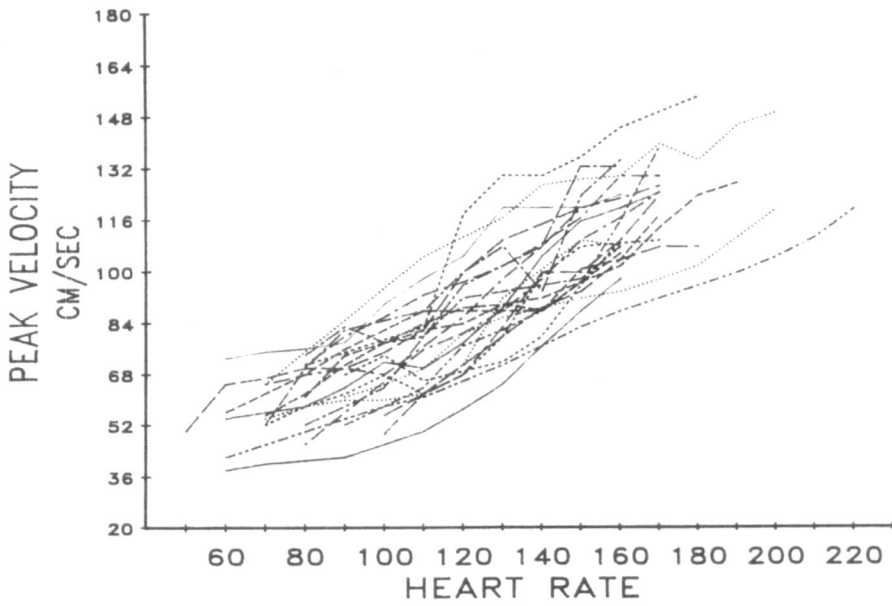

Figure 8. The relationship of peak ejection velocity to heart rate during treadmill exercise as measured from the suprasternal notch in 34 subjects with normal coronary angiograms. Notice the quasilinear relationship between peak ejection velocity and heart rate.

Recently, we took the posture that there was no reason to ignore the stress electrocardiographic information nominally obtained during Doppler stress testing. We combined the degree of ST segment depression recorded during exercise with the degree of Doppler ejection augmentation during the exercise stress. A quotient was formed with the change in Doppler maximal acceleration (MA) from rest to peak exertion as the numerator divided by the maximal ST segment depression recorded during exercise as the denominator. A low index returned from a stress testing procedure would imply poor augmentation of ejection dynamics and/or development of significant ST segment depression, while an excellent augmentation of Doppler maximal acceleration without ST segment depression would return a high index. In 135 male patients undergoing coronary angiography and treadmill exercise, we found a MA/ST index decision threshold of 17 m/s/s/mm highly sensitive (0.91) and specific (0.94) for coronary disease. Further work will be required to validate this analytical approach during pharmacologic stress testing and during exercise testing of females with coronary artery disease.

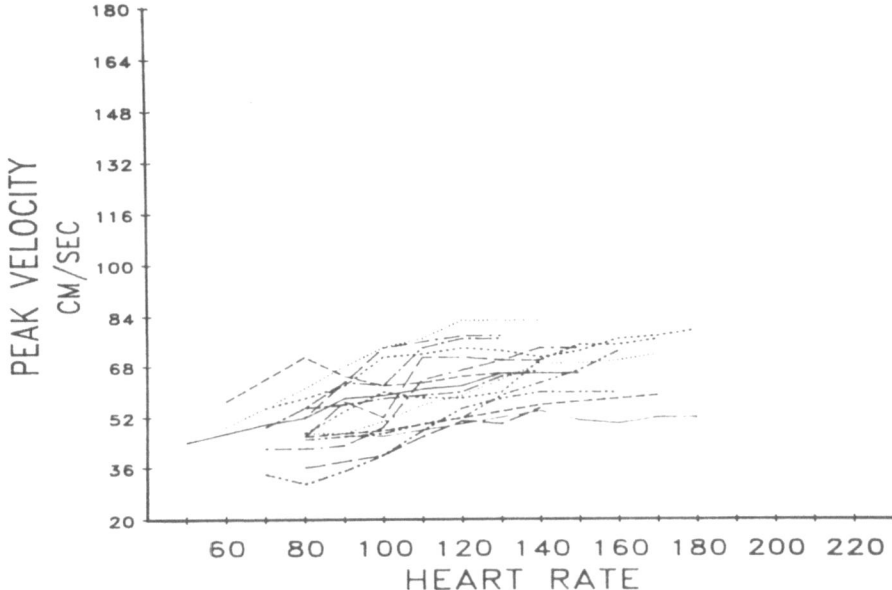

Figure 9. Twenty-eight coronary patients underwent treadmill exercise under a protocol identical to that described in Figure 6. Notice the flat trajectory between peak velocity and heart rate in these individuals with an angiographic average of 2.1 ± 0.9 stenosed proximal coronary arteries.

5.10 Summary

With proper equipment, appropriate probe maneuvers, and methods of data analysis, Doppler stress testing affords an excellent, inexpensive, noninvasive means for the evaluation of ventricular stress responses and the identification of patients with coronary disease. This chapter has addressed practical and procedural issues necessary for a successful study. It should be possible to reproduce the clinical results reported in other chapters of this book if these issues are kept in mind.

References

1. Ishikawa K, Buggs H, Sarma R, *et al.* Blood flow velocity in the carotid artery as a measure of myocardial contractility. Jap Heart J 1975; 16:22–35.
2. Segadal L, Matre K. Blood velocity distribution in the human ascending aorta. Circula-

58

tion 1987; 76:90–100.

3. Bernstein DP. Noninvasive cardiac output, Doppler flowmetry, and gold-plated assumptions. Critical Care Medicine 1987; 15:886.

4. Hohinger C. Method and system for unambiguous measurement of volume flow. U.S. Patent # 4,067,236, 1978.

5. Skidmore R, Evans JM, Baker JD, Wells PNT. An angle and diameter independent method of measuring noninvasive cardiac output by Doppler ultrasound. Circulation 1970; 76 (Suppl IV):97 (abstract).

6. Looyenga DS, Liebson RP, Bone RC, et al. Determination of cardiac output in critically ill patients by dual beam Doppler echocardiography. J Am Coll Cardiol 1989; 13:340–347.

7. Gardin JM, Tobis JM, Dabestani A, Smith C, Elkayam U, Castleman E, White D, Allfie A, Henry WL. Superiority of two-dimensional measurement of aortic vessel diameter in Doppler echocardiographic estimates of left ventricular stroke volume. J Am Coll Cardiol 1985; 6:66–74.

8. Labovitz AJ, Buckingham TA, Habermehl K, Nelson J, Kennedy HL, Williams GA. The effect of sampling site on the two-dimensional echo Doppler determination of cardiac output. Am Heart J 1985; 109:327–332.

9. Buggs H, Balguma FB, Johnson PE, Printup CA, Penido JRF. Transcutaneous bidirectional carotid artery blood flow velocity monitored before, during and after cardiopulmonary bypass at openheart surgery. Chest 1973; 63:607.

10. Elkayam U, Gardin JM, Berkley R, Hughes CA, Henry WL. The use of Doppler flow velocity measurement to assess the hemodynamic response to vasodilators in patients with heart failure. Circulation 1983; 67:377–383.

11. Keren G, Bier A, Strom AJ, Laniado S, Sonnenblick EH, LeJemtel TH. Dynamics of mitral regurgitation during nitroglycerin theraphy: A Doppler Echocardiographic study. Am Heart J 1986; 112:517–525.

12. Teague SM, Heinsimer JA, Williams RS. Doppler left ventricular ejection dynamics: influence of afterload, exercise, and inotropy. Circulation 1986; 74 (Suppl II):12.

13. Mehta N, Bennett D, Mannering D, Dawkins K, Ward DE. Usefulness of noninvasive Doppler measurement of ascending aortic blood velocity and acceleration in detecting impairment of the left ventricular functional response to exercise three weeks after acute myocardial infarction. Am J Cardiol 1986; 58:879–884.

14. Teague SM, Corn C, Sharma M, Prasad R, Burow R, Voyles WF, Thadani U. A comparison of Doppler and radionuclide ejection dynamics during ischemic exercise. Am J Cardiac Imaging 1987; 1:145–151.

15. Harrison MR, Smith MD, Friedman BJ, DeMaria AN. Uses and limitations of exercise Doppler echocardiography in the diagnosis of ischemic heart disease. J Am Coll Cardiol 1987; 10:809–817.

16. Bryg RJ, Labovitz AJ, Mehdirad AA, Williams GA, Chaitman BR. Effect of coronary artery disease on Doppler-derived parameters of aortic flow during upright exercise. Am J Cardiol 1986; 58:14–19.

17. Klocke FJ. Coronary blood flow in man. Prog Cardiovasc Dis 1976; 19:117.

18. Scott JC. Physical activity and the coronary circulation. Can Med Assoc J 1967; 96:853.

19. Sarnoff SJ, et al. Hemodynamic determinants of oxygen consumption of the heart with special reference to the tension-time index. In: Rosenbaum FF (Ed). Work and the heart. Paul B. Hoeber, Harper & Bros., New York, 1959.

20. Gobel FL, et al. The rate-pressure product as an index of myocardial oxygen consumption during exercise in patients with angina pectoris. Circulation 1978; 57:549.

21. Sonnenblick EH, Ross J, Braunwald E. Oxygen consumption of the heart. Newer concepts of its multifunctional determination. Am J Cardiol 1968; 22:328.

22. Taylor HL, Buskirk E, Henschel A. Maximal oxygen intake as objective measurement of cardiorespiratory performance. J Appl Physiol 1955; 8:73.

23. Teague SM, Mark DB, Radford M, *et al.* Doppler velocity profiles reveal ischemic exercise responses. Circulation 1984; 70 (Suppl II):185 (abstract).
24. Mehdirad AA, Williams GH, Labovitz AJ, Bryg RJ, Chaitman BR. Evaluation of left ventricular function during upright exercise: correlation of exercise Doppler with post exercise two-dimensional echocardiographic results. Circulation 1987; 75:413–419.
25. Daley PJ, Sagar KB, Collier BD, Kalbfleisch J, Wann LS. Detection of exercise induced changes in left ventricular performance by Doppler echocardiography. Br Heart J 1987; 58:447–454.
26. Mahn T, Sagar KB, Wann LS. Exercise Doppler echocardiography for evaluating coronary artery disease. Am J Cardiac Imaging 1987; 1:97–102.
27. Bryg RJ, Labovitz AJ. Exercise pulsed wave Doppler in the evaluation of coronary artery disease: Importance of peak ejection velocity. Am J Cardiac Imaging 1987; 1:207–214.

6. Effects of age and gender upon Doppler stress measurements at rest and during exercise in normal subjects

FARSHAD J. NOSRATIAN and JULIUS M. GARDIN

Division of Cardiology, Department of Medicine, California College of Medicine, 101 City Drive South, University of California, Irvine, California, 72668–3297, U.S.A.

As Doppler echocardiography becomes more popular as a non-invasive tool to assess left ventricular function, the need to develop a body of normal reference measurements becomes more important. In particular, it is crucial to define the effects on Doppler measurements of variables such as age, gender, body surface area, heart rate, loading conditions and contractility. For example, using M-mode echocardiography, investigators have previously demonstrated [1–4] a relationship between both age and body surface area and measurements of left ventricular, left atrial and aortic root dimensions, and left ventricular wall thickness. Body surface area, of course, has a close relationship to gender, males usually having larger body surface areas than females. Heart rate and loading conditions have also been documented to be related to cardiac chamber dimensions [5]. The purpose of this chapter is to assess in normal subjects the relationships, during both rest and exercise, between Doppler systolic flow velocity measurements and age, gender, and body surface area.

6.1 Doppler flow velocity measurements in the aorta and pulmonary artery at rest

To try to assess the impact of age, gender and body surface area on normal resting Doppler aortic and pulmonary measurements, Gardin *et al.* [6] evaluated 97 adults, ages 21–78 years, who had no history of hypertension or heart disease. Forty-five were men and fifty-two were women. All subjects had a normal chest x-ray, electrocardiogram, and M-mode and two-dimensional echocardiograms.

Doppler studies at rest were performed using an ultrasound instrument combining a mechanical sector scanner for two-dimensional imaging, with a spectrum analyzer-based pulsed Doppler velocimeter [7–10] for blood flow velocity recording. In both the ascending aorta and main pulmonary artery, a sample volume of approximately 10 millimeters in axial extent was used to record flow velocity. Ascending aortic flow velocity recordings were performed using a 2.25 MHZ modified right-angle M-mode transducer positioned in the suprasternal notch. At each sample volume depth, the transducer was angulated until the maximum aortic

Steve M. Teague (ed.) Stress Doppler Echocardiography, 61–78.
© 1990 *Kluwer Academic Publishers.*

62

flow velocity was recorded [7, 8, 10]. Doppler flow velocity was recorded in the proximal main pulmonary artery utilizing the two-dimensional parasternal short-axis echocardiographic image at the level of the great arteries to position the sample volume parallel to the presumed long-axis of pulmonary blood flow. In addition, the transducer was angulated to insure that maximum PA flow velocity was recorded. In both the aorta and the pulmonary artery, beats used for analysis in each subject were those that demonstrated the greatest Doppler peak flow velocity, since this assumes that ultrasound beam is nearly parallel to the long axis of blood flow [11].

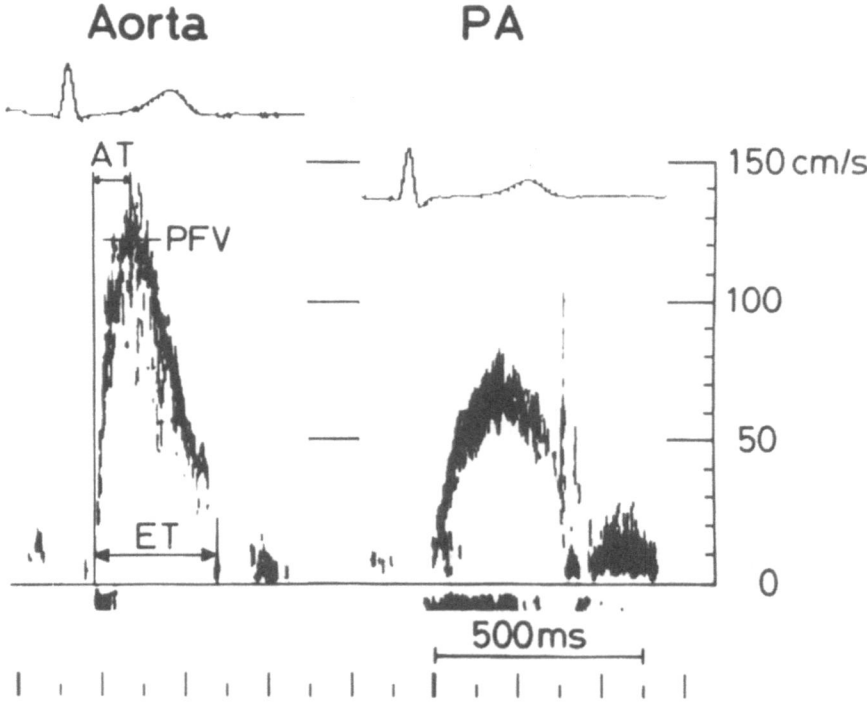

Figure 1. Doppler aortic and pulmonary artery flow velocity recordings from a normal subject. Measurements made in both great arteries included peak flow velocity (PFV) in cm/sec, ejection time (ET) in msec, acceleration time (AT) in msec, and average acceleration (AA) in cm/sec^2 (calculated by dividing PFV by AT). In addition, the aortic flow velocity integral, or area under the aortic flow velocity curve, was estimated. (See text for details.) (Reprinted from: Gardin JM, Burns CS, Childs WJ, Henry WL. Evaluation blood flow velocity in the ascending aorta and pulmonary artery of normal subjects by Doppler echocardiography. Am Heart J 1984; 107:310–319.)

Figure 1 demonstrates the method for making Doppler measurements from aortic and pulmonary artery flow velocity recordings in a normal subject [10]. Doppler flow velocity in centimeters per second is displayed on the vertical axis and time in seconds on the horizontal axis.

Table 1. Age, gender distribution, heart rate, and body surface area in adult normal subjects.

		No. of subjects		HR		BSA	
Group	Age decade	Men	Women	Men	Women	Men	Women
I	21–30	13	5	58 ± 10	62 ± 9	1.9 ± 0.1	1.7 ± 0.1
II	31–40	6	6	64 ± 10	66 ± 9	1.9 ± 0.2	1.9 ± 0.2
III	41–50	8	10	64 ± 13	61 ± 11	12.1 ± 0.2	1.7 ± 0.2
IV	51–60	10	17	69 ± 15	67 ± 12	1.9 ± 0.2	1.7 ± 0.1
V	61–70	7	13	71 ± 7	70 ± 9	2.0 ± 0.1	1.7 ± 0.1
		44 (total)	51 (total)	65 ± 11 (mean ± SD)	66 ± 10 (mean ± SD)	2.0 ± 0.2 (mean ± SD)	1.7 ± 0.2 (mean ± SD)

HR = heart rate; BSA = body surface area.

Table 2. Relationship of age to aortic flow velocity measurements in adult normal population.

Group	Age (yr)	PFV (cm/sec)	PFV corr (cm/sec)	ET (msec)	ET corr (msec)	FVI (cm)	FVI corr (cm)
		n 80	80	83	82	79	80
I	21–30	93 ± 11	92 ± 14	297 ± 19	293 ± 22	13.8 ± 2.1	13.7 ± 2.2
II	31–40	87 ± 14	91 ± 18	304 ± 20	315 ± 24	13.1 ± 2.2	13.7 ± 2.7
III	41–50	78 ± 17	81 ± 20	315 ± 37	324 ± 38	12.3 ± 3.0	12.7 ± 3.1
IV	51–60	80 ± 13	85 ± 15	313 ± 32	326 ± 23	12.7 ± 2.5	13.2 ± 2.3
V	61–70	65 ± 12	71 ± 13	296 ± 43	321 ± 46	9.5 ± 2.3	10.4 ± 2.5

Group	Age (yr)	FVI Actual (cm)	AT (msec)	AT corr (msec)	AA (cm/sec²)	AA corr (cm/sec²)
		n 79	82	80	78	77
I	21–30	15.8 ± 2.4	100 ± 10	99 ± 12	939 ± 157	930 ± 190
II	31–40	15.0 ± 2.5	106 ± 14	110 ± 15	854 ± 220	895 ± 261
III	41–50	14.1 ± 3.4	103 ± 23	106 ± 24	794 ± 242	822 ± 273
IV	51–60	14.5 ± 2.8	104 ± 16	110 ± 19	765 ± 133	801 ± 158
V	61–70	10.8 ± 2.6	103 ± 32	112 ± 35	695 ± 254	761 ± 291

Abbreviations: n = number of subjects; corr = corrected for heart rate by dividing measurement by the square root of the R–R interval; PFV = peak flow velocity; ET = ejection time; FVI = flow velocity integral; AT = acceleration time; AA = average acceleration. Values are expressed as mean ± standard deviation. (Reprinted from: Gardin *et al.* Relationship between age, body size, gender and blood pressure and Doppler flow measurement in the aorta and pulmonary artery. Am Heart J 1984; 113:101.)

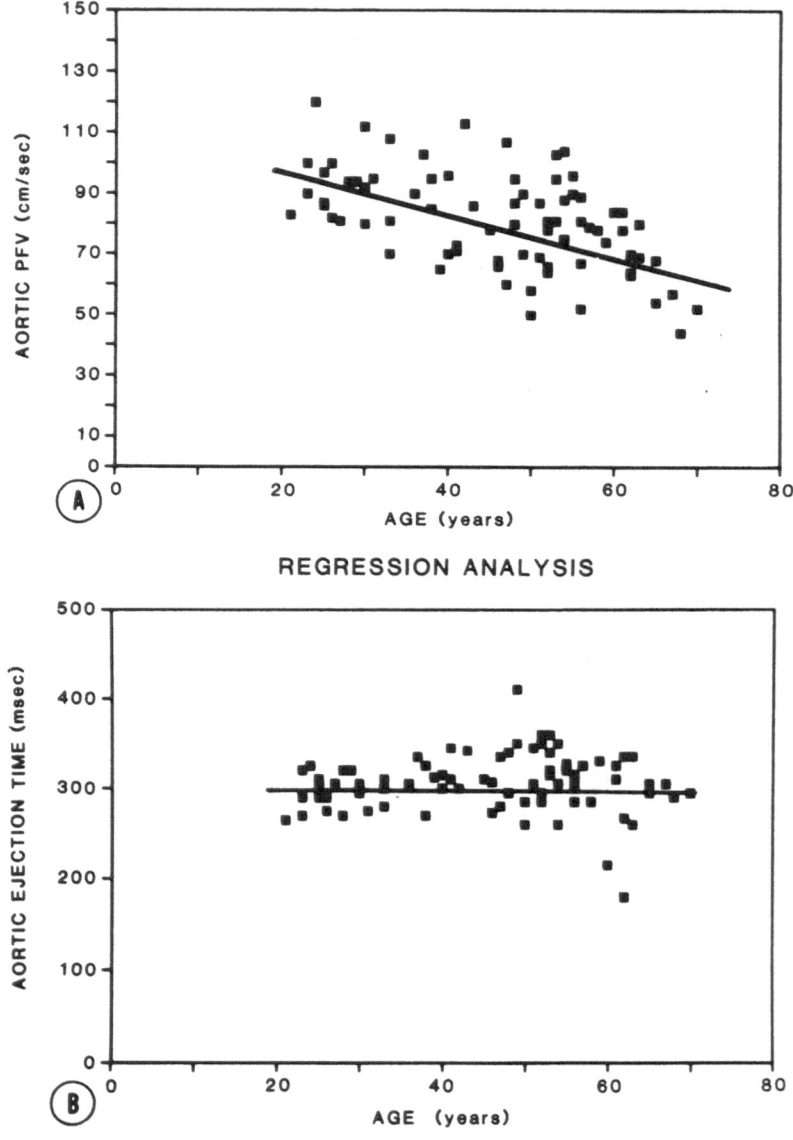

Figure 2. A) Relationship between aortic peak flow velocity (in cm/sec) and age (in years) in the 80 subjects in whom aortic peak flow velocity measurements were available. The solid line represents the line of regression. Note the negative slope of the relationship between the two parameters (r = 0.54). Aortic PFV is significantly lower in the 61- to 70-year age group (mean = 65 cm/sec) than in the 21- to 30-year age group (mean = 93 cm/sec). B) Relationship between aortic ejection time (in msec) and age, displayed in the format of A. Note that there is no significant difference in the mean ejection time in the 61 to 70 year age group (296 msec) compared with the 21 to 30 year age group (297 msec). (Reprinted from: Gardin *et al.* Relationship between age, body size, gender and blood pressure and Doppler flow measurement in the aorta and pulmonary artery. Am Heart J 1984; 113;101.)

Peak flow velocity (PFV) in centimeters per second was measured at the mid-point of the darkest area of the spectrum at the time of maximum flow velocity [7, 8, 10]. Ejection time (ET) was measured in milliseconds from the onset of the systolic flow velocity curve, to the time the curve crossed the zero-flow line at end-systole. In the aorta, the flow velocity integral (FVI, in centimeters) which represents the area under the flow velocity curve, was estimated by the following formula: $FVI = 0.5 \times PFV \times ET$ [8]. This simplified formula underestimates the actual FVI by approximately 16% in normal subjects. Consequently, aortic FVI (actual) in centimeters was estimated by the formula FVI (actual = 1.14 (aortic FVI) + 0.3 [8]. Acceleration time (AT) in milliseconds was measured from the onset of ejection to the mid-point of the Doppler spectrum at the time of peak flow velocity. Average acceleration was calculated by dividing the PFV by the AT and was expressed in centimeters per second. In addition, heart rate-corrected values for ET, AT, and AA were derived by dividing the appropriate time-based measurements by the square root of the RR interval.

Data was analyzed using stepwise linear and multiple regression analysis to assess the effects of age, body surface area, and gender on each of the Doppler measurements. For each of five age decades (Groups I–V), the mean ± standard deviation (S.D.) for heart rate, blood pressure, and body surface area, as well as for each aortic and pulmonary artery Doppler flow parameter, was computed (See Tables 1 and 2).

Table 1 displays the mean ± S.D. for heart rate and body surface area in each of the five age decades for men and women. There was a modest but significant increase in heart rate with increasing age ($r = 0.31$, $p < 0.01$), with the mean (± S.D.) heart rate being 59 (± 9) beats/minute in Group I (the youngest age group) as compared with 69 (± 7) beats/minute in Group V (the oldest age group). Although there was no significant relationship between body surface area and age, note that in each age group the women had smaller body surface areas than the men. The mean (± S.D.) for body surface area was 2.0 ± 0.2 m^2 for all men and 1.7 ± 0.2 m^2 for all women ($p < 0.001$).

Incidentally, blood pressure was also studied in this population, and while systolic blood increased slightly with age ($p < 0.05$), there was no significant relationship between age and diastolic blood pressure in this selected normal population.

6.2 Influence of age

Table 2 displays the relationship between age and aortic Doppler flow velocity measurements. Multiple linear regression analysis revealed that age was significantly correlated with aortic peak flow velocity (PFV), average acceleration, and flow velocity integral (all $p < 0.001$). Figure 2A depicts the overall relationship between aortic PFV (in cm/sec) and age (in years). The two parameters were related by the regression equation:

Aortic PFV = –0.64 (age) + 110 ($r = -0.54$, $p = 0.001$).

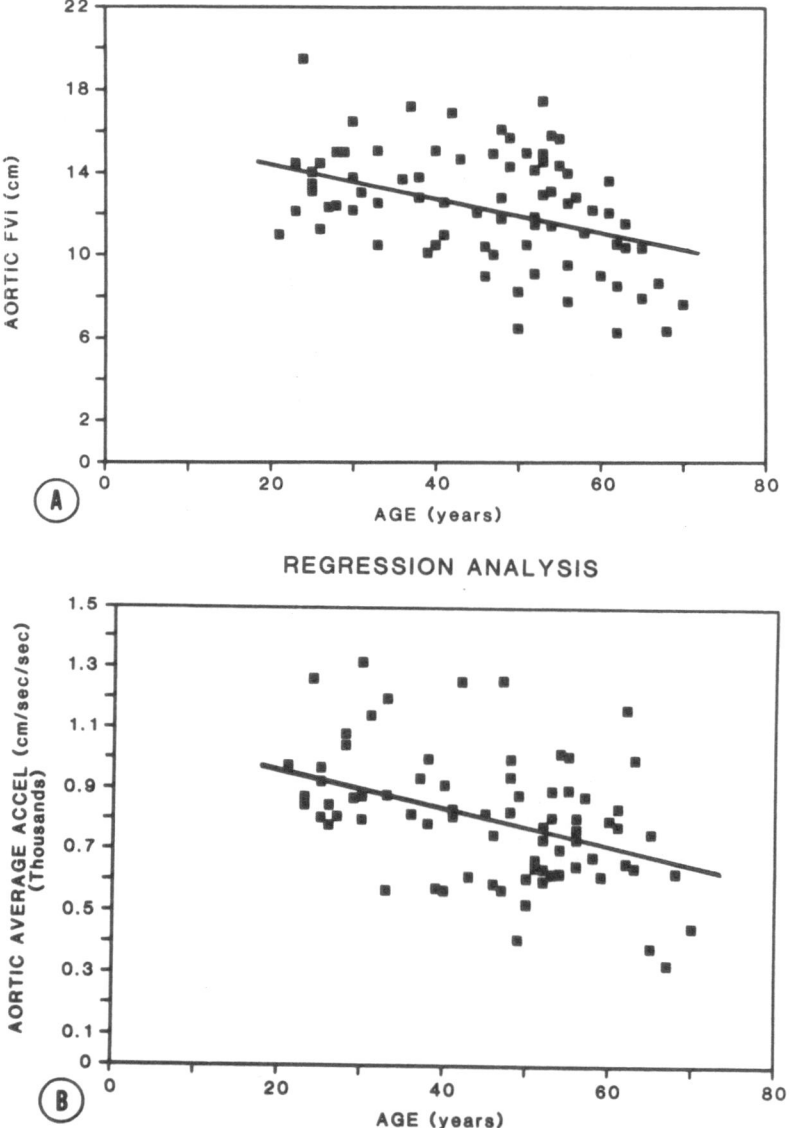

Figure 3. A) Relationship between aortic flow velocity integral (in cm) and age (in years). Note the significantly lower flow velocity integral in the 61 to 70 year age group (mean ± S.D. = 9.5 ± 2.3) than in the 21 to 30 year age group (13.9 ± 2.1 cm) p < 0.001). B) Relationship between aortic average acceleration (in cm/sec²) and age. Note the significantly lower average accleration in the 61 to 70 year decade (mean = 695 cm/sec²) as compared to the 21 to 30 year age group (939 cm/sec², p < 0.005). (Reprinted from: Gardin *et al.* Relationship between age, body size, gender and blood pressure and Doppler flow measurement in the aorta and pulmonary artery. Am Heart J 1984; 113:101.)

Aortic PFV was significantly lower in Group V than in Group I. The correlation of aortic PFV with age remains significant ($p < 0.001$) after division of peak flow velocity by the square root of the RR interval. Figure 2B displays the data for relationship between aortic ejection time (ET) and age. While there was no significant correlation between ejection time and age, ET divided by the square root of the RR interval (ET corr.) increased significantly with increasing age, as expressed by the regression equation:

Aortic ET corr. = 0.78 (age) + 280 ($r = 0.33$, $p < 0.001$).

Figure 3A depicts the relationship between aortic flow velocity integral (FVI) and age. Note that aortic FVI is significantly lower for Group V than for Group I ($p < 0.001$). Aortic FVI and age were related by the regression equation:

Aortic FVI = –0.01 (age) + 16.5 ($r = -0.44$, $p < 0.001$).

There was no significant relationship ($p > 0.05$) between aortic acceleration time and age.

Figure 3B displays the relationship between aortic average acceleration (AA) and age. Note the significantly lower ($p < 0.005$) aortic AA in Group V as compared to Group I. AA in the aorta and age were related by the regression equation

Aortic AA = –6.55 (age) + 1109 ($r = -0.42$ $p < 0.001$).

This correlation remained significant ($r = -0.29$, $p < 0.02$) after dividing AA by the square root of the RR interval.

In summary, Gardin et al. [6] demonstrated that ascending aortic peak flow velocity, flow velocity integral and average acceleration decreased progressively with age, whereas acceleration time remained unchanged. Aortic ejection time (ET) did not change with age, but ET divided by the square root of RR interval increased significantly with increasing age. Light et al. [13] have also shown a decrease in aortic peak flow velocity in normal subjects from the ages of 20–60 years. The decrease in aortic peak flow velocity and flow velocity integral noted with increasing age are probably due, at least in part, to the increase in aortic root diameter (and cross-sectional area) noted with aging [1, 3, 4]. Resting stroke volume [3, 4] and cardiac output [14] do not change significantly with age. Since Doppler stroke volume can be estimated by multiplying the aortic flow velocity integral (FVI) by the aortic root area, a decrease in FVI must be accompanied by an increase in aortic root area (and diameter) to maintain a constant stroke volume. Furthermore, since aortic FVI is approximately equal to one-half the peak flow velocity (PFV) multiplied by the ejection time (ET) [8], and since no change in aortic ET was found with aging by Gardin et al. [10], aortic PFV would be expected to decrease with aging.

As in the aorta, there was no significant relationship between age and ejection time or acceleration time in the pulmonary artery (PA). However, in contrast to the decrease in peak flow velocity (PFV) noted with increasing age in the aorta, there was no significant relationship between PFV in the pulmonary artery and age. Therefore, the pulmonary artery flow velocity integral, which is related to the

68

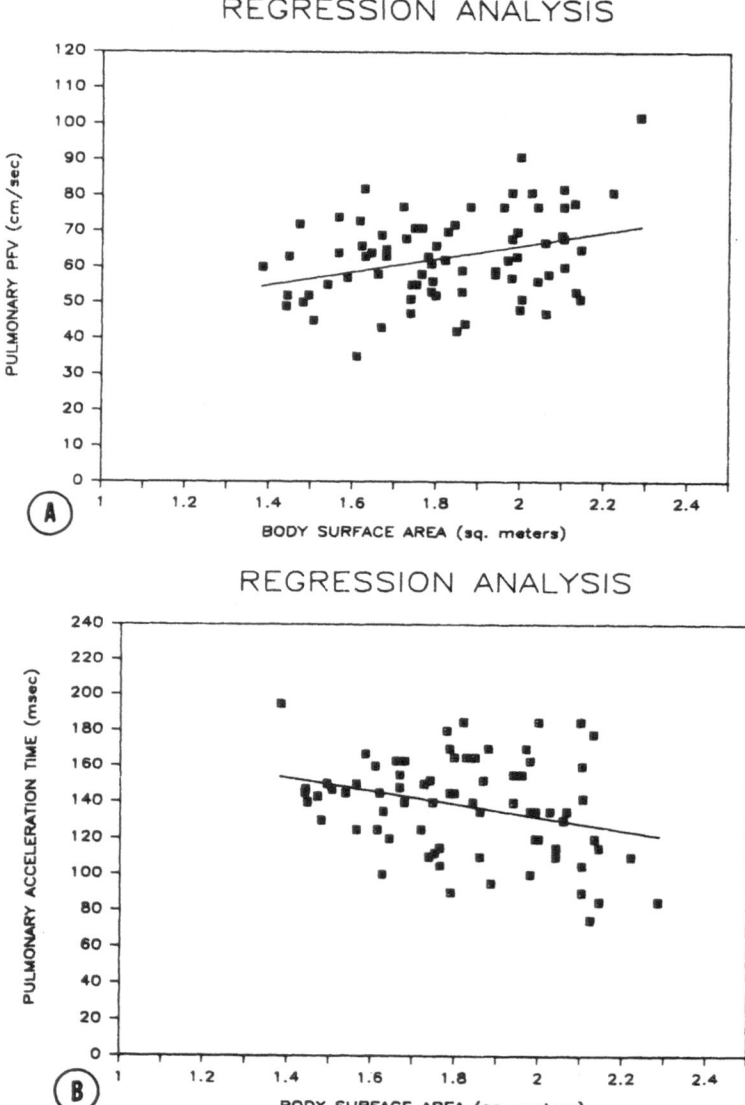

Figure 4. A) Relationship between P peak flow velocity (in cm/sec) and body surface area (in m², n = 76). Note the positive slope of the relationship between the two parameters (r = 0.32, p < 0.02). B) Relationship between PA acceleration time and BSA (r = 0.50, p < 0.002). (Reprinted from: Gardin *et al.* Relationship between age, body size, gender and blood pressure and Doppler flow measurement in the aorta and pulmonary artery. Am Heart J 1984; 113:110.)

product of pulmonary peak flow velocity and ejection time does not change with aging. If PA stroke volume, as is true for aortic stroke volume, also does not change with aging, the area and diameter of the pulmonary artery (unlike ascending aorta) would not be expected to change with aging.

There was no significant correlation between peak flow velocity (PFV) in the pulmonary artery and age. PFV in Group V was 58 cm/sec (mean) and in Group I was 64 cm/sec (mean). Similarly, the correlation between pulmonary artery, average acceleration (or between pulmonary artery, average acceleration corrected for heart rate) and age did not attain statistical significance ($p > 0.05$). Finally, there was no significant correlation between PA ejection time and age, or between PA ejection time divided by the square root of the RR interval and age. Therefore, in contrast to its effects on Doppler *aortic* flow velocity parameters, age had no sig-- nificant influence on any of the Doppler *PA* flow velocity measurements.

6.3 Influence of body surface area (Table 3)

There was no significant relationship ($p > 0.05$) between body surface and any of the Doppler *aortic* flow measurements. In contrast, body surface area was related to various Doppler *pulmonary artery* measurements. Figure 4A depicts the relationship between pulmonary artery peak flow velocity (in cm/sec) versus body surface area (in square meters, range 1.44 to 2.29). Note that mean pulmonary artery peak flow velocity increased from 57 cm/sec at a body surface are of $1.5m^2$ to 71 cm/sec on a body surface area of 2.25 m^2. Pulmonary artery peak flow velocity (PFV) and body surface area were related by the following regression equation:

Pulmonary Artery PFV = 1.86 (BSA) + 29 ($r = 0.33$, $p < 0.01$).

This correlation with body surface area remains significant ($r = 0.34$) after correction of pulmonary artery PFV for the square root of the RR interval. There was no significant relationship between either PA ejection time or PA ejection time corrected for the square root of the RR interval, and body surface area.

Figure 4B depicts the relationship between pulmonary artery acceleration time (AT) (in milliseconds) and body surface area. Note that in going from a body surface area of 1.5 m^2 to 2.25 m^2, AT decreases from 150 to 123 milliseconds. The following regression equation relates PA AT to body surface area:

Pulmonary AT = –35.6 (BSA) + 203 ($r = -0.29$, $p < 0.02$).

This relationship remains significant after correction of AT for the square root of the R–R interval.

Pulmonary artery average acceleration (AA) (in cm/sec/sec) and body surface area (in m^2) were related by the following regression equation:

Pulmonary AA = 322 (BSA) – 107 ($r = 0.41$, $p < 0.002$).

Mean pulmonary artery AA increased significantly from 376 cm/sec^2 at a body surface area of 1.5 m^2 to 617 cm/sec^2 at a body surface area of 2.25 m^2. The correlation between pulmonary artery AA and body surface area remains significant after correction for the square root of the R–R interval.

Table 3. Relationship of body surface area to pulmonary artery flow velocity measurements in adult normal subjects.

BSA (m^2)		PFV (cm/sec)	PFV corr (cm/sec)	ET (msec)	ET corr (msec)
	n	67	67	68	68
1.40–1.75		60 ± 11	63 ± 13	323 ± 23	335 ± 24
1.76–2.00		61 ± 9	63 ± 10	334 ± 21	345 ± 29
2.01 ± 2.25		67 ± 12	72 ± 12	309 ± 35	334 ± 30
BSA (m^2)		AT (msec)	AT corr (msec)	AA (cm/sec^2)	AA corr (cc/sec^2)
	n	67	67	66	66
1.40–1.75		143 ± 20	149 ± 18	429 ± 114	450 ± 141
1.76–2.00		149 ± 27	154 ± 28	425 ± 109	441 ± 125
2.01–2.25		124 ± 31	132 ± 27	561 ± 162	607 ± 196

Abbreviations: n = number of subjects; corr = corrected for heart rate by dividing measurement by the square foot of the R–R interval; PFV = peak flow velocity; ET = ejection time; AT = acceleration time; AA = average acceleration; BSA = body surface area. (Reprinted from: Gardin *et al*. Relationship between age, body size, gender and blood pressure and Doppler flow measurement in the aorta and pulmonary artery. Am Heart J 1984; 113:101.)

6.4 Summary

Influence of gender. This study showed that there was no significant difference in values for Doppler aortic or pulmonic artery flow velocity parameters between men and women of the same age and body surface area. The differences between men and women in pulmonary artery Doppler measurements could, in general, be explained by differences in body surface area.

Influence of Body Surface Area (BSA). There was no significant relationship between BSA and any of the Doppler aortic measurements over a range of body surface areas from 1.44 to 2.29 m^2. However, in the pulmonary artery, there were significant increases in peak flow velocity and average acceleration and a decrease in acceleration time with increasing BSA, primarily over the range of larger body surface areas seen in men. The reason for this relationship is not readily apparent, and may be due to differences in lifestyle factors such as daily activities or smoking, but this hypothesis requires further investigation.

Influence of blood pressure. While there was no significant relationship between BP and any of the aortic or pulmonary artery flow velocity in these normal subjects, it is certainly possible that abnormalities in systolic or disastolic BP may have an effect on Doppler flow velocity parameters. In fact, studies [15–17] have shown tha elevated mean pulmonary artery (PA) pressure results in a shortening of PA acceleratin time.

6.5 Doppler flow velocity measurements in the aorta during upright treadmill exercise

Studies by Lazarus *et al.* [18] evaluated the possible effects of age and gender on Doppler aortic blood flow velocity measurements in 60 normal subjects aged 15–74 years, who underwent upright treadmill exercise tests. Subjects had no evidence of previous cardiovascular disease and were divided into three groups, based on their age (Table 4). Group I was composed of 20 subjects aged 15 to 29 (mean ± SD = 21 ± 4); Group II consisted of 20 subjects aged 30 to 49 years (mean ± SD = 36 ± 5); Group III included 20 subjects aged 50 to 74 year (mean ± SD = 58 ± 7). Subjects were studied using the Bruce protocol at rest and during exercise. A non-imaging, continuous wave ultrasound transducer interfaced to a dedicated Doppler velocimeter (ExerDop, Quinton Instruments, Co.) was used to record ascending aortic flow from the suprasternal notch [18].

Statistical analysis of Doppler flow velocity measurements in the three age groups was performed using an analysis of variance and the Tukey-A test. Linear regression analysis was used to compare changes in heart rate and blood pressure with Doppler aortic peak velocity and peak acceleration. To evaluate the role of physical conditioning on the response of Doppler measurements to exercise, two groups were defined. Group A was composed of 23 subjects (mean age 37.5 years) who were not involved in any routine exercise, while Group B consisted of 21 subjects (mean age 38.5 years) who routinely exercised on two or more days per week.

Table 4. Subject profile for the 60 healthy participants in the exercise study.

Group	Subjects (n)	Male (n)	Female (n)	Age (yrs)
1	20	14	6	21 ± 4
2	20	13	7	36 ± 5
3	20	12	8	58 ± 7

Values are mean standard deviation. (Reprinted from: Lazarus *et al.* Evaluation of age, gender, heart rate, and blood pressure changes and exercises conditioning on Doppler measured aortic blood flow acceleration and velocity during upright treadmill testing. Am J Cardiol 1988; 62:439.)

72

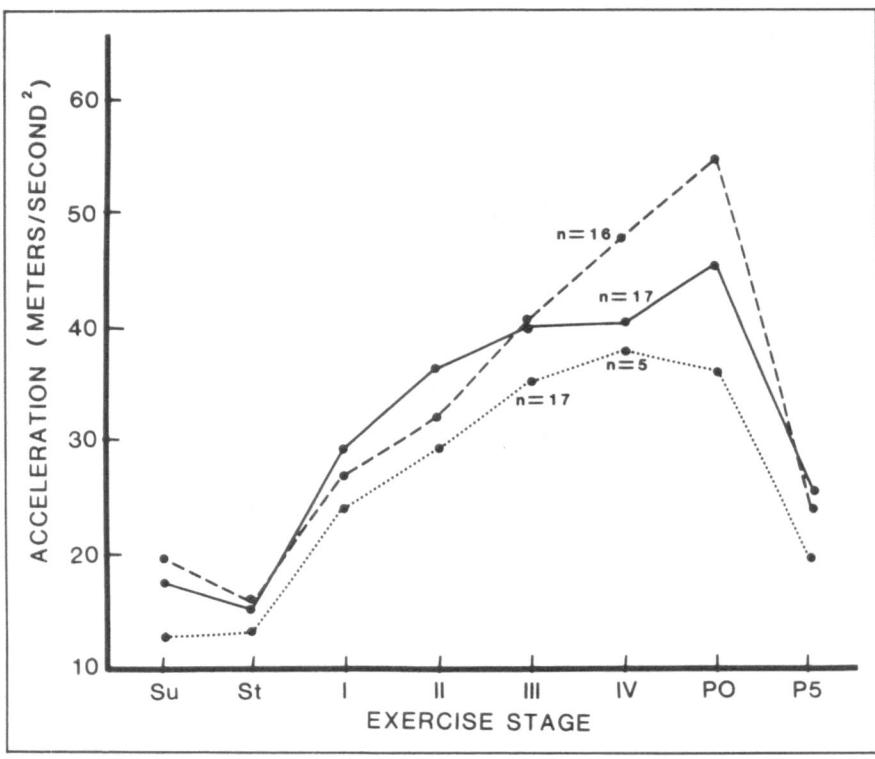

Figure 5. Doppler peak acceleration measurements before, during and immediately after exercise testing as recorded by continuous wave Doppler from the suprasternal notch. St = standing; Su = supine; Po = immediate post exercise; PS = 5 minutes after exercise. Data are shown on the mean for 20 subjects in each group except as noted by "n" value in exercise Stage III and IV. (Reprinted from: Lazarus *et al.* Evaluation of age, gender, heart rate, and blood pressure changes and exercise conditioning on Doppler measured aortic blood flow acceleration and velocity during upright treadmill testing. Am J Cardiol 1988; 62:439.)

6.6 Influence of age

Peak acceleration. As seen in Figure 5, peak acceleration measured at rest in the supine position was found to be significantly higher in the youngest age group (Group I, $p < 0.01$). During exercise, blood flow acceleration increased in all age groups over the respective baseline values in the standing position, before starting exercise. In the immediate post-exercise period (standing position), peak aortic blood flow acceleration decreased in Group III below the value recorded during stage 4 exercise, while it continued to rise for the younge age groups. A statistically significant difference between the groups was found only during the immediate post-exercise period ($p < 0.05$).

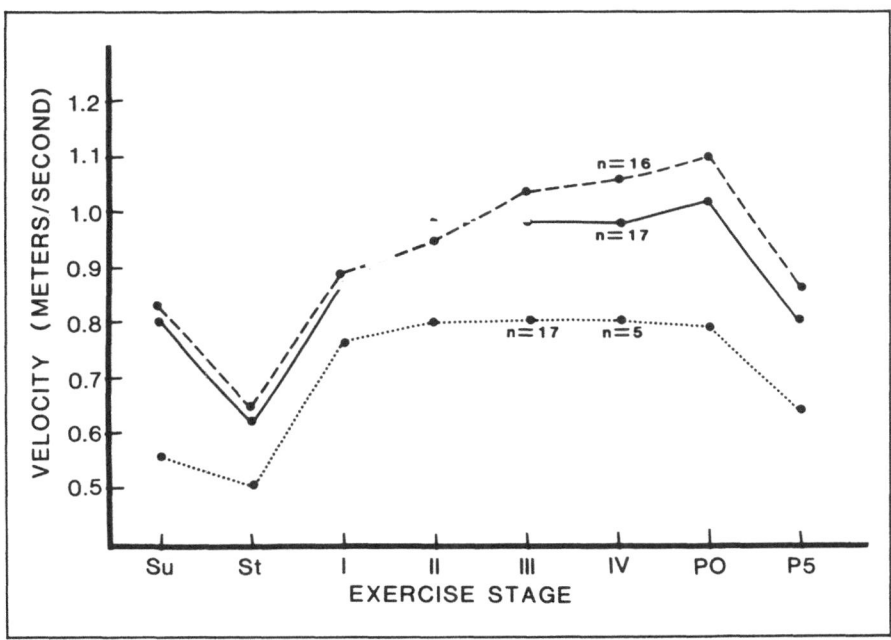

Figure 6. Doppler peak aortic velocity measurements before, during and immediately after exercise testing as recorded by continuous wave Doppler. Format and abbreviations are as in Figure 5 (Reprinted from: Lazarus *et al.* Evaluation of age, gender, heart rate and blood pressure changes and exercise conditioning on Doppler measured aortic blood flow acceleration and velocity during upright treadmill testing. Am J Cardiol 1988; 62:439.)

This study demonstrated that peak acceleration of blood flow was inversely related to age, but not related to gender or changes in heart rate or blood pressure. The data are consistent with previous aortic Doppler measurements in resting normal subjects [6]. With increasing exercise time, peak acceleration increased for Group I and II into the immediate post-exercise period, but not for the oldest subjects (Group III), in whom immediate post-exercise peak acceleration decreased compared with the stage 4 value. A similar decrease in peak velocity (and velocity) occurred in Group III in the immediate post-exercise period compared with peak exercise.

Peak velocity. Data for aortic peak velocity in the three age groups are shown in Figure 6. Age was also inversely related to resting and exercise aortic peak velocity. Peak velocity was higher at rest, throughout exercise, and in the recovery period, for the two younger age groups than for Group III. A statistical difference between the groups was found only in the standing position during the immediate post-exercise state (Group I, 1.1 ± 0.2; Group 2, 1.0 ± 0.2; Group III, 0.8 ± 0.2

meters per second, p < 0.01). In all three age groups, velocity increased with exercise. For the youngest subjects, peak velocity increased throughout exercise into the immediate post-exercise period. In Groups II and III, peak velocity reached a maximum in the earliest stages (two and three) of exercise and levelled off as exercise continued.

It is unknown whether the decreased peak velocity in Group III during exercise is related to silent ischemia or merely to the increased aortic root area known to occur with aging [3, 6]. Although motion artifact during exercise might potentially be a source for erroneous and non-reproducible Doppler measurements, previous studies with the ExerDop instrument have shown good correlation of Doppler peak velocity and acceleration with invasive measurements [19, 20].

6.7 Influence of gender and physical conditioning

Gender did not affect aortic peak acceleration and peak velocity at rest or during exercise. Level of exercise conditioning was also not significantly related to heart rate (between immediate post-exercise and stnading pre-exercise), peak aortic acceleration, or peak velocity (Table 5).

Table 5. Heart rate, Doppler peak aortic acceleration and peak velocity responses.

Exercise Program	Maximum exercise time (min)	Δ Peak acceleration (m/s^2)	Δ Peak velocity (m/s)	Δ Heart rate (bpm)
Yes (n = 23)	13.2	32.8	0.37	89
No (n = 21)	10.5	30.5	0.38	95

bpm = beats/min. Subjects participating in regularly scheduled exercise programs (n = 23) compared with those subjects (n = 21) not exercising on a routine basis. Delta values are calculated as the difference between immediate post-exercise and standing preexercise data. (Reprinted from: Lazarus *et al*. Evaluation of age, gender, heart rate, and blood pressure changes and exercise conditioning on Doppler measured aortic blood flow acceleration and velocity during upright treadmill testing. Am J Cardiol 1988: 6⌐·439.)

6.8 Doppler flow velocity measurements in the aorta during supine bicycle exercise

Doppler aortic flow velocity signals were recorded during supine bicycle exercise in 17 normal subjects by Gardin, *et al*. [21]. Seven men and ten women, aged 17 to 24 years, were evaluated. All subjects were normal in weight; none were trained athletes. Similar inclusion criteria were used in these subjects as described above for the Doppler studies at rest [6, 1, 18]. These subjects performed supine exercise using an adjustable, horizontal table equipped with a bicycle ergometer (W.E. Collins, Inc.) [21] Pulsed Doppler recordings of aortic velocity were performed in the ascending aorta. (See Table 6.) The method for performing Doppler aortic flow velocity measurements, including positioning the nonimaging Doppler transducer in the suprasternal notch, was similar to that used in previous studies [7, 8, 10].

Table 6. Changes in Doppler aortic flow velocity parameters during exercise.

	PFV (cm/s)	ET (ms)	HR (beats/min)	FVI (cm)	HR X FVI (cm/min)
Control	109 ± 16	294 ± 30	69 ± 13	18.2 ± 2.9	$1,239 \pm 226$
Early exercise	$124 \pm 13^*$	$269 \pm 23^*$	$99 \pm 12^*$	19.1 ± 2.6	$1,863 \pm 269^*$
Late exercise	$140 \pm 19^*$	$218 \pm 29^*$	$138 \pm 16^*$	17.0 ± 2.9	$2,335 \pm 379^*$
Peak exercise	$147 \pm 23^*$	$194 \pm 22^*$	$159 \pm 14^*$	$16.1 \pm 2.5^{\ddagger}$	$2,567 \pm 441^*$
Early recovery	$158 \pm 21^*$	$204 \pm 24^*$	$129 \pm 15^*$	18.3 ± 2.6	$2,310 \pm 424^*$
Late recovery	$123 \pm 21^*$	$274 \pm 27^{\dagger}$	$90 \pm 16^{\dagger}$	19.1 ± 3.4	$1,684 \pm 302^*$

Levels of significance when compared to control values: $*$ $p<0.005$; $\dagger$ $p<0.01$; $\ddagger$ $p<0.05$; all others not significant. ET = ejection time; FVI = flow velocity integral; HR = heart rate; PFV = peak flow velocity. (Reprinted from: Lazarus *et al.* Evaluation of age, gender, heart rate, and blood pressure changes and exercise conditioning on Doppler measured aortic blood flow acceleration and velocity during upright treadmill testing. Am J Cardiol 1988; 62:439.)

As shown in Table 6 and Figure 7, this study demonstrated the feasibility of making the Doppler aortic peak flow velocity measurements during exercise using pulsed Doppler echocardiography. On average, aortic PFV increased by a maximum of 45% during supine bicycle exercise. Aortic peak velocity reached its maximum at two minutes after exercise, rather than at peak exercise, probably due to a normal vasodilator response of peripheral resistance vessels immediately after exercise. Aortic ejection time decreased by 34% during exercise, and was shortest at peak exercise. Since heart rate was maximal (130% above control), and R–R interval lowest at peak exercise, it is understandable that ejection time was shortest at peak exercise.

Neither peak flow velocity, nor ejection time, nor heart rate had returned to control by ten minutes after exercise. Aortic flow velocity integral decreased by 10% at peak exercise, but since aortic diameter was not measured at the site of Doppler recording, flow velocity integral data could not be directly translated into absolute stroke volume changes. Nevertheless, since aortic root size was not felt to change significantly during exercise, aortic flow velocity integral probably provides a reasonable measure of stroke volume during exercise.

6.9 Summary

Doppler echocardiography has become a useful tool in assessing left ventricular function. Changes in Doppler aortic peak ejection velocity or acceleration have shown good correlation with changes in left ventricular ejection fraction during exercise [22–25] with ejection fraction as determined by left ventricular angio-

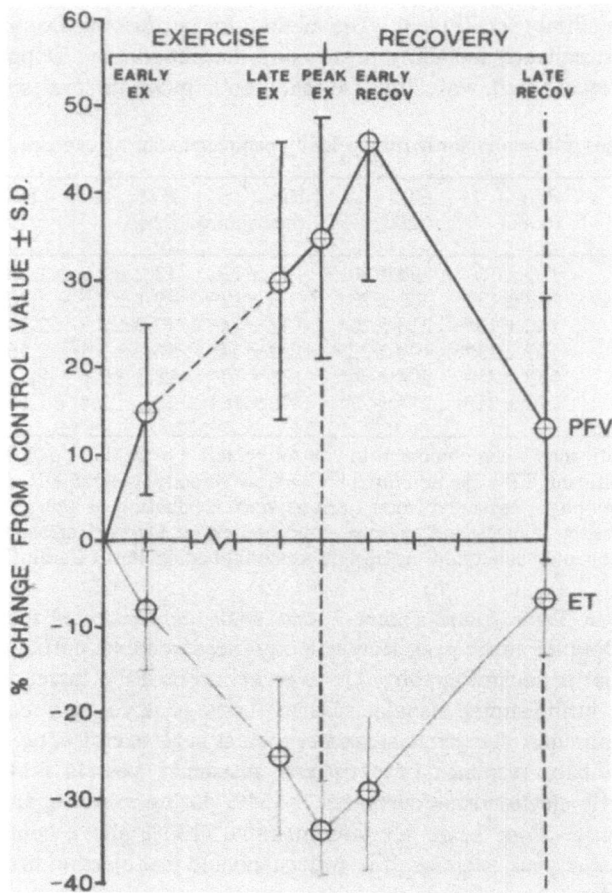

Figure 7. Percent changes (mean ± standard deviation [S.D.]) from control values for peak flow velocity (*PFV*) and ejection time (*ET*) at early exercise (EX), 2 minutes before peak exercise, peak exercise, 2 minutes after exercise, and 10 minutes after exercise. Peak flow velocity reached a maximal level of 45% above control at 2 minutes after exercise and is still elevated at 10 minutes after exercise. Ejection time decreases progressively with exercise, being 34% less than control at peak exercise and remaining abnormal at 10 minutes after exercise. (Reprinted from: Gardin *et al.* Studies of Doppler aortic flow velocity during supine bicycle exercise. Am J Cardiol 1986; 57:327.)

graphy [25, 26], with cardiac output as determined by the thermodilution technique [27], and with left ventricular ischemia produced by coronary artery ligation in anesthetized dogs [28]. Doppler aortic ejection phase measurements have also been of value in predicting the presence of ischemic myocardium in human subjects during routine treadmill testing [29, 30].

To use Doppler aortic flow measurements meaningfully, one must consider the effects on these measurements of the normal aging process and gender, as well as of resting and exercise blood pressure, heart rate, and loading factors. In this chapter, we have reviewed studies that address some of these factors.

It is clear that both at rest and during exercise, aortic peak flow velocity, flow velocity integral (reflecting stroke volume), and average acceleration all decrease with aging. Ejection time (corrected for heart rate) increases and there is no change in acceleration time. Aortic peak flow velocity is not significantly affected by gender or body surface area. Doppler pulmonary artery peak flow velocity, on the other hand, is apparently not affected by the aging process, while it shows an increase, as does average acceleration with increased body surface area. With exercise, peak velocity and peak acceleration do increase in younger adults, while they decrease in older normal subjects in immediate post-exercise period. This discrepancy is the result of multiple factors affecting older subjects such as aortic stiffening and uncoiling, Doppler angle, and possibility of silent ischemia.

References

1. Krovetz J. Age-related changes in size of the aortic valve anulus in man. Am Heart J 1975; 90:569–574.
2. Gerstenblith G, Frederiksen J, Yin FCP, Fortui NJ, Lakatta EG, Wiesfeldt ML. Echocardiographic assessment of a normal aging population. Circulation 1977; 56:273–8.
3. Gardin JM, Henry WL, Savage DD, Ware JH, Burn C, Borer JS. Echocardiographic measurement in normal subjects: Evaluation of an adult population without clinically apparent heart disease. J Clin Ultrasound 1978; 7:439–47.
4. Henry WL, Gardin JM, Ware JH. Echocardiographic measurement in normal subject from infancy to old age. Circulation 1980; 62:1054–61.
5. DeMaria AN, Neumann A, Schubert PJ, Lee G, Mason DT. Systematic correlation of cardiac chamber size and ventricular performance determined with echocardiography and alterations in heart rate in normal persons. Am J Cardiol 1979; 43:1–9.
6. Gardin JM, Davidson DM, Rohan MK, Butman S, Knoll M, Garcia R, Dubrai S. Relationship between age, body size, gender, and blood pressure and Doppler flow measurements in the aorta and pulmonary artery. Am Heart J 1987; 113:101–109.
7. Gardin JM, Iseri LT, Elkayam U, Tobis J, Child W, Burn CS, Henry WL. Evaluation of dilated cardiomyopathy in pulsed Doppler echocardiography. Am Heart J 1983; 106:1057–65.
8. Elkayam U, Gardin JM, Berkley R, Hughes C, Henry WL. The use of Doppler flow velocity measurement to assess the hemodynamic response to vasodilator in patients with heart failure. Circulation 1983; 67:377–83.
9. Griffith JM, Henry WL. An ultrasound system for combined cardiac imaging and Doppler blood flow measurements in man. Circulation 1978; 57:925–30.
10. Gardin JM, Burn CS, Childs JT, Henry WL. Evaluation of blood flow velocity in the ascending aorta and main pulmonary artery of normal subjects by Doppler echocardiography. Am Heart J 1984; 107:310–9.
11. Steingart RM, Miller J, Barovick, J, Patterson R, Herman M, Teichholz LE. Pulsed Doppler echocardiographic measurements of beat-to-beat changes in stroke volume in dogs. Circulation 1980; 62:542–48.
12. Snedecor GW, Cochran WC. Statistical methods (7th ed.). Iowa State University Press, Ames, Iowa 1980; 215–237, 334–364.
13. Light LH, Cross G. Convenient monitoring of cardiac output and global left-ventricular function by transcutaneous aortovelography – an effective alternative to cardiac output measurements. In: Spencer M (ed.). Cardiac Doppler diagnosis. Martinus Nijhoff,

Boston, 1983; 69–80.

14. Rodeheffer RJ, Gerstenblith G, Becker LC, Fleg JL, Weisfeldt ML, Lakatta EG. Exercise cardiac output is maintained with advanced age in healthy human subjects: Cardiac dilation and increased stroke volume compensate for a diminished heart rate. Circulation 1984; 69:203–13.

15. Dabestani A, Mahan G, Gardin JM, Takenaka K, Burn C, Allfie A, Henry WL. Evaluation of pulmonary artery pressure and resistance by pulsed Doppler echocardiography. Am J Cardiol (In press).

16. Kitabatake A, Inoue M, Asao M, Masuyama A, Tanouci J, Morita T, Mishima A, Uematsu M, Shimazu T, Hori M, Abe H. Non-invasive evaluation of pulmonary hypertension by pulsed Doppler techniques. Circulation 1983; 68:302–9.

17. Kosturakis D, Goldberg SJ, Allen HD, Loeber C. Doppler-echocardiography prediction of pulmonary arterial hypertension in congenital heart disease. Am J Cardiol 1984; 53:1110–1115.

18. Lazarus M, Dang T, Gardin JM, Allfie A, Henry WL. Evaluation of age, gender, heart rate, and blood pressure changes and exercise conditioning on Doppler measured aortic blood flow acceleration and velocity during upright treadmill testing. Am J Cardiol 1988; 62:439–43.

19. Stein PD, Sabbah HN, Albert DE, Snyder JE. Blood velocity and acceleration: Comparison of continuous wave Doppler with electromagnetic flowmetry (abstract). Fed Proc 1985; 44:1565.

20. Mehta N, Noble MIM, Mills CJ, Pugh S, Drake Holland A, Bennett ED. Validation of Doppler measured ascending aortic blood velocity and acceleration in humans against an electromagnetic cetheter-tip system (abstract). Med Res Soc 1986; AHR–4858.

21. Gardin JM, Kozlowski J, Dabestani A, Murphy M, Kusnick C, Allfie A, Russel D, Henry WL. Studies of Doppler aortic flow velocity during supine bicycle exercise. Am J Cardiol, 1986; 57:327–32.

22. Mehdirad AA, Williams GA, Labovitz AJ, Bryg RJ, Chaitman BR. Evaluation of left ventricular function during upright exercise: Correlation of exercise Doppler with post-exercise two-dimensional echocardiographic results. Circulation 1987; 40:413–419.

23. Teague SM, Corn C, Sharma M, Prasad R, Burrow R, Voyles WF, Thadand U. A comparison of Doppler and radionuclied ejection dynamics during ischemic exercise. Am J Cardiac Imaging 1987; 1:145–51.

24. Bryg RJ, Labovitz AJ, Mehdirad AA, Williams GA, Chaitman BR. Effect of coronary artery disease on Doppler-derived parameters of aortic flow during upright exercise. Am J Cardiol 1986; 58:14–19.

25. Sabbah HN, Khaja F. Bryman JF, McFarland TM, Albert DE, Stein PD. Non-invasive measurement of peak aortic blood acceleration with continuous wave Doppler for the assessment of left ventricular performance in patients (abstract). JACC 1986; 7:11A.

26. Sabbah HN, Khaja F, Brymer JF, McFarland TM, Albert DE, Snyder JE, Goldstein S, Stein PD. Non-invasive evaluation of left ventricular performance based on peak aortic blood acceleration measured with a continuous wave Doppler velocity meter. Circulation 1986; 74:323–29.

27. Nishimura RA, Callahan MJ, Schaff HV, Ilstrup DM, Miller FA, Tajik AJ. Non-invasive measurement of cardiac output by continuous wave Doppler echocardiography: Initial experience and review of the literature. Mayo Clinic Proc. 1984; 59:484–489.

28. Sabbah HN, Przybysiski J, Albert DE, Stein PD. Peak aortic blood acceleration reflects the extent of left ventricular ischemic mass at risk. Am Heart J 1987; 113:885–890.

29. Teague SM, Mark DB, Bradford M, Robertson J, Albert D, Porter JA, Waugh RA. Doppler velocity profiles reveal ischemic exercise response (abstract). Circulation 1984; 70 (suppl):II–185.

30. Williams, GA, Labovitz AJ, Byers SL, Windhorst DM, Chaitman BR. Change in cardiac output with exercise in patients with and without CAD as measured by Doppler echocardiography (abstract). Clin Res 1985; 33:328A.

7. Exercise Doppler in coronary artery disease: Correlation with thallium-201 perfusion scintigraphy

ROBERT M. ROTHBART and ROBERT S. GIBSON
Cardiac Noninvasive Laboratory – Division of Cardiology, University of Virginia Health Sciences Center, Charlottesville, Virginia, U.S.A.

7.1 Introduction

During the past 12 years, more than 15,000 exercise thallium-201 scintigraphic studies have been performed in the Cardiac Noninvasive Laboratory of the University of Virginia. Although thallium perfusion imaging has been extremely useful for the evaluation of myocardial blood flow reserve in our institution, we recognize the considerable technical difficulties associated with its implementation and optimal use in clinical laboratories whose previous experience in Nuclear Cardiology is limited. Accordingly, we have been intrigued by the development of Doppler instruments with the potential to assess cardiac ischemia by the measurement of aortic ejection phase parameters during exercise. In this chapter we summarize our experience with suprasternal Doppler aortic blood flow measurements during treadmill exercise testing in a large population of normal patients and compare stress Doppler results to thallium-201 scintigraphy in a cohort of patients referred for evaluation of suspected or known coronary artery disease.

7.2 Value and limitations of exercise thallium-201 testing

Electrocardiographic stress testing has dominated the assessment of coronary artery disease during most of the 60 years that have elapsed since Feil and Siegel's description of exercise-induced ST segment depression [1] and Master's initial report of formal exercise testing [2]. Despite improvements in electrocardiographic quality, lead systems and test interpretation, the diagnostic accuracy of standard stress testing continues to be suboptimal. Sensitivity is limited, particularly for patients with single vessel coronary artery disease in whom values of 0.60–0.70 have commonly been reported [3, 4]. Specificity has tended to be somewhat better; nonetheless, most studies have found an undesirably high 10–20% prevalence of false positive tests. The diagnostic accuracy of exercise testing can be significantly improved if performed in conjunction with any one of a number of cardiac imaging techniques developed during the past 2 decades. Most widely used among these is thallium-201 scintigraphy, whose diagnostic [5–16] and prognostic [17–21] capabilities in patients with coronary artery disease have been extensively validated.

Steve M. Teague (ed.) Stress Doppler Echocardiography, 79–94.
© 1990 *Kluwer Academic Publishers.*

Thallium-201 imaging is particularly valuable for diagnosis of coronary artery disease in individuals with single vessel disease [3] and in patients who fail to achieve an adequate work level [8, 14], manifest substantial abnormalities on their resting electrocardiographic tracings [13, 15] or have a high likelihood for false positive electrocardiographic responses during exercise [12, 15]. However, considerably more than dichotomous diagnostic information is provided by these studies. They can be used to evaluate the extent of coronary disease [6, 10, 11] and the significance of individual stenoses [16] as well as to provide important prognostic data in patients with chest pain [19, 20], symptomatic ischemic heart disease [18] or prior myocardial infarction [21]. Exercise-induced lung uptake of thallium is a powerful predictor of subsequent cardiac events and death [17]. Thallium imaging has also been effective in the evaluation of revascularization therapies including coronary artery bypass grafting [22], percutaneous coronary angioplasty [23] and thrombolysis [24, 25].

The aforementioned advantages of thallium-201 scintigraphy must be balanced against its drawbacks. Highly trained technicians and impeccable quality control are mandatory if results reported in the literature are to be equaled in clinical practice. Thallium-201 is a relatively expensive radiopharmaceutical that must be generated in a cyclotron, transported promptly and used soon after delivery. Additional expense accrues from the purchase and maintenance of gamma cameras and the labor intensive process of image acquisition and analysis. Thallium scintigraphy prolongs and complicates stress testing and results in significant radiation exposure to the patient. Moreover, a number of other problems including disposal of radioactive wastes and licensure of laboratory personnel are inherent in the use of this technology. Finally, even after extensive training, inter-reader variability in the interpretation of thallium images remains considerable; a consensus interpretation from multiple readers is desirable if diagnostic accuracy is to be optimized [26].

The difficulties associated with thallium-201 have precluded its routine use during stress testing in many laboratories. Exercise Doppler, as a simpler, safer and less expensive test offers major potential advantages in comparison to radionuclide studies; however, Doppler's role in the assessment of coronary disease has not yet been adequately explored. In the remainder of this chapter, we will describe initial studies from our laboratory and others investigating to what extent, if any, suprasternal Doppler recordings of ascending aortic blood flow might replace thallium-201 scintigraphy as an adjunct to exercise testing.

7.3 Exercise Doppler studies at the University of Virginia

We performed exercise testing on a treadmill using the standard Bruce protocol, obtaining 12 lead electrocardiograms and blood pressure determinations at baseline, at 1 minute intervals throughout exercise and during the initial 5 minutes of recovery. Tests were terminated for limiting symptoms of angina, dyspnea or fatigue, for ventricular tachycardia or for symptomatic exercise-induced hypotension. Electrocardiographic responses were regarded as abnormal if 1 mm or more

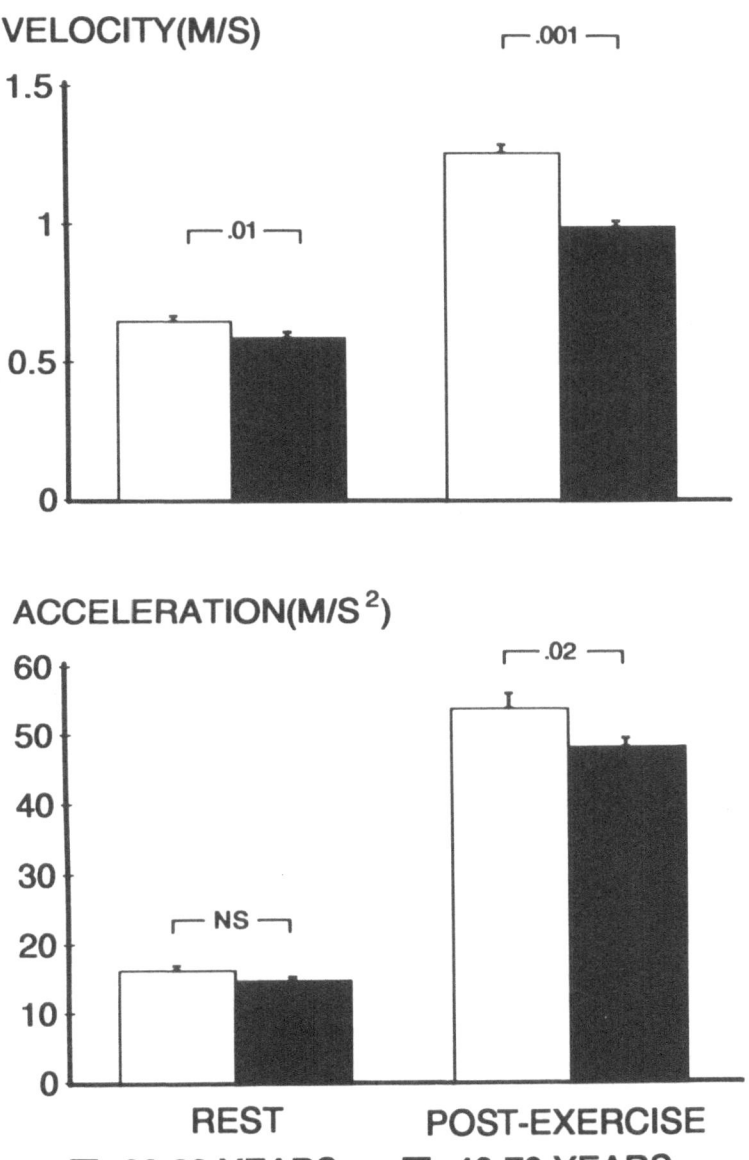

Figure 1. Mean velocity and acceleration at rest and immediately post-exercise for all subjects with a probability of coronary artery disease < 5%. Data is displayed for 2 age ranges, 20–39 years and 40–70 years. In this and all subsequent figures, the numeric values and associated brackets refer to the p values for the indicated comparisons of means. The error bars denote standard errors of the mean. NS = no statistical significance.

82

% INCREASE

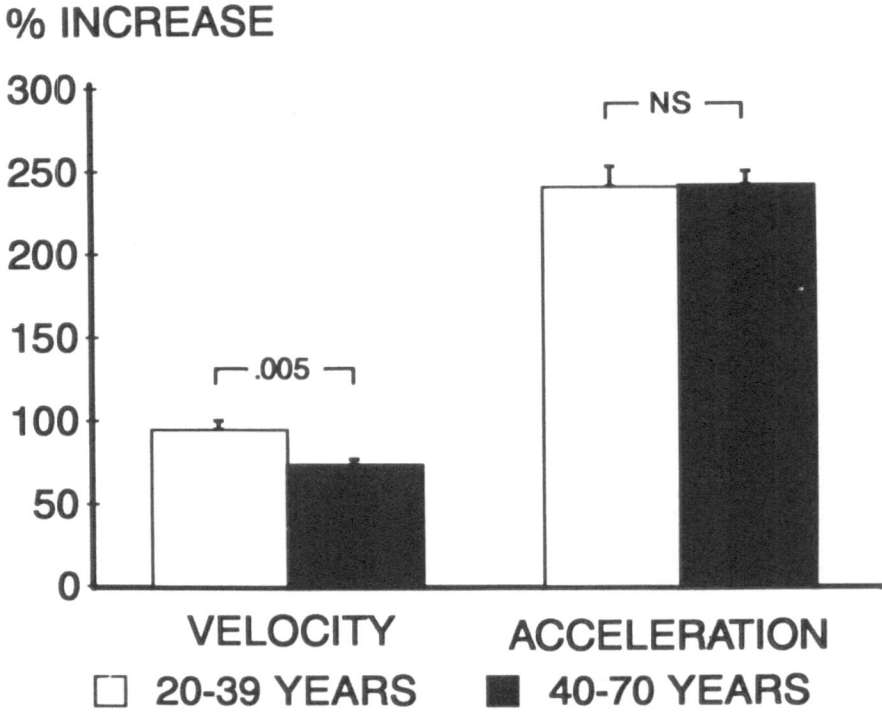

Figure 2. Percent increase from resting to immediate post-exercise Doppler measurements of velocity and acceleration in subjects with a < 5% probability of coronary artery disease in the age ranges 20–39 years and 40–70 years.

of ST segment depression occurred 80 ms after the J point in 3 consecutive complexes.

For blood flow measurements, we utilized a continuous wave Doppler device with a non-imaging 3 MHz transducer specifically designed for suprasternal interrogation of the ascending aorta during exercise (Exerdop, Quinton Instrument Company, Seattle, Washington, U.S.A.). With the patient in the standing position, 10 consecutive systolic flow signals were recorded at rest, at the end of each stage of exercise and immediately post-exercise from which the Doppler instrument automatically derived measurements of peak modal velocity and maximal acceleration. We adjusted transducer angulation prior to Doppler recording until optimal signals with the purest auditory components and maximal velocity readings were obtained.

Our procedures for thallium-201 myocardial scintigraphy have been previously described [8, 21, 22]. Each patient received an intravenous dose of 1.8–2.1 mCu of thallium-201 at peak exercise and continued exercising for 30–60 additional seconds. Imaging utilizing a gamma camera with an all purpose collimator com-

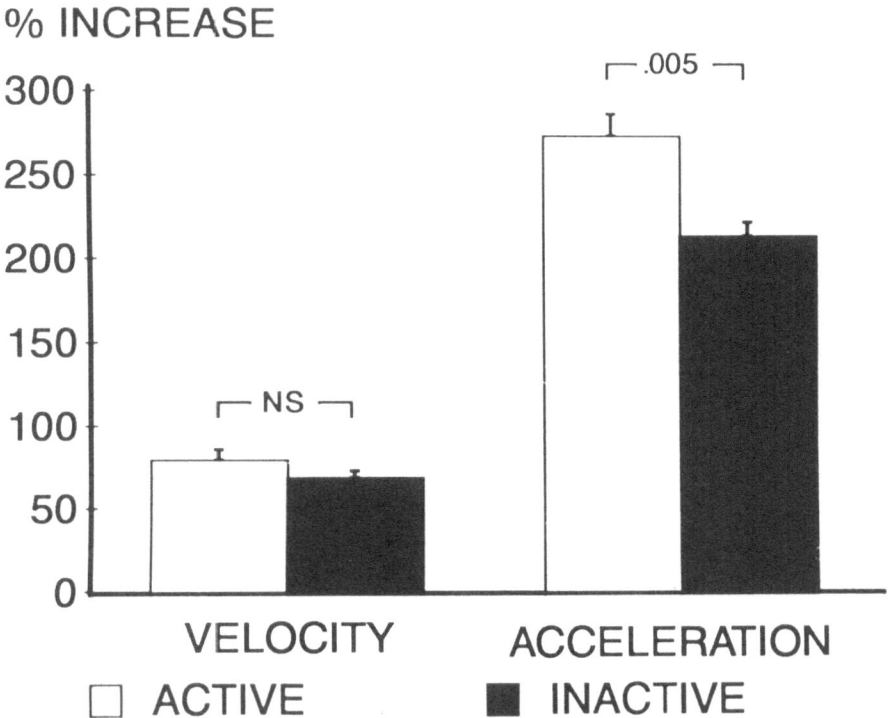

Figure 3. Percent increase during exercise of velocity and acceleration in subjects 40–70 years of age with < 5% probability of coronary artery disease. Active individuals reported aerobic exercise periods exceeding 20 minutes 3 or more times per week. Inactive subject exercised less frequently.

menced within 10 minutes following isotope injection. Anterior, 45 degree and 70 degree left anterior oblique projections as well as delayed images in these same views at 2–3 hours were obtained. Background subtraction and quantitative analysis of regional myocardial uptake and washout were undertaken via computer algorithms developed in our laboratory [8]. Scintigrams were interpreted by two experienced observers and were classified as abnormal if a numerically significant defect was identified in the initial images. The presence or absence of redistribution was also specified.

7.4 Normal Doppler response to exercise

As discussed in previous chapters, limited data concerning Doppler measurements of ascending aorta blood flow during exercise in individuals without cardiovascular disease are available. In order to compare the diagnostic capabilities of stress thallium studies with exercise Doppler, we found it necessary first to define the normal aortic blood flow response to exercise. Accordingly, we tested 185 subjects without cardiovascular symptoms and with normal resting electrocardiograms [< 5% probability for coronary artery disease [27]]. None of these individuals were receiving beta blockers, calcium channel antagonists or other medications with vasoactive or cardiac effects.

To determine whether age significantly affected our Doppler parameters, we compared the 60 younger individuals aged 20–39 years (mean 30 ± 6 years) to the 125 older subjects whose ages ranged from 40 to 70 years (mean: 47 ± 6 years). Technically adequate resting and peak exercise Doppler studies were obtained in 181 (98%) of these exercise tests. Mean Doppler velocities and accelerations from this normal population grouped by age are presented in Figure 1. At rest, peak velocity was significantly greater in the younger cohort (0.65 ± 0.02 vs. 0.59 ± 0.02 m/s*; $p = 0.01$) despite an insignificant difference in resting heart rates (83 ± 2 vs. 79 ± 1 bpm; $p = 0.01$) and a lower resting systolic blood pressure (119 ± 2 vs. 129 ± 1 mmHg; $p = 0.0001$). Resting acceleration was similar between the two age groups (16.2 ± 0.7 vs. 14.7 ± 0.5 m/s/s; $p = NS$). With exercise, aortic flow velocity and acceleration increased progressively. Immediate post-exercise mean velocity and acceleration values in younger individuals significantly exceeded those for the older subjects (1.26 ± 0.03 vs. 0.99 ± 0.02 m/s:$p = 0.001$ and 53.7 ± 2.2 vs. 48.1 ± 1.2 m/s/s; $p = 0.02$, respectively). When the data were recast as percentage change from resting measurements (Figure 2), the acceleration increase of 250% during exercise was most dramatic. In contrast, average velocities increased by less than 100%. The younger subjects experienced a greater percentage increase in peak velocity but not acceleration when compared to the older age group ($95 \pm 5\%$ vs. $74 \pm 3\%$; $p = 0.001$ and $240 \pm 12\%$ vs. $241 \pm 8\%$; $p = NS$, respectively).

We also assessed the relationship between level of conditioning and Doppler indices of left ventricular performance during exercise in our older patients. The active subgroup ($n = 55$) of these 121 individuals reported moderate or strenuous aerobic activity at least 3 times per week while those who were inactive ($n = 66$) exercised less. As expected, the conditioned individuals had a lower resting heart rate (74 ± 2 vs. 83 ± 2 bpm; $p = 0.0004$, and a lower diastolic blood pressure (82 ± 1.1 vs. 86 ± 1.0 mmHg; $p = 0.02$). Immediately after exercise there were no significant differences in heart rate, blood pressure or rate pressure product. Figure 3 depicts the percentage change of velocity and acceleration during exercise testing in these subgroups. Active individuals had a significantly greater increase in acceleration with exercise ($274 \pm 13\%$ vs. $214 \pm 8\%$; $p = 0.005$). Velocity also increased to a greater extent in the active group ($80 \pm 6\%$ vs. $69 \pm 4\%$), but this difference did not reach statistical significance.

---

* These and all subsequent numeric values are expressed as mean ± standard error of the mean.

7.5 Exercise Doppler versus thallium-201 scintigraphy

In this phase of our investigation, 144 patients referred for the evaluation of known or suspected coronary artery disease underwent both suprasternal exercise Doppler and thallium-201 scintigraphy in conjunction with treadmill exercise testing. We limited our data analysis to the 136 patients (94%) with technically adequate Doppler studies, 66 of whom were receiving no medication at the time of exercise testing while 70 were being treated with either beta blocking agents or calcium channel antagonists. Since these drugs impair left ventricular contractile function, we examined their effects on Doppler ejection indices.

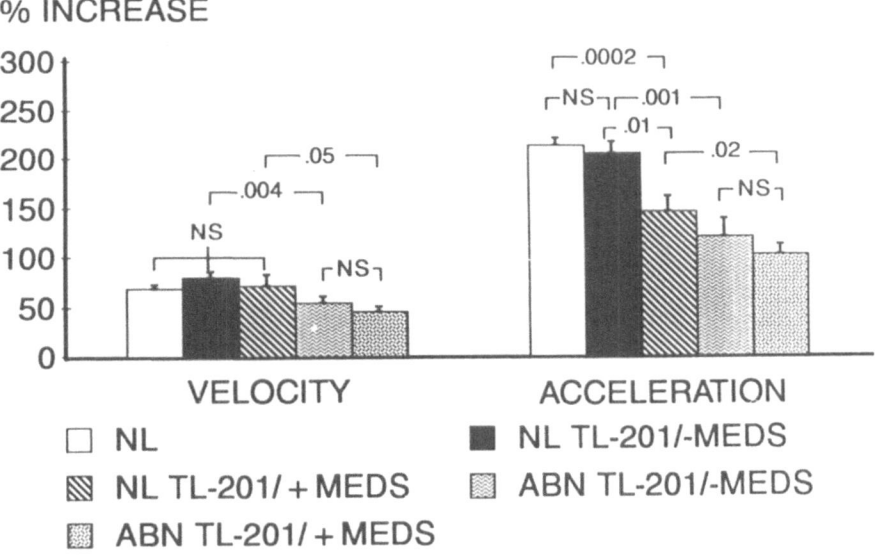

Figure 4. Percent increase in velocity and acceleration during exercise for the 40–70 year old inactive patients with a < 5% probability of coronary artery disease (NL), patients with normal and abnormal thallium studies not receiving beta blocking agents or calcium channel antagonists (NL TL–201)/–MEDS and ABN TL–201/–MEDS, respectively) and patients with normal and abnormal thallium studies receiving such medications (NL TL–201/+MEDS and ABN TL–201/+MEDS, respectively).

In Figure 4, percentage increases in velocity and acceleration are plotted for patient subgroups defined on the basis of thallium scintigraphic results and the use of negative inotropic medications. Data for age and activity-matched controls with < 5% probability of ischemic heart disease are also included. Velocity was unaffected by medication use whether thallium studies were normal (no medication: $80 \pm 6\%$ vs. + medication: $72 \pm 11\%$) or abnormal (no medication: $55 \pm 6\%$ vs. + medication: $46 \pm 5\%$).

Acceleration measurements, however, were depressed by these drugs. Significantly greater acceleration increases were recorded in both our normal controls and medication-free patients with normal thallium studies when compared to patients with negative scintigrams receiving medication ($214 \pm 8\%$ vs. $147 \pm 15\%$; $p = 0.0002$ and $206 \pm 12\%$ vs. $147 \pm 15\%$; $p = 0.01$, respectively). Acceleration gains during exercise were substantially lower in patients with abnormal thallium studies; the use of negative inotropic agents resulted in an additional decrement that was not statistically significant.

The data in Figure 4 also permit analysis of the effects of ischemia on mean exercise Doppler aortic flow measures. Patients with chest pain syndromes but normal thallium findings did not differ significantly from their age-matched controls. In contrast, the percentage increase in both velocity and acceleration measurements during exercise was lower in patients with abnormal thallium studies not receiving medication. In the patients treated with beta adrenergic blockers or calcium channel antagonists, similar significant differences, but of a smaller absolute magnitude, were noted. Therefore, velocity and acceleration normally increase during exercise whether or not negative inotropic medications are being used. Ischemia impairs this normal increase in Doppler parameters.

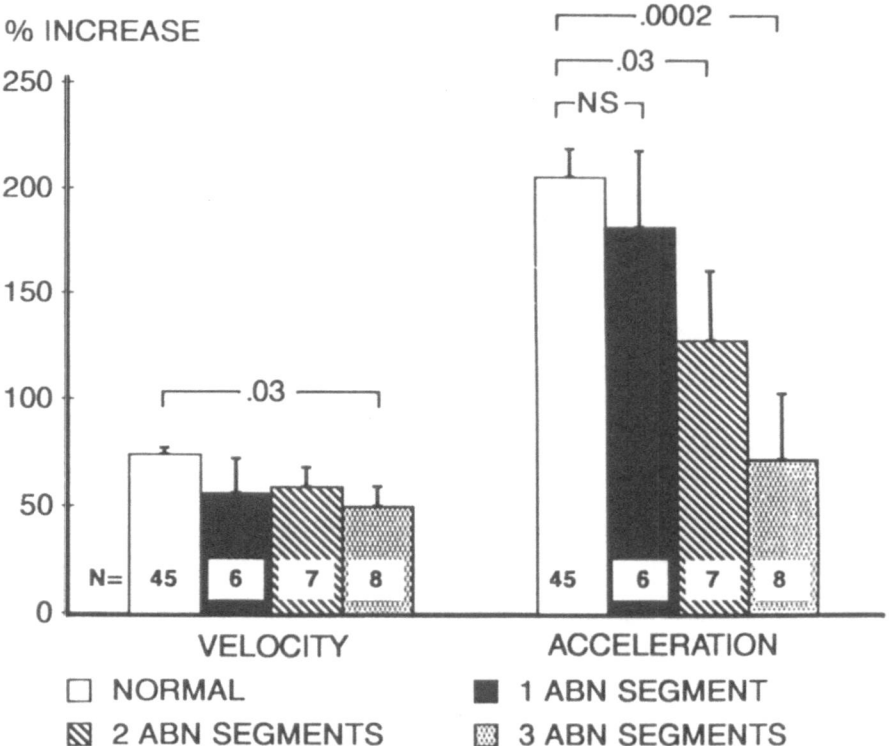

Figure 5. Percent increase in velocity and acceleration during exercise for patients undergoing thallium scintigraphy and not receiving negative inotropic medication. Data are presented for patient groups with normal scintigraphic studies, and 1, 2 or ≥3 abnormal segments.

Previous experiments in both animal models and humans have demonstrated a direct relationship between the magnitude of left ventricular systolic dysfunction and the resultant abnormalities in aortic ejection parameters measured either by invasive techniques [28–30] or by Doppler ultrasound [31, 32]. We therefore sought to determine whether the extent of ischemia as assessed by thallium scintigraphy would correlate with exercise Doppler findings. In Figure 5, the percentage changes in velocity and acceleration are plotted versus the number of myocardial segments with abnormal thallium-201 uptake. Although relatively few patients are included in each group, greater impairment of the Doppler response to exercise is apparent in patients with more numerous thallium defects. Mean percentage increases in acceleration and velocity are insignificantly lower when patients with normal thallium images are compared to those with a single abnormal scan segment ($74 \pm 3\%$ vs. $56 \pm 16\%$ and $206 \pm 13\%$ vs. $182 \pm 36\%$, respectively); however, progressively larger and significant differences in acceleration are present in the group with 2 abnormal segments and those with 3 or more segmental defects ($206 \pm 13\%$ vs. $128 \pm 33\%$; $p = 0.03$ and vs. $70 \pm 31\%$; $p = 0.0002$ for 0 vs. 2 and 0 vs. ≥ 3 abnormal segments). Velocity was only significantly depressed in patients with ≥ 3 abnormal segments compared to normals ($50 \pm 9\%$ vs. $74 \pm 3\%$; $p = 0.03$).

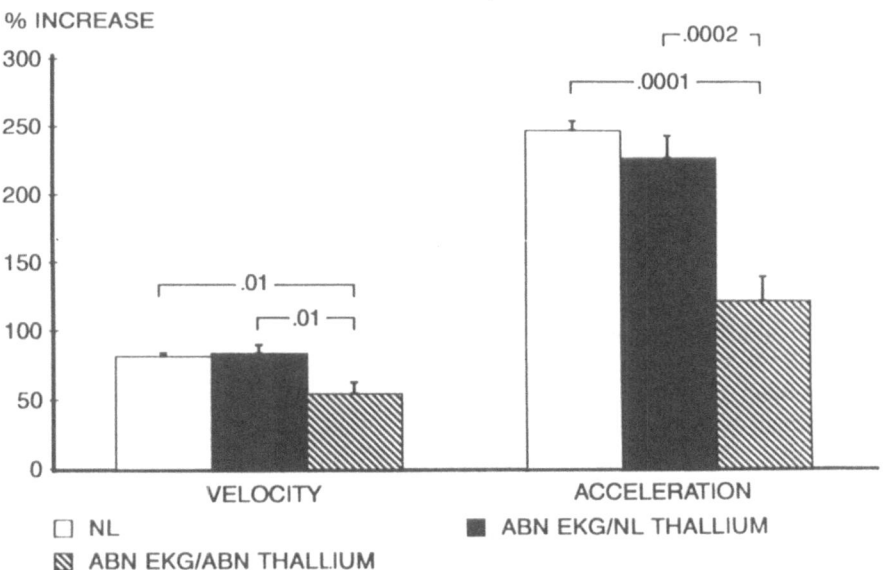

Figure 6. Percent increase in velocity and acceleration during exercise for inactive older subjects with a < 5% likelihood for coronary artery disease (NL), patients with false positive exercise tests (ABN EKG/NL THALLIUM) and patients with true positive exercise tests (ABN EKG/ABN THALLIUM).

7.6 The false positive stress test.

We also examined the potential diagnostic value of exercise Doppler in patients with false positive stress tests, defined for this analysis as tests in which significant ST segment depression occurred despite normal thallium scintigraphy. Previous work from our laboratory and others indicates that cardiac death or non-fatal myocardial infarction occurs rarely in patients with these findings; their risk is comparable to that of individuals with angiographically normal coronary arteries [20].

Twenty-six patients not receiving beta blocking agents or calcium antagonists at the time of study had false positive electrocardiographic responses to exercise by our criteria. An additional 14 medication-free patients had ischemia documented by abnormal thallium scintigraphy. Figure 6 depicts the Doppler parameters in these 2 groups of patients compared to age and activity-matched normals. No significant differences in Doppler velocity or acceleration were noted between the normal group and the patients with false positive stress tests; however, significantly lower velocities and accelerations were recorded in the patients with ischemia. Thus, Doppler measurements of velocity and acceleration during exercise are normal in patients with positive stress tests and normal thallium images but abnormal in patients with ischemia demonstrated by concordant findings from exercise electrocardiography and thallium scintigraphy. Accordingly, exercise Doppler may be useful in distinguishing false positive from true positive standard stress tests.

7.7 Exercise Doppler in individual patients

While the foregoing analyses document that Doppler-determined aortic ejection parameters reflect physiologic differences between groups of patients during exercise, they fail to assess the diagnostic utility of exercise Doppler in individual cases. As a result, we examined the frequency distributions of the percentage increases in velocity and acceleration during exercise in 3 of our patient subgroups: 1) those aged 40–70 years with a < 5% probability of coronary disease, 2) those with normal thallium scintigraphy and thus without demonstrable myocardial ischemia and 3) those with physiologically significant ischemic heart disease documented by abnormal thallium scintigraphy. As can be seen in Figure 7, despite marked differences in parameter distributions between the 2 normal groups on one hand and the patients with abnormal thallium studies on the other, considerable overlap in the Doppler velocity and acceleration measurements was present. Percentage increase in acceleration was superior to velocity in distinguishing between patients with and without coronary artery disease; however, diagnostic accuracy was still limited. Defining an abnormal test as one in which peak acceleration failed to increase by at least 150% at maximal exercise yielded the best total predictive accuracy (0.80) for any single Doppler measurement in our population. Using this criterion, a moderately high specificity of 0.82 was calculated, but sensitivity was only 0.57.

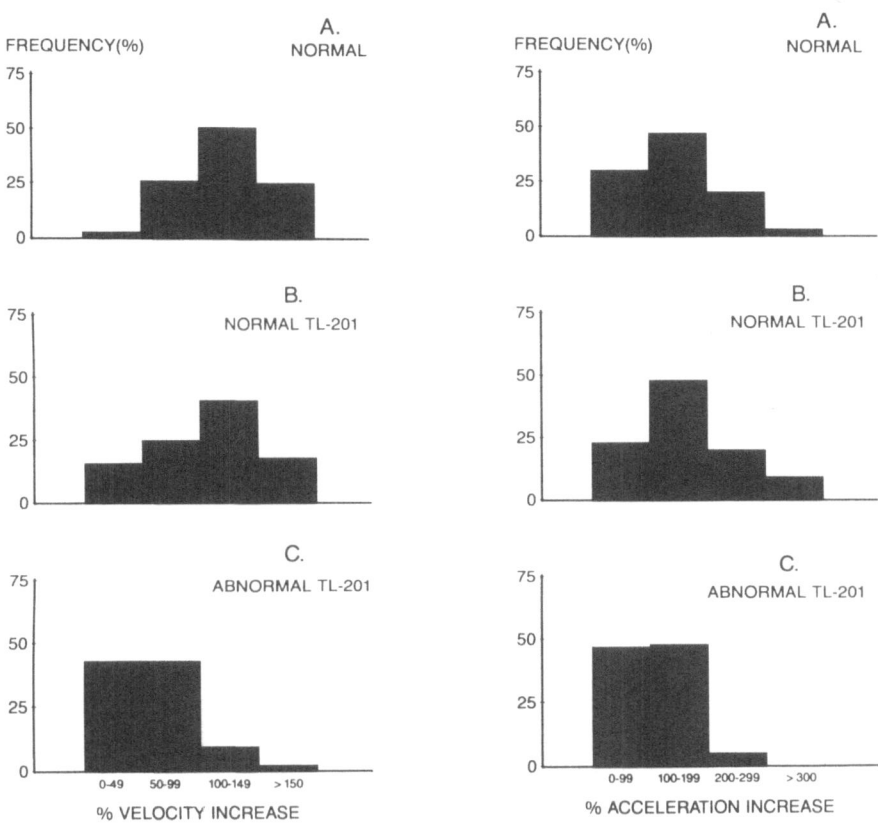

Figure 7. Frequency distributions of the percent increase in velocity and acceleration during exercise for (A) the older inactive subjects with a < 5% likelihood of coronary artery disease, (B) patients with normal thallium scintigraphy or (C) abnormal thallium studies. None of the patients respresented in this figure were receiving beta blocking agents or calcium channel antagonists.

Thus, if analyzed as an isolated test, the diagnostic capabilities of exercise Doppler do not compare to the reported values for stress thallium scintigraphy [3, 15]. Nonetheless, might Doppler importantly improve the overall accuracy of exercise electrocardiography by providing useful information in a subset of patients? In Figure 8, we depict the percentage change of acceleration during exercise for the 40 patients with abnormal electrocardiographic responses during exercise who were receiving neither beta blockers nor calcium channel antagonists. Abnormal thallium scintigrams were recorded in 14 (presumed true positive exercise EKG) while normal thallium images were present in 26 (presumed false positive EKG). The increase in acceleration exceeded 220% in 18 of the 26 patients with false positive exercise tests (69%), but in only 1 of the 14 patients (7%) with true positive stress electrocardiograms. This patient with ischemia by thallium but no abnormality in acceleration by Doppler had only a single small redistribution defect in the scintigraphic images.

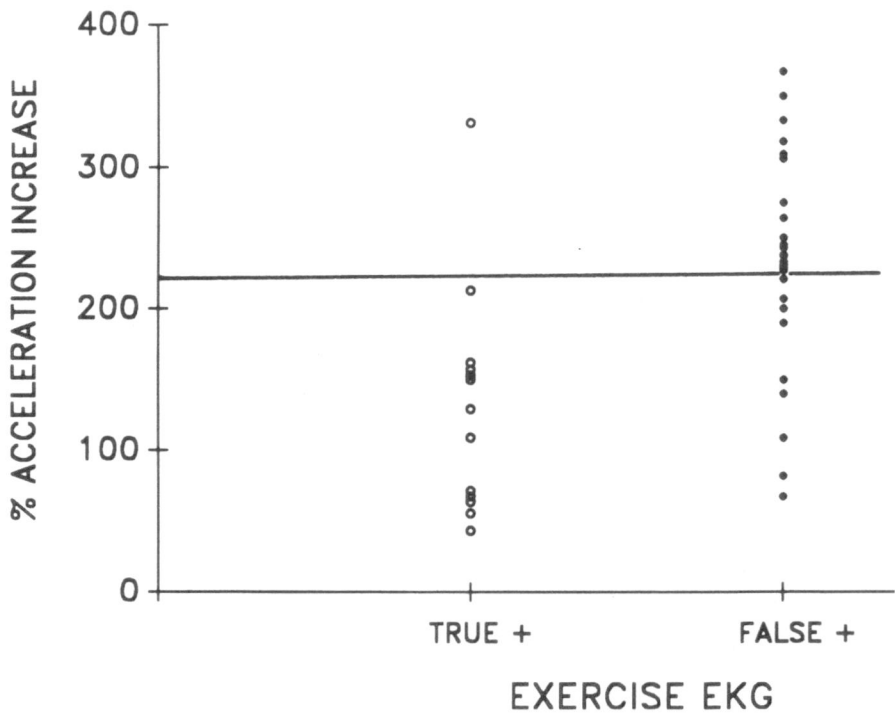

Figure 8. Scatter plot of percent increase in acceleration for patients with either false positive or true positive electrocardiographic responses to exercise. None of these individuals were receiving negative inotropic medication.

Based upon these findings, a possible strategy for the diagnostic use of Doppler aortic flow measurements emerges. In patients with equivocal electrocardiographic responses to exercise or those in whom a false positive test is likely, the group with an unimpressive increase in blood flow acceleration (< 220%) would include all or nearly all of the patients with significant ischemic heart disease as well as a considerable number of normals. Additional testing, perhaps thallium scintigraphy, would be needed to distinguish between those patients with and without important obstructive coronary artery disease. However, the remaining individuals with marked exercise-induced increases in acceleration would have a low probability for critical coronary stenosis and might not require additional studies to exclude this diagnosis. Due to the small size of our study, this finding concerning the diagnostic utility of exercise Doppler should not be considered conclusive. It will be necessary to study a larger number of patients, obtaining both angiographic assessment of coronary disease and adequate clinical outcome data, in order to verify our preliminary results.

7.8 Comparison of stress thallium scintigraphy with exercise Doppler in other laboratories

Harrison [33] (see chapter 10 – ed.) has reported on aortic Doppler studies performed during upright exercise in 28 young normal volunteer subjects and 74 older patients referred for stress thallium scintigraphy. Maximal acceleration and velocity of aortic blood flow increased progressively during exercise in most individuals. Velocity and acceleration at peak exercise in young normals exceeded values in older subjects without scintigraphic evidence for coronary artery disease. Peak velocities were similar in patients with abnormal and normal thallium studies, but acceleration was significantly lower in patients with scintigraphic evidence of ischemia. These investigators also found progressively more impressive abnormalities in Doppler parameters with increased severity of coronary artery disease and concluded that while exercise Doppler failed to duplicate the diagnostic accuracy of thallium scintigraphy, it might have a role in identifying a subset of patients with more extensive coronary artery disease. All of these findings are similar to our observations; however, percentage change in acceleration, which was the most sensitive diagnostic parameter in our studies, was not examined by Harrison and coworkers. Moreover, they failed to control adequately for the important effects of treatment with beta adrenergic blocking drugs and calcium channel antagonists.

Another group of investigators has explored the usefulness of Doppler mitral flow measurements during exercise and compared their results to thallium scintigraphy [34]. In this study, diastolic function was assessed by measurement of mean transmitral velocity. Velocity increased during exercise but to a lesser extent in patients with abnormal thallium images. Defining an abnormal test as one with a 50% or lesser increase in velocity yielded a specificity of 0.90 and sensitivity of 0.83 in the 28 patients studied. Although these findings suggest that exercise induced abnormalities in diastolic as well as systolic properties of the left ventricle might be profitably assessed by Doppler, experimental design problems limit the certainty with which conclusions can be drawn from this data. First, use of medications with the potential to modify left ventricular diastolic properties was not controlled. Moreover, a large proportion of the patients (82%) had segmental wall motion abnormalities at rest and thus presumed previous myocardial infarction. Additional investigation involving a larger number of patients will be required to adequately evaluate this promising Doppler technique. Such a study should control for medications which might affect left ventricular diastolic or systolic properties, include a baseline assessment of left ventricular systolic function by two dimensional echocardiography and of diastolic function by Doppler and incorporate high quality quantitative thallium scintigraphy for accurate identification of ischemic and infarcted myocardium.

7.9 Summary and conclusions

Exercise Doppler is a safe and relatively simple examination that can be performed with inexpensive equipment after a brief period of training. Technical feasibility in our hands has been excellent with adequate Doppler signals obtained from 97% of 325 consecutive patients.

The typical response to exercise in normal individuals is a progressive increase in velocity to a maximum of nearly 200% of resting values and a more profound increase of approximately 350% in peak acceleration. Velocity and acceleration changes with exercise are less impressive in older individuals, inactive subjects and patients receiving beta blocking agents or calcium channel antagonists. The normal increase in these Doppler parameters during exercise is also impaired in patients with myocardial ischemia or infarction documented by abnormal thallium scintigraphy.

Our initial studies indicate that the diagnostic accuracy of exercise Doppler for coronary artery disease is inferior to that of stress thallium-201 imaging. Normal individuals frequently have relatively modest increases in aortic blood flow velocity and acceleration during exercise, findings indistinguishable from those that occur in many patients with significant coronary artery disease. Thus, if normality is defined in the standard fashion to include 95% of the test responses in subjects without significant ischemic heart disease, many patients with important disease will be inappropriately identified as 'normal', and sensitivity will be low. However, patients without coronary artery disease frequently manifest increases in acceleration exceeding those seen in nearly all patients with coronary artery disease. Thus, exercise Doppler may serve as a useful adjunct to standard stress testing by identifying a subset of patients with positive or equivocal electrocardiographic responses to exercise in whom normal Doppler findings suggest a low probability of significant ischemia. These patients would be spared the need for additional diagnostic testing. Moreover, markedly abnormal stress Doppler responses may select patients with a high probability for severe coronary artery disease.

References

1. Feil H, Siegel ML. Electrocardiographic changes during attacks of angina pectoris. Am J Med Sci 1928; 175:255–60.
2. Master AM, Oppenheimer EJ. A simple exercise tolerance test for circulatory efficiency and standard tables for normal individuals. Am J Med Sci 1929; 177:223–42.
3. Gibson RS, Beller GA. Should exercise electrocardiographic testing be replaced by radioisotope methods? In: Rahimtoola SH, Brest AN (eds.). Controversies in Coronary Artery Disease. F.A. Davis, Philadelphia, 1982; p. 1–32.
4. Chaitman BR. The changing role of the exercise electrocardiogram as a diagnostic and prognostic test for chronic ischemic heart disease. J Am Coll Cardiol 1986; 8:1195–1210.
5. Beller GA, Gibson RS. Sensitivity, specificity and prognostic significance or noninvasive testing for occult or known coronary artery disease. Prog Cardiovasc Dis 1987; 29:241–70.

6. Dash H, Massie BM, Botvinick EH, Brundage BH. The noninvasive identification of left main and three vessel coronary artery disease by myocardial stress perfusion scintigraphy and treadmill exercise testing. Circulation 1979; 60:276–84.

7. Iskandrian AS, Wasserman LA, Anderson GS, et al. Merits of stress thallium-201 myocardial perfusion imaging in patients with inconclusive exercise electrocardiograms: Correlation with coronary angiograms. Am J Cardiol 1980; 46:553–558.

8. Berger BC, Watson DD, Taylor GJ, et al. Quantitative thallium-201 exercise scintigraphy for detection of coronary artery disease. J Nucl Med 1981; 22:585–593.

9. Nohara R, Kambara H, Suzuki Y, et al. Stress scintigraphy using single-photon emission computed tomography in the evaluation of coronary artery disease. Am J Cardiol 1984; 53:1250–1254.

10. Nygaard TW, Gibson RS, Ryan JM, et al. Prevalence of high-risk thallium-201 scintigraphic findings of left main coronary artery stenosis: Comparison with patients with multiple- and single-coronary artery disease. Am J Cardiol 1984; 53:462–469.

11. Maddahi J, Abdulla A, Garcia EV, et al. Noninvasive identification of left main and triple vessel coronary artery disease: Improved accuracy using quantitative analysis of regional myocardial stress distribution and washout of thallium-201. J Am Coll Cardiol 1986; 7:53–60.

12. Guiney TE, Pohost GM, McKusick KA, et al. Differentiation of false- from true-positive ECG responses to exercise stress by thallium-201 perfusion imaging. Chest 1981; 80:4–10.

13. McCarthy DM, Blood DK, Sciacca RR, Cannon PJ. Single dose myocardial perfusion imaging with Thallium-201: Application in patients with non-diagnostic electrocardiographic stress tests. Am J Cardiol 1979; 43:899–905.

14. Iskandrian AS, Segal BL. Value of exercise thallium-201 imaging in patients with diagnostic and non-diagnostic exercise electrocardiograms. Am J Cardiol 1981; 48:233–8.

15. Botvinick EH, Taradash MR, Shames DM, Parmley WW. Thallium-201 myocardial perfusion scintigraphy for the clinical clarification of normal, abnormal and equivocal electrocardiographic stress tests. Am J Cardiol 1978; 41:43–51.

16. Wijns W, Serruys PW, Reiber JHC, et al. Quantitative angiography of the left anterior descending coronary artery: correlations with pressure gradient and results of exercise thallium scintigraphy. Circulation 1985; 71:273–279.

17. Gill JB, Ruddy TD, Newell JB, Finkelstein DM, Strauss HW, Boucher CA. Prognostic importance of thallium uptake by the lungs during exercise in coronary artery disease. N Engl J Med 1987; 317:1485–9.

18. Koss JH, Kobren SM, Grunwald AM, Bodenheimer MM. Role of exercise thallium-201 myocardial perfusion scintigraphy for predicting prognosis in suspected coronary artery disease. Am J Cardiol 1987; 59:531–4.

19. Pamelia FX, Gibson RS, Sirowatka J, Gascho J, Watson DD, Beller GA. The prognostic value of normal exercise thallium-201 scintigraphy in patients presenting for evaluation of chest pain. Am J Cardiol 1985; 55:920–926.

20. Wackers FJ, Russo DJ, Russo D, Clements JP. Prognostic significance of normal quantitative planar thallium-201 stress scintigraphy in patients with chest pain. J Am Coll Cardiol 1985; 6:27–30.

21. Gibson RS, Watson DD, Craddock GB, et al. Prediction of cardiac events after uncomplicated myocardial infarction: A prospective study comparing predischarge exercise thallium-201 scintigraphy and coronary angiography. Circulation 1983; 68:321–336.

22. Gibson RS, Watson DD, Taylor GJ, Crosby IK, Wellons HL, Holt ND, Beller GA. Prospective assessment of regional myocardial perfusion before and after coronary revascularization surgery by quantitative Thallium-201 scintigraphy. J Am Coll Cardiol 1983; 1:804–15.

23. Breisblatt WM, Barneo JV, Weiland F, Spaccavento LJ. Incomplete revascularization in multivessel percutaneous transluminal coronary angioplasty: The role for stress

Thallium-201 imaging. J Am Coll Cardiol 1988; 11:1183–90.

24. Schwartz JS, Ponto R, Carlyle P, *et al.* Early redistribution of thallium-201 after temporary ischemia. Circulation 1982; 57:332–335.

25. Melin JA, De Coster PM, Renkin J, *et al.* Effect of intracoronary thrombolytic therapy on exercise-induced ischemia after acute myocardial infarction. Am J Cardiol 1985; 56:705–711.

26. Okada RD, Boucher CA, Kirshenbaum HK, *et al.* Improved diagnostic accuracy of thallium-201 stress test using multiple observers and criteria derived from interobserver analysis of variance. Am J Cardiol 1980; 46:619–624.

27. Diamond GA, Forrester JS. Analysis of probability as an aid in the clinical diagnosis of coronary artery disease. N Engl J Med 1979; 300:1350–1357.

28. Jewitt D, Gabe I, Mills C, Mauren B, Thomas M, Shilling Ford J. Aortic velocity and acceleration measurements in the assessment of coronary artery disease. Eur J of Cardiol 1974; 1:299–305.

29. Stein PD, Sabbah HN. Ventricular performance measured during ejection. Studies in patients of the rate of change of ventricular power. Am Heart J 1976; 91:599–606.

30. Bennett ED, Else W, Miller GA, Sutton GC, Miller HC, Noble MI. Maximum acceleration of blood from the left ventricle in patients with ischemic heart disease. Clin Sci Mol Med 1974; 46:49–59.

31. Sabbah HN, Khaja F, Brymer JF *et al.* Noninvasive evaluation of left performance based on peak aortic blood acceleration measured with a continuous-wave Doppler velocity meter. Circulation 1986; 74:323–329.

32. Bennett ED, Barclay SA, Davis AL, Mannering D, Mehta N. Ascending aortic blood velocity and acceleration using Doppler ultrasound in the assessment of left ventricular function. Cardiovasc Res 1984; 18:632–638.

33. Harrison MR, Smith MD, Friedman BJ, DeMaria AN. Uses and limitations of exercise Doppler echocardiography in the diagnosis of ischemic heart disease. J Am Coll Cardiol 1987; 10:809–17.

34. Mitchell GD, Brunken RC, Schwarger M, Donohue BC, Krivokajnick J, Child JS. Assessment of mitral flow velocity with exercise by an index of stress-induced left ventricular ischemia in coronary artery disease. Am J Cardiol 1988; 61:536–40.

8. Doppler left ventricular ejection dynamics: Correlation with nuclear ejection indices during exercise

CAROLYN R. CORN and STEVE M. TEAGUE
University of Oklahoma Health Sciences Center, Room 5 SP 300, P.O. Box 26901, Oklahoma City, OK 73190, U.S.A.

8.1 Exercise testing in the diagnosis of coronary artery disease

Exercise testing is commonly used in both the diagnosis of coronary artery disease and in assessment of its physiological significance. Stress electrocardiography has a diagnostic sensitivity and specificity of 64% and 93% [1], respectively, using 1.0 mm depression as an ischemic threshold. The sensitivity of exercise testing can be significantly increased by adding radionuclide angiography [2], but exercise nuclear ventriculography is expensive and technically difficult to perform. Two dimensional echocardiography has been used to detect ischemic wall motion abnormalities occurring with exercise, but the success rate of obtaining an optimal study has been disappointing. The use of Doppler echocardiography to interrogate flow in the ascending aorta offers the advantage of a high success rate (81–100%) [3, 4], except in obese subjects and those with hypertrophied neck muscles. In addition, Doppler echocardiography entails little equipment, and can be performed at relatively low cost. Both pulsed and continuous wave systems can be used to analyze maximal acceleration, peak velocity, and systolic velocity integral.

A number of studies in humans have demonstrated the usefulness of Doppler echocardiography in the noninvasive evaluation of global left ventricular function, but have not correlated Doppler parameters with left ventricular ejection fraction (LVEF) during exercise, or attempted to define Doppler criteria for an ischemic response. Since the normal augmentation of maximal acceleration (MA) and peak velocity (PV) during exercise is diminished roughly in proportion to the extent of coronary artery disease [5, 6, 7], it is reasonable that exercise induced changes in Doppler derived values might be similar to changes in nuclear ejection indices during supine bicycle exercise in patients with atherosclerotic coronary disease.

8.2 Correlation of radionuclear left ventricular ejection fraction with simultaneous Doppler derived parameters.

Invasive studies have shown maximal acceleration and peak velocity to be closely related to left ventricular function, and have demonstrated that this relationship is

Steve M. Teague (ed.) Stress Doppler Echocardiography, 95–105.

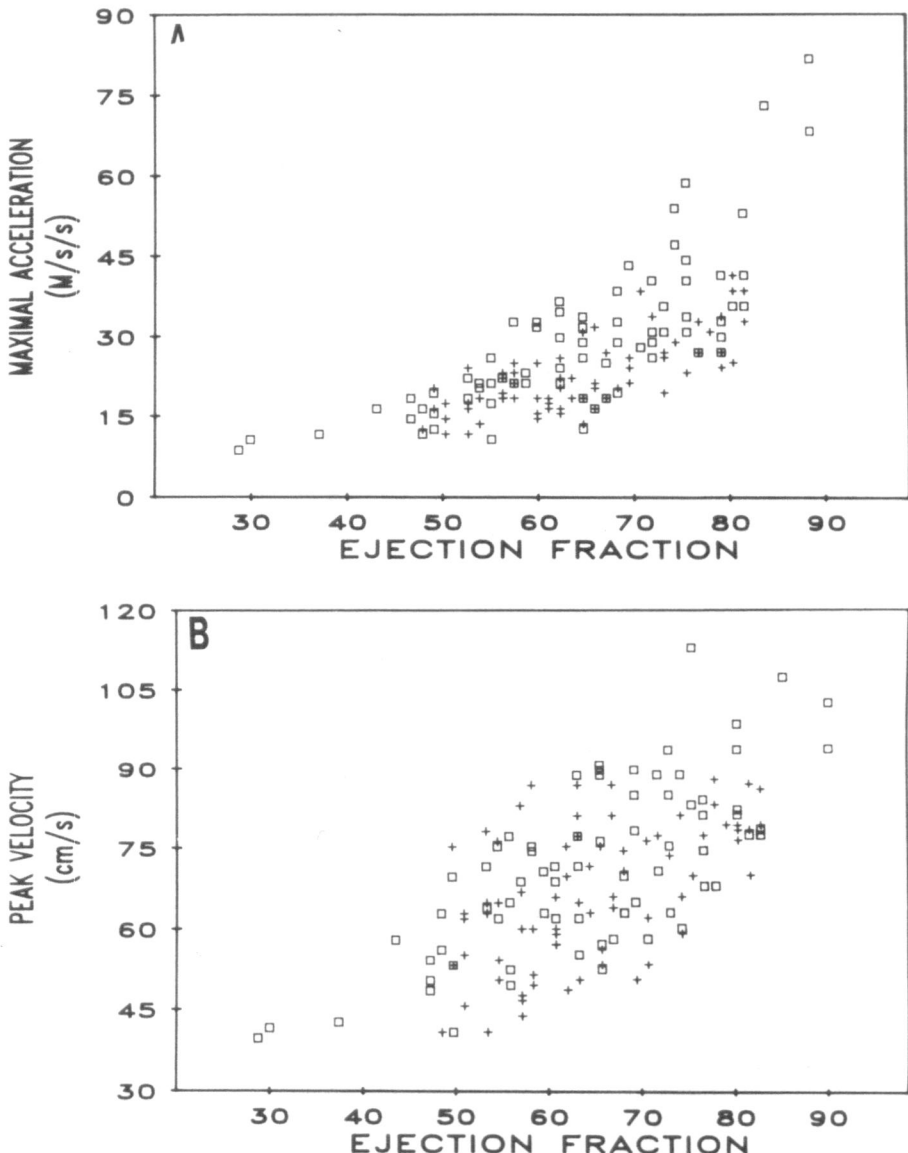

Figure 1. Nuclear ejection fractions at rest (+) and peak exertion (□) are correlated with maximal acceleration (A) and peak modal velocity (B). Maximal acceleration was related to ejection fraction in a curvilinear manner, while the relationship with peak velocity was linear. The relationship between MA and LVEF was best described by the equation: MA = 7.5 + 0.0002 [(LVEF–25)³], r = 0.89, SEE = 8.4. The relationship between peak velocity and LVEF was best described by the equation PV = 1.1 (LVEF+3.9), r = 0.67, SEE = 11.5. (Reproduced with permission from: Teague, *et al.* A comparison of Doppler and radionuclide ejection dynamics during ischemic exercise. Am J Cardiac Imaging 1987; 1:145–151).

relatively insensitive to variations in preload and afterload [8, 9]. Maximal acceleration has been found to be sensitive to alterations in inotropic state and to have a close relationship with LVEF [10]. Sabbah [11] and co-workers found a strong ($r = 0.93$) curvilinear relationship between maximal acceleration (MA) and LVEF at rest described by the formula MA = 0.3 (LVEF$^{0.93}$).

We prospectively compared Doppler and nuclear indices of left ventricular function in 73 patients with chest pain undergoing elective coronary artery angiography [12]. All subjects were male with an average age of 58 ± 14 years, and none had significant valvular disease or evidence of prior infarction. Thirty-nine percent were taking calcium channel antagonists at the time of the study, while 38% were using beta blockers. The drugs were not discontinued during the study. Supine bicycle exercise testing was performed with simultaneous radionuclide imaging and Doppler echocardiography utilizing a 3 mHz continuous wave Doppler transducer with a dedicated microprocessor (Exerdop, Quinton Instruments). Fifty-five patients had significant disease (> 70% stenosis), and the remainder had either normal coronary arteries (N = 16) or insignificant (< 40% stenosis) disease. Patients with and without coronary artery disease achieved a similar level of exercise as measured by heart rate and workload, and only three patients reached 85% of age-predicted maximum heart rate.

Combining both rest and exercise data, we found a curvilinear relationship between simultaneously measured values of Doppler derived maximal acceleration and nuclear ejection fraction (Figure 1). The least squares best fit to the data was described in the form MA = A + B[(LVEF–C)^3] where A is 7.5, B is 0.0002, and C is 25, ($r = 0.89$, SEE = 8.4). Resting and peak exercise data for modal ejection velocity and LVEF are also shown in Figure 1, and were linearly related by the equation PV = 1.1(LVEF + 3.9), $r = 0.67$, SEE = 11.5). Although both correlations are highly significant, there is considerable scatter in the data points, especially between PV and LVEF.

These observations confirm the curvilinear relationship between LVEF and MA reported by Sabbah [11], and extend it to include data obtained during exercise.

8.3 Changes in Doppler indices during exercise compared to changes in radionuclide LVEF

Numerous radionuclide studies in normals have demonstrated a minimal increase of 0.05 in the left ventricular ejection fraction during supine or upright bicycle exercise [13]. This is largely due to an increase in stroke volume coupled with a decrease in end systolic volume. End diastolic volume does not consistently increase during supine exercise, although it typically increases by 20% or so during upright stress [2]. Failure of the LVEF to increase by 0.05 with exercise is considered evidence of coronary artery disease, and the decrement in LVEF with exercise is roughly proportional to the anatomic extent of coronary disease [14]. To determine whether exercise induced changes in Doppler indices of ejection might have similar diagnostic utility, we compared Doppler echocardiographic responses

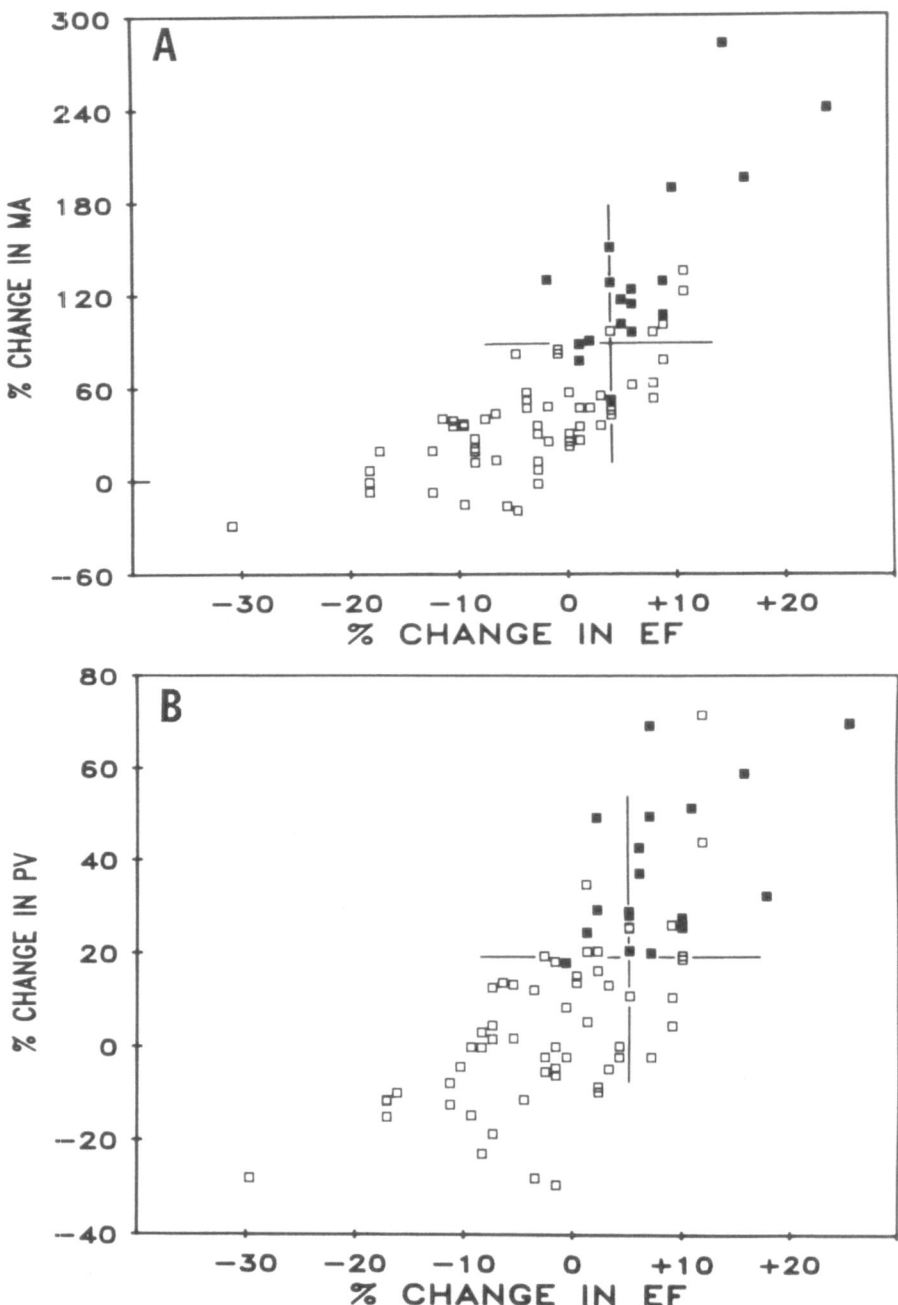

Figure 2. The change in ejection fraction from rest to peak exertion is compared with the corresponding change in maximal acceleration (A), peak modal velocity (B), or stroke distance (C). Eighteen patients free of significant coronary disease are indicated by solid squares, while 55 with coronary disease are indicated by open squares. The vertical cross hair is drawn at the radionuclear threshold for coronary disease (+0.05) while horizontal cross hairs are drawn to best separate normal and coronary patients by the Doppler indices (80% MA, 20% PV, 2% SD). (Reproduced with permission from: Teague, *et al.* A comparison of Doppler and radionuclide ejection dynamics during ischemic exercise. Am J Cardiac Imaging 1987; 1:145–151.)

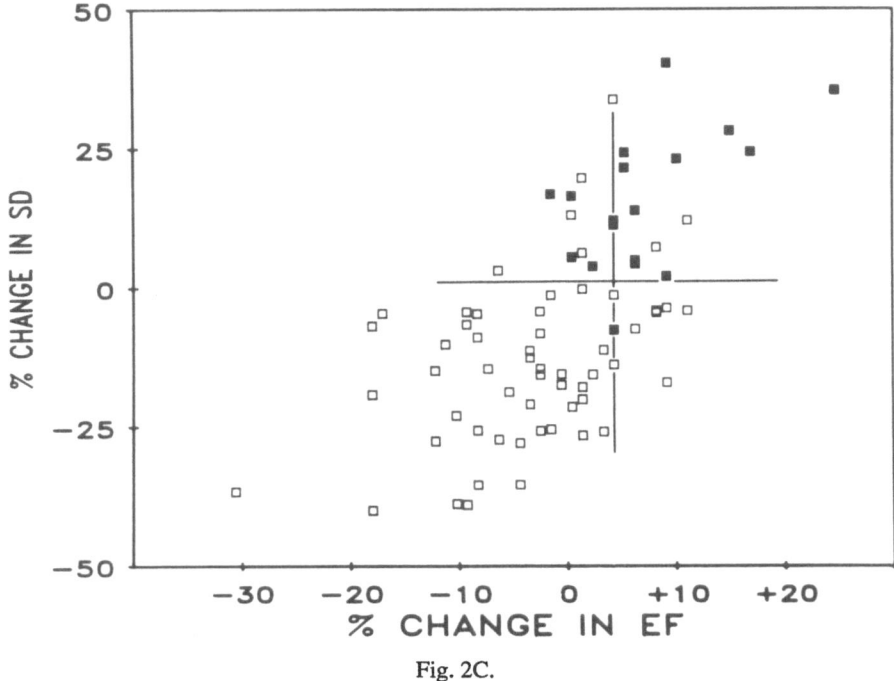

Fig. 2C.

to the change in LVEF during supine bicycle exercise using an increase of 0.05 in the LVEF as the criterion for a normal response. Changes in left ventricular end systolic volume and regional wall motion were not considered for analytic purposes.

Resting values for maximal acceleration, peak modal velocity, and stroke distance were not significantly different for patients with and without coronary artery disease. Those with normal coronary arteries were able to augment Doppler indices of left ventricular function during exercise. Maximal acceleration averaged 18 ± 6 m/s^2 at rest, and rose to 38 ± 14 m/s^2 (P = 0.0003) during supine bicycle exercise. Similarly, peak velocity rose from 65 ± 14 cm/s at rest to 83 ± 12 cm/s during exercise (P = 0.05). In contrast, patients with coronary artery disease failed to increase either parameter significantly during exercise. Maximal acceleration averaged 16 ± 4m/s^2 at rest and 22 ± 8 m/s^2 during exercise, whereas peak velocity averaged 62 ± 14 cm/s and 65 ± 16 cm/s. Stroke distance appeared to rise slightly in normals with exercise (9.2 ± 3 to 9.8 ± 2 cm) and to decrease with exertion in patients with coronary artery disease (10 ± 3 to 8.8 ± 3 cm), but these small differences did not achieve statistical significance.

The percent change in LVEF versus the percent change in Doppler derived maximal acceleration, peak velocity, and stroke distance are shown in Figure 2. In order to establish a threshold for the diagnosis of impaired ventricular response, a horizontal cross hair was drawn in each panel at a level that gave the best separation between patients with and without coronary artery disease. These values were +80 percent increase for maximal acceleration, +20 percent increase for peak velocity, and +2 percent increase for stroke distance. The vertical cross hair was drawn at the conventional nuclear threshold for identification of an ischemic response (0.05 increase in ejection fraction). The cross hair in each plot divides the graph into four quadrants. The upper right quadrant and lower left quadrant contain stress responses that are concordant by Doppler and nuclear techniques; patients in the right upper quadrant are declared free of disease by both noninvasive modalities. In the lower left quadrant, both techniques identify impaired ventricular responses to exercise. In the upper left and lower right quadrants, responses are discordant. The greatest concordance between change in ejection fraction and change in Doppler indices was found with maximal acceleration, followed by peak velocity and then stroke distance.

Sensitivity, specificity, and predictive accuracy of stress electrocardiographic ST segment responses were 0.64, 0.89, and 0.94, respectively. Identification of coronary artery disease by ejection fraction criteria yielded a sensitivity, specificity, and predictive accuracy of 0.85, 0.78, and 0.92. Corresponding values for Doppler parameters were 0.90, 0.88, and 0.96 for maximal acceleration, 0.83, 0.94, and 0.97 for peak modal velocity, and 0.85, 0.94, and 0.97 for stroke distance. Thus, sensitivity, specificity, and predictive accuracy of Doppler ejection variables are comparable to the values obtained from nuclear ejection fraction responses, and superior to those of electrocardiographic ST segment responses in the identification of patients with angiographically proven coronary artery disease. Furthermore, the three Doppler parameters had comparable discriminative ability to identify coronary patients. However, the thresholds used to separate normals from diseased patients are retrospectively chosen, and must be subjected to prospective validation before they can be generally accepted.

Daley et al. [15] compared exercise induced changes in nuclear left ventricular ejection fraction to maximal acceleration, peak velocity, and stroke volume measured by a 2 mHz continuous wave transducer in 38 patients (mean age 56) who were undergoing evaluation for suspected ischemic heart disease. Twenty-six of the patients underwent coronary angiography, and two of these had evidence of cardiomyopathy. Medications were not stopped prior to exercise testing. The overall level of exercise attained was low in these patients, with a mean exercise heart rate of 114. Patients were divided into four groups according to resting LVEF and change in LVEF with exercise. Group 1 had a normal resting LVEF that increased appropriately with exercise. Group 2 had a normal resting LVEF that failed to increase at least 0.05 with stress. Groups 3 and 4 had an abnormal resting LVEF which increased normally in group 3 but rose by less than 0.05 in group 4. Acceleration, peak velocity, and stroke volume increased during exercise in group 1. In group 2, acceleration also increased with exercise, while peak velocity and stroke volume failed to increase significantly. Acceleration and velocity both increased in group 3, although to a lesser extent than in group 1, while stroke volume was unchanged. Peak velocity increased somewhat in group 4, while acceleration and stroke volume remained the same. The magnitude of the changes in Doppler

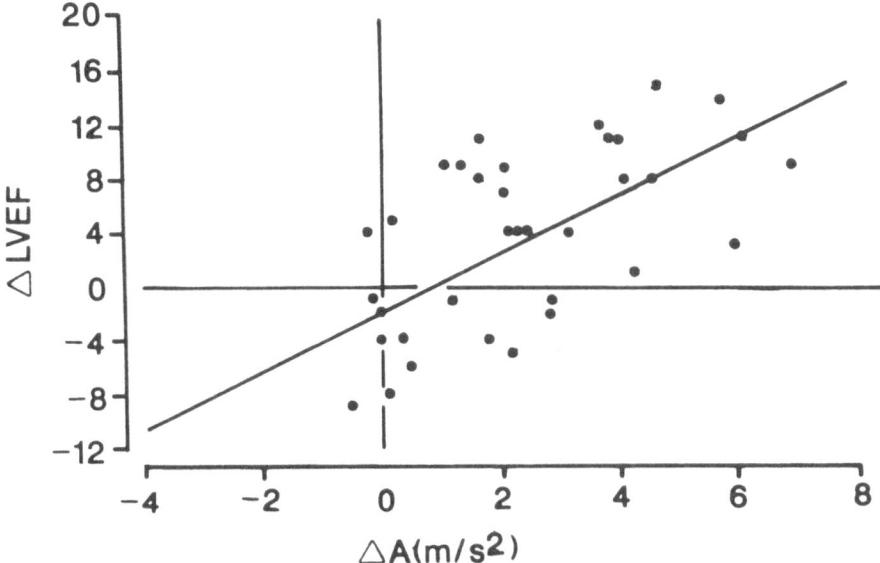

Figure 3. Change in ejection fraction (ΔLVEF) from rest to exercise compared with the change in acceleration (ΔMA). p < 0.001, SEE = 5.16. (Reproduced with permission from: Daley, *et al.* Detection of exercise induced changes in left ventricular performance by Doppler echocardiography. Br Heart J 1987; 58:447–54.)

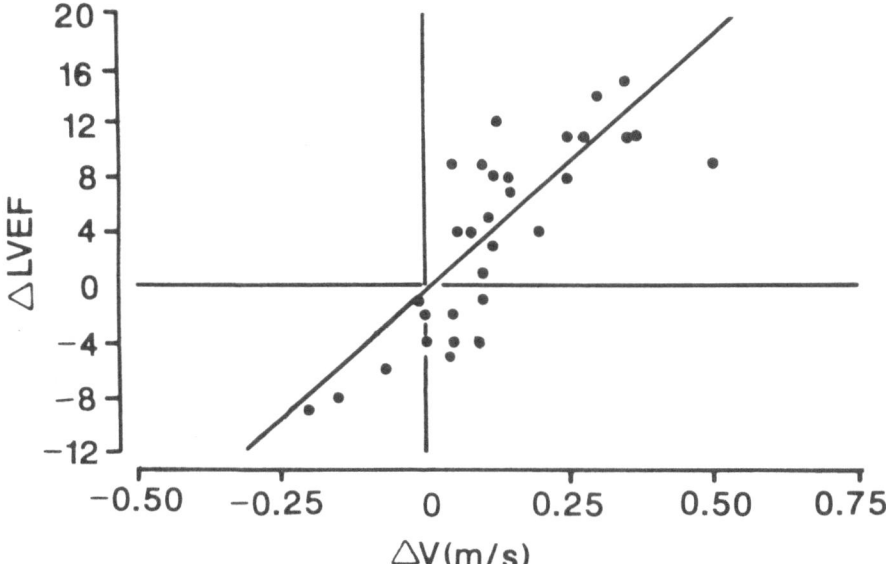

Figure 4. Change in ejection fraction (ΔLVEF) from rest to exercise compared with the change in peak velocity (ΔPV). p < 0.001, SEE = 4.08. (Reproduced with permission from: Daley, *et al.* Detection of exercise induced changes in left ventricular performance by Doppler echocardiography. Br Heart J 1987; 58:447–54.)

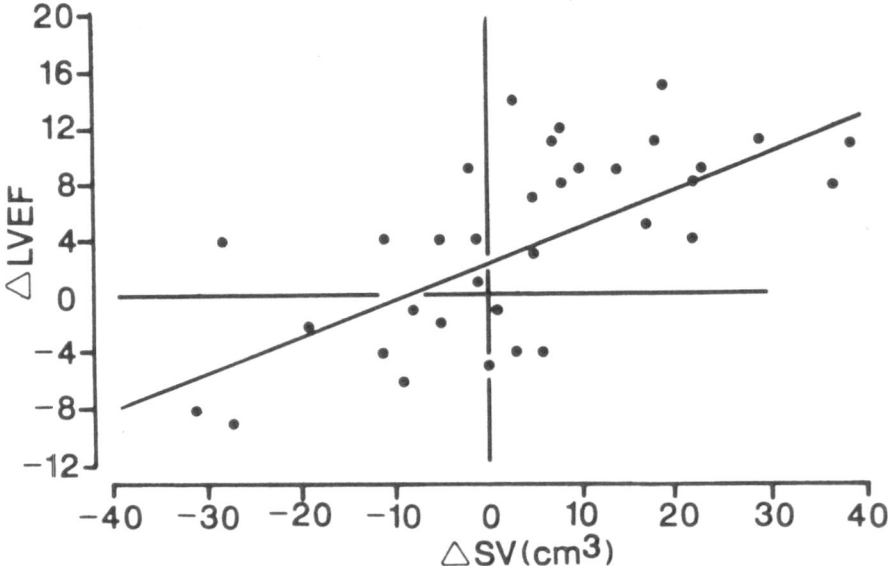

Figure 5. Change in ejection fraction (ΔLVEF) from rest to exercise compared with the change in stroke volume (ΔSV). p < 0.001, SEE = 4.95. (Reproduced with permission from: Daley, *et al.* Detection of exercise induced changes in left ventricular performance by Doppler echocardiography. Br Heart J 1987; 58:447–54.

derived values varied with the divisions according to ejection fraction; the increase in acceleration and velocity was greatest in group 1, less in group 2, and smaller still in groups 3 and 4.

The relationship between the change in LVEF and the change in maximal acceleration from the study by Daley, *et al.* [15] is shown in Figure 3. The data show a linear relationship between change in velocity and change in LVEF was also observed (Figure 4), with a correlation coefficient of 0.79. A lesser correlation between change in LVEF and change in stroke volume was found (Figure 5), with a correlation coefficient of 0.67. The authors concluded that the best correlations were found between the change in acceleration or peak velocity and the change in ejection fraction, but cautioned that LVEF and ascending aortic flow are 'different manifestations of left ventricular performance'.

8.4 Factors affecting the correlation between left ventricular ejection fraction and Doppler ejection parameters

Several studies have reported the change in maximal acceleration and velocity occurring with exercise. Unlike the change in ejection fraction, the magnitude of the Doppler responses is heavily dependent upon position. In the studies of Teague [12] and Daley [15], mean increases in maximal acceleration of 111% and 56% respectively were found during supine bicycle exercise in normals. In these same studies, the average increase in maximal acceleration was 38% [12] and 18% [15] in subjects with coronary artery disease. In contrast, others [4, 16, 17, 18] have observed an average increase in maximal acceleration ranging from 144% to 250% during upright exercise. Teague [12] and Daley [15] found average increases of 45% and 28% respectively for peak velocity in normals exercising in the supine position, but only a 13% and 5% average increment in patients with coronary disease. Increases in peak velocity in normal subjects are larger when measured in the upright position, with mean values from several studies ranging from 59 to 78% [4, 5, 16, 17, 18].

In addition to patient position, other factors may have contributed to the lower values for Doppler indices found in our study. Our patients developed symptoms at relatively low workloads and heart rates; similar limitations were observed in the subjects reported by Daley *et al.* [15]. Beta blocking and calcium antagonist drugs may well have reduced the magnitude of exercise induced changes in the Doppler indices [16, 17], although there is some controversy regarding this point [6]. Doppler derived parameters decrease with age [16, 17], and the older population studied by both Teague [12] and Daley [15] may account in part for the somewhat lower values measured for maximal acceleration and peak velocity. Technical considerations also play a role in the measurement of peak velocity. Prior studies have reported the peak velocity envelope, or the highest velocity seen free of background noise. The Doppler device used in our study [12] calculates peak modal velocity, which represents the velocity of the majority of the reflecting red cells, rather than the small population with the highest velocity. It should be noted that different instruments and recording techniques were used in the studies of Teague [12] and Daley [15].

The rise in left ventricular ejection fraction with stress evaluates left ventricular physiology, and may not reflect coronary anatomy when percent vascular stenosis is used as a reference [19, 20]. The same considerations may affect Doppler ejection parameters when they are employed for the diagnosis of coronary artery disease. Both Doppler and radionuclide methods might have a relatively low specificity for the diagnosis of coronary artery disease when prospectively applied, not only due to post test referral bias [21], but also because left ventricular impairment from any etiology would be reflected in the results. Accuracy of exercise radionuclide angiography can be improved with the additional analysis of exercise induced regional wall motion abnormalities and the change in end systolic volume with stress. It remains to be seen if additional Doppler parameters, or some combination of existing measures, will yield improvements in the diagnostic use of Doppler echocardiography. Furthermore, age, and possibly, sex matched reference values for maximal acceleration, peak velocity, and stroke distance may be necessary before these values can be used diagnostically. The 'control' groups used in both the studies of Teague [12] and Daley [15] were patients undergoing evaluation for chest pain syndromes and thus, do not constitute a true normal reference group.

Finally, despite the concordance obtained between Doppler indices of aortic flow and radionuclide left ventricular ejection fraction with exercise, these are fundamentally different measures and may be affected dissimilarly by changes in inotropic state, preload, and afterload. Teague [22] has recently demonstrated that both maximal acceleration and peak velocity are dependent upon heart rate and geometric aspects of ventricular ejection (Chapter 19). Using a mathematical model of left ventricular ejection, he showed that ventricles of disparate ejection fractions and systolic radii could yield similar values for maximal acceleration and peak velocity, and that heart rate alone could substantially alter measurement of acceleration and velocity in ventricles with no change in LVEF or chamber size. Thus, comparing the results of exercise radionuclide angiography and Doppler echocardiography may not always yield very close correlations.

The studies by Teague [12] and Daley [15] comparing LVEF response to exercise with Doppler ejection parameters have shown that both measures change in a similar manner with exercise induced left ventricular dysfunction. Thus, assessment of exercise related changes in Doppler indices of aortic ejection offers a potentially cost-effective method for the noninvasive detection of coronary artery disease. The Doppler test can be performed with inexpensive equipment by personnel requiring minimal training and with no radiation exposure to the patient. Further work will be needed to prospectively evaluate diagnostic Doppler criteria and to establish the range of normal responses, but these studies have verified the utility of Doppler testing in the assessment of global left ventricular function with exercise.

References

1. Goldschlager N, Selzer A, Cohn K. Treadmill stress tests as indicators of presence and severity of coronary artery disease. Ann Internal Med 1976; 85:277–286.
2. Boucher C. Radionuclide imaging. In: Morganroth, Parsi, Prohost (eds.). Noninvasive Cardiac Imaging. Year Book Medical Publishers, Inc. Chicago, 1983.
3. Marx G, Hicks R, Allen H, Kinzer S. Measurement of cardiac output and exercise factor by pulsed Doppler echocardiography during supine bicycle ergometry in normal young adolescent boys. J Am Coll Cardiol 1987; 10:430–434.
4. Harrison M, Smith M, Friedman B, DeMaria A. Uses and limitations of exercise Doppler echocardiography in the diagnosis of ischemic heart disease. J Am Coll Cardiol 1987; 10:809–817.
5. Bryg R, Labovitz A, Mehdirad A, Williams G, Chaitman B. Effect of coronary artery disease on Doppler-derived parameters of aortic flow during upright exercise. Am J Cardiol 1986; 58:14–19.
6. Mehta N, Bennett D, Mannering D, Dawkins K, Ward D. Usefulness of noninvasive Doppler measurement of ascending aortic blood velocity and acceleration in detecting impairment of the left ventricular functional response to exercise three weeks after acute myocardial infarction. Am J Cardiol 1986; 58:879–884.
7. Teague S, Mark D, Radford M, Robertson J, Albert D, Porter J, Waugh R. Doppler ejection dynamics during ischemic exercise responses. Circulation 1985; 72; Supp III:448.
8. Stein P, Sabbah H. Rate of change of ventricular power. An indicator of ventricular performance during ejection. Am Heart J 1976; 91:219–227.

9. Wallmeyer K, Wann S, Sagar K, Kalbfleisch J, Klopfenstein S. The influence of preload and heart rate on Doppler echocardiographic indexes of left ventricular performance: Comparison with invasive indexes in an experimental preparation. Circulation 1986; 74:181–186.

10. Bennett E, Else W, Miller G, Sutton G, Miller H, Noble N. Maximum acceleration of blood from the left ventricle in patients with ischemic heart disease. Clin Sci Mol Med 1974; 46:49–56.

11. Sabbah H, Khaja F, Brymer J, McFarland T, Albert D, Snyder J, Goldstein S, Stein P. Noninvasive evaluation of left ventricular performance based on peak aortic blood acceleration measured with a continuous-wave Doppler velocity meter. Circulation 1986; 74:323–329.

12. Teague S, Corn C, Sharma M, Prasad R, Burow R, Voyles W, Thadani U. A comparison of Doppler and radionuclide ejection dynamics during ischemic exercise. Am J Cardiac Imaging 1987; 1:145–151.

13. Iskandrian A, Hakki A, DePace N, *et al.* Evaluation of left ventricular function by radionuclide angiography during exercise in normal subjects and in patients with chronic coronary heart disease. J Am Coll Cardiol 1981; 1:518–529.

14. Leong K, Jones R. Influence of the location of left anterior descending coronary artery stenosis on left ventricular function during exercise. Circulation 1982; 65:109–114.

15. Daley P, Sagar K, Collier B, Kalbfleisch J, Wann S. Detection of exercise induced changes in left ventricular performance by Doppler echocardiography. Br Heart J 1987; 58:447–454.

16. Lazarus M, Dang T, Gardin J, Allfie A, Henry W. Evaluation of age, gender, heart rate and blood pressure changes and exercise conditioning on Doppler measured aortic blood flow acceleration and velocity during upright treadmill testing. Am J Cardiol 1988; 62:439–443.

17. Kelly T, Patrone V, Rothbart R, Moore J, Watson D, Weltman A, Gibson R. The utility of exercise Doppler in normals and patients with coronary artery disease. Circulation 1986; 74; Supp II:230.

18. Gardin J, Kozlowski J, Dabestani A, Murphy M, Kusnick C, Allfie A, Russell D, Henry W. Studies of Doppler aortic flow velocity during supine bicycle exercise. Am J Cardiol 1986; 57:327–332.

19. White C, Wright C, Doty D, Hiratza L, Eastham C, Harrison D, Marcus M. Does visual interpretation of the coronary arteriogram predict the physiologic importance of a coronary stenosis? N Eng J Med 1984; 310:819–823.

20. Osbakken M, Boucher C, Okada R, Bingham J, Strauss H, Pohost G. Spectrum of global left ventricular responses to supine exercise: limitation in the use of ejection fraction in identifying patients with coronary artery disease. Am J Cardiol 1983; 51:28–35.

21. Rozanski A, Diamond G, Berman D, Forrester J, Morris D, Swan H. The declining specificity of exercise radionuclide ventriculography. N Engl J Med 1983; 309:518–522.

22. Teague S, Burow R, Voyles W. A mathematical model that couples Doppler ejection indices to ventricular contraction. Circulation 1988; 78; Supp II:549.

9. Doppler treadmill studies in coronary patients: Angiographic correlates

ROBERT J. BRYG[1] and ARTHUR J. LABOVITZ[2]

[1]*University of Nevada, and Veterans Affairs Hospital, Reno, Nevada, U.S.A.*
[2]*St. Louis University, St. Louis, Missouri, U.S.A.*

9.1 Introduction

Doppler echocardiography in the 1980's has become one of the cornerstones of noninvasive testing in the evaluation of valvular heart disease. Because more of the population has coronary artery disease than valvular heart disease, investigators have searched for a use of Doppler echocardiography in this population. In addition, there has been a continuing search for improved sensitivity and specificity of exercise testing the diagnosis of coronary artery disease. Because of these combined needs, investigators have used Doppler derived parameters of aortic flow to assess for abnormalities during exercise.

Resting cardiac output is similar for both normal subjects as well as patients with a variety of cardiac conditions with normal or nearly normal left ventricular function, including coronary artery disease. Oftentimes, therefore, an intervention such as exercise is necesary to separate normal subjects from those with coronary artery disease.

The relationship between left ventricular function and Doppler derived parameters of aortic flow were validated at rest prior to applications in the exercise laboratory. At rest, there is a good correlation between the Doppler derived stroke volume and cardiac output compared to both Fick and thermodilution methods [1–4]. Further studies have validated this technique during exercise [5, 6].

It was with this background, that further studies were initiated to demonstrate the response to exercise of the Doppler derived parameters: peak ejection velocity, acceleration, stroke volume and cardiac output, in both normal subjects and patients with coronary artery disease.

9.2 Doppler examination

Aortic flow during exercise is most commonly interrogated from the suprasternal notch because of the relative ease with which the data can be acquired from this location. In general, it is difficult to obtain aortic flow from either the cardiac apex or right parasternal region during exercise.

Steve M. Teague (ed.) Stress Doppler Echocardiography, 107–119.
© 1990 *Kluwer Academic Publishers*.

Usually a dedicated Doppler transducer is placed in the suprasternal notch to obtain the aortic flow. The tonal quality and the velocity spectrum are both utilized to obtain the maximal velocity in the ascending aorta. If pulsed Doppler is used, the depth of the sample volume is maintained at that level for the duration of the exercise protocol.

During exercise, we have normally obtained the Doppler waveforms during the last 30 seconds of each stage of exercise, acquiring on hardcopy at a rapid paper speed to most accurately determine the velocity and timing of the flow profile.

Time intervals, such as the left ventricular ejection time and acceleration time, can be measured directly from the velocity tracings. The flow velocity integral is the area under the flow velocity curve. The darkest aspect of the profile is normally used for this determination. Peak ejection velocity (PEV) is the velocity obtained at the midpoint of the darkest portion of the velocity curve.

The cardiac output can then be calculated as the product of the flow velocity integral, the aortic cross sectional area and the heart rate. The determination of the aortic root diameter for the calculation of the cross sectional area is potentially a major source of error in the calculation of stroke volume and cardiac output. In measuring the diamter of the aortic root, different investigators have used a variety of measurements including the A-mode measurement of the aortic root, M-mode measurement of the aorta and aortic leaflet separation, and two dimensional measurement of the aorta and left ventricular outflow tract. The measurement that has proven to be the most reliable is the measurement of the left ventricular outflow tract obtained from the 2-dimensional parasternal long axis view just below the aortic valve and the ascending aorta just distal to the sinus of Valsalva [4, 7]. Using these measurements of the diameter and assuming a circular orifice, the area of the aorta can be calculated by the equation: Aortic area $= \pi * (D/2)^2$. The stroke volume is then: aortic area * FVI, and the cardiac output is the stroke volume multiplied by the heart rate. In view of the difficulty in determining the aortic root diameter at rest and during exercise, it may be preferable to simply compare PEV and FVI.

Some investigators have studied peak and mean accelerating during exercise to ascertain whether this adds to our understanding of ejection dynamics during exercise. Because of the high heart rates and difficulty obtained high quality Doppler signals, these are difficult to obtain manually, though there is an automated device (Exerdop, Quinton Corp.) which provides reproducible measurements of aortic acceleration during exercise.

9.3 Response to exercise (Table 1)

Normal subjects

The initial studies on normal subjects used supine and upright bicycle exercise [8–11]. At rest, lying in the left lateral decubitus position, with a normal heart rate of 60–80 beats per minute, the normal stroke volume index is 50–55 ml/min/m^2, the cardiac index is approximately 3 L/min/m^2, and the peak aortic flow velocity is

0.86 to 1.09 m/sec. When a normal subject assumes the standing position, the heart rate increases by approximately 10 beats per minute, the stroke index drops by 1/3 to approximately 33 ml/min/m^2, and the peak aortic velocity falls to a mean of 0.71 m/sec.

Table 1. Changes in aortic flow parameters with exercise.

		Rest	Moderate	Peak exercise	Recovery
Sitting	HR (beats/min)	67 ± 13	127 ± 21	152 ± 20	NA
Exercise (9)	CO (L/min)	4.6 ± 1.0	11.8 ± 1.3	14.7 ± 1.3	NA
	PEV (cm/sec)	71 ± 10	117 ± 16	128 ± 12	NA
Treadmill	HR (beats/min)	72 ± 13	121 ± 21	177 ± 26	94 ± 16
Exercise (14)	CI (L/min/m^2)	2.3 ± 0.7	6.7 ± 2.3	8.6 ± 2.5	5.2 ± 2.4
(normal)	PEV (cm/s)	72 ± 12	118 ± 21	156 ± 32	113 ± 26
Treadmill	HR (beats/min)	78 ± 18	118 ± 21	129 ± 19	82 ± 11
Exercise (14)	CI (1/min/m^2)	2.3 ± 0.7	5.1 ± 1.9	5.6 ± 2.2	3.8 ± 1.1
(CAD)	PEV (cm/s)	61 ± 14	85 ± 25	89 ± 26	81 ± 21
Treadmill	HR (beats/min	80 ± 20	NA	117 ± 23	NA
post MI (20)	PEV (cm/s)	41 ± 10	NA	45 ± 11	NA
(– TMST)	MA (m/s/s)	16 ± 3	NA	21 ± 5	NA
Treadmill	HR (beats/min)	81 ± 19	NA	121 ± 22	NA
post MI (20)	PEV (cm/s)	40 ± 8	NA	40 ± 11	NA
(+TMST)	MA (m/s/s)	15 ± 3	NA	18 ± 4	NA

The changes in aortic flow parameters during upright bicycle exercise, treadmill exercise in normal subjects, treadmill exercise in patients with coronary artery disease, and treadmill exercise post myocardial infarction with negative and positive treadmill exercise tests in three different studies are shown. The resting parameters were obtained in the upright position. The levels of moderate exertion are not at the same workload and direct comparison should not be made. In addition, the last study was performed with a continuous wave Doppler probe, and the peak velocities are lower than with a pulsed Doppler device. Abbreviations: CAD = coronary artery disease, CI = cardiac index, CO = cardiac output, HR = heart rate, MA = maximal acceleration, MI = myocardial infarction, PEV = peak ejection velocity, TMST = Treadmill ST segment response, (+) or (–) for ischemia. NA = not available.

During supine exercise, the stroke volume remains unchanged or falls slightly. At the same time, because of the marked increase in heart rate, the cardiac output increases 2–4 fold. The peak injection velocity increases approximately 20% during early exercise, and continues to progressively increase throughout exercise, with a net increase of approximately 50% to 1.4–1.6 m/sec. These values then return to baseline during recovery.

The response to upright exercise is slightly different. Initially, there is a significant decrease in stroke volume with standing compared with the supine position. With the initiation of exercise, the stroke volume rises rapidly to, or slightly above, the supine resting level before falling slightly at peak exercise. The cardiac output, because of the marked increase in heart rate and the increase in stroke volume, has a more marked change than seen with supine exercise, increasing 3–5

110

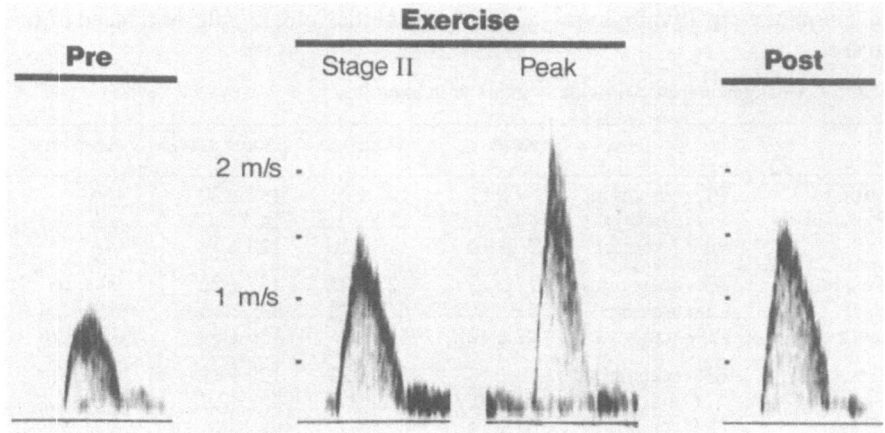

Figure 1. Typical pulsed Doppler aortic flow tracings during exercise in a normal subject. The peak velocity continues to increase during exercise. (Reprinted with permission of the American College of Cardiology: Chaitman BR. The changing role of exercise electrocardiogram as a diagnostic and prognostic test for chronic ischemic heart disease. J Am Coll Cardiol 1986; 8:1200.

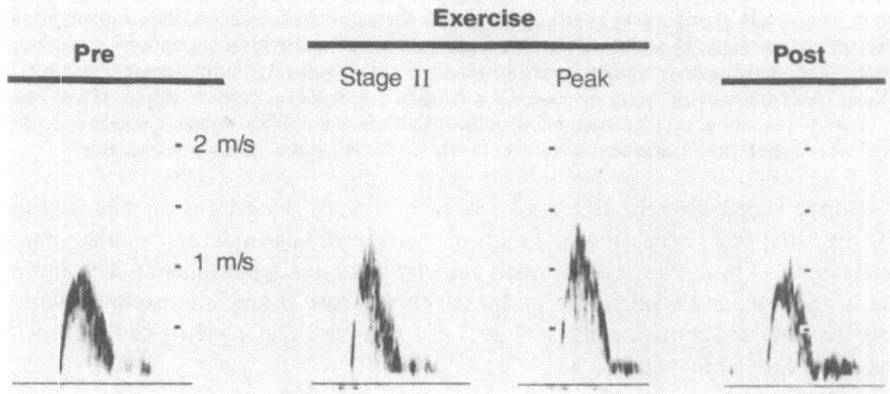

Figure 2. Typical pulsed Doppler aortic flow tracings during exercise in a patient with coronary artery disease. The peak velocity remains fairly constant through the various stages of exercise. (Reprinted with permission: Labovitz and Williams. *Doppler Echocardiography: The Quantitative Approach.* Lea and Febiger, 1987, Second Edition.

fold. Peak ejection velocity rises progressively, once again reaching a level of 1.4–1.6 m/sec at maximal exercise (Figure 1). There is no difference in responses seen between bicycle and treadmill exercise. In addition, the stroke volume, cardiac output, and peak velocity attained at maximal exercise are similar between supine and upright exercise.

Age has been shown to effect the responses seen in normal subjects. Using a continuous wave device that produces lower peak modal velocity than seen with pulsed Doppler examination, both Lazarus and Mehta have assessed the effect of age and sex on normal subjects [12, 13]. Mehta studied 96 normal volunteers and demonstrated that the increase in stroke volume is smaller in subjects over age 40. Peak velocity obtained at maximal exercise was approximately 100 cm/sec in those over 40, and was significantly higher at 118 cm/sec in those under 40. Even more striking was the response in maximal acceleration between these two groups. The maximal acceleration at peak exercise (Bruce stage 5) was 57 m/s/s in the younger group and only 42 m/s/s in those over 40. Gardin demonstrated similar findings. Both authors demonstrated that sex did not affect the peak velocity or maximal acceleration attained during exercise.

Coronary artery disease (Figure 2)

In the initial report on the use of Doppler echocardiography in the evaluation of coronary artery disease, we evaluated 20 normal subjects and 17 patients with coronary artery disease with treadmill exercise [14]. In the group with coronary artery disease, 8 had single vessel coronary artery disease, 4 had double vessel disease, while 5 had three vessel disease. All subjects were studied while performing a Bruce exercise protocol. There were marked differences between the two groups of patients. Normal subjects had a decrease in the stroke volume by 33% when arising to the standing position. This then increased rapidly during exercise, and in stage 2 of the Bruce protocol, the stroke volume was slightly greater than at rest while supine. The stroke volume did not change significantly for the remainder of exercise. In the patients with coronary artery disease, the initial stroke volume while supine was slightly lower, but fell by a similar percentage when standing. During exercise, the stroke volume only rose to the level of supine rest, and once again fell slightly at maximal exercise. There was a large amount of overlap between the normal group and the patients with coronary artery disease with this parameter, and there was no significant difference between the two groups.

The cardiac output in the group of patients with coronary artery disease started at 2.3 ± 0.7 L/min/m^2 and rose rapidly through exercise. By stage 2 of exercise, the mean cardiac index was lower than in the normal subjects, primarily because of the smaller increase in stroke volume. The heart rate at this stage was similar between the two groups. The maximal cardiac output only reached 5.6 ± 2.2 L/min/m^2, significantly lower than that reached by the normal subjects (8.6 ± 2.5 L/min/m^2) ($P < 0.001$). There was significant overlap in the calculated cardiac output between the normal subjects and those with coronary artery disease, and so this parameter,

112

like stroke volume, could not be used to independently differentiate between a normal and abnormal response.

The parameter that was able to separate the normal subjects from those with coronary artery disease was the peak ejection velocity (Figure 2, 3). Peak ejection velocity in the patients with coronary artery disease started at 79 cm/sec while supine and fell to 61 cm/sec when they assumed the upright position (p < 0.05). The peak velocity then climbed at a much lower rate, so that in Bruce stage II, the peak ejection velocity was 85 cm/sec (p < 0.001) and only rose to 89 cm/sec at maximal exercise. This is markedly lower than the 156 cm/sec seen in the normal subjects (p < 0.001). The peak velocity then fell slowly during the recovery period.

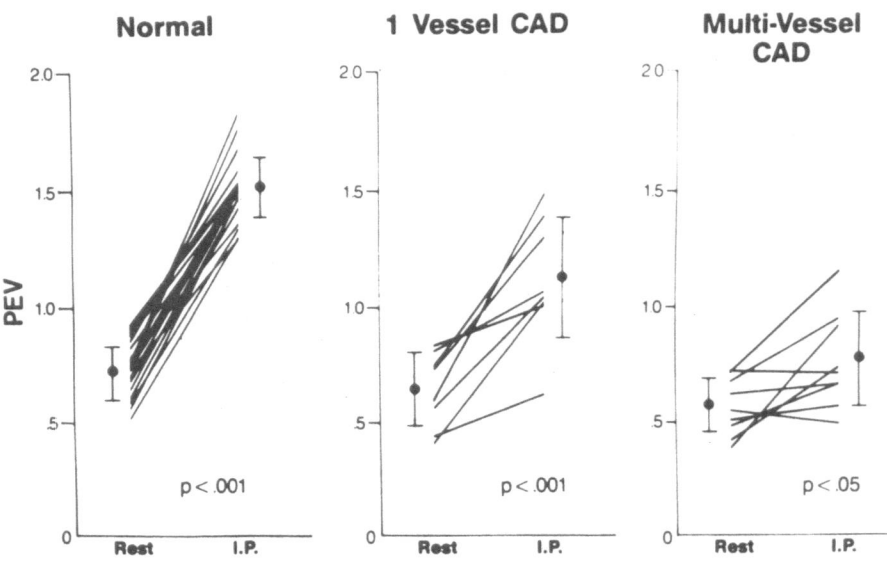

Figure 3. The change in peak ejection velocity (PEV) from rest to maximal exercise is shown in the normal subjects (left), patients with single vessel coronary artery disease (CAD (center) and with multivessel coronary artery disease (right). (Reprinted with permission [14].)

The patients with coronary artery disease could be divided into three different groups based on the response of the peak ejection velocity to exercise (Figure 4). The first group, those with single vessel coronary artery disease of a noncritical nature (70% stenoses) had a response similar to that seen in the normal subjects (type 1). The peak velocity increased at least 80% from the resting upright value and attained a maximal value of at least 100 cm/sec. The second response (type 2) was an increase in peak velocity, but less than 80% of the resting upright value. This second group, which consisted of eight patients, had an increase in peak velocity of only 25 ± 23% by stage II of the Bruce protocol, and only 29 ± 23% at maximal exercise. Three of the eight patients had single vessel coronary artery disease, three had 2 vessel coronary artery disease, while only 2 had 3 vessel CAD. There was little or no systolic dysfunction at rest in 6/8 of these patients.

The third response (type 3) was defined as a decrease in the peak velocity at maximal exercise. The peak velocity in the 6 patients with this response increased 54 ± 54 at Bruce stage II, but then fell to a difference of only 34 ± 45% at maximal exercise. In this group, 2 patients had single vessel coronary artery disease, 1 had double vessel disease, while 3 had 3 vessel CAD. Only 2 of the patients had a normal resting left ventriculogram.

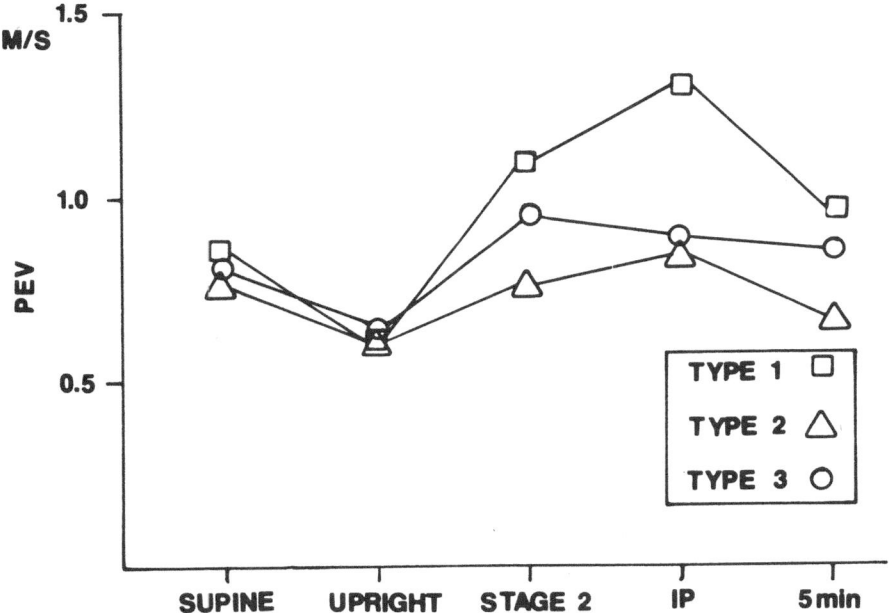

Figure 4. The three responses in peak ejection velocity response in patients with coronary artery disease are demonstrated. (Square = type 1, triangle = type 2, circle = type 3) at rest, supine and upright, at stage 2 of a Bruce protocol, immediately postexercise (IP) and 5 minutes after the cessation of exercise. (Reprinted with permission [14].)

9.4 2–Dimensional echocardiographic correlates

In a subsequent study, we compared the change in the peak ejection velocity during exercise to the change in echocardiographic ejection fraction [15, 16]. In this report, 14 normal subjects, and 14 patients with documented coronary artery disease were studied. The changes in heart rate and peak ejection velocity in both the normal subjects and those with coronary artery disease were similar to that of the previous study. The echocardiographic ejection fraction increased from a mean of 51% to 61% with exercise in the normal subjects. The ejection fraction at rest in those with coronary artery disease was similar to the normal subjects at rest at 49%. There was a slight fall in the ejection fraction during exercise to 48% in those with coronary artery disease. There was a good correlation between the percentage change in ejection fraction between rest and peak exercise and the percentage change in peak ejection velocity in this study ($r_s = 0.64$) (Figure 5). When the data from the 14 patients with coronary artery disease was analyzed separately, the correlation was even better ($r_s = 0.84$). There was, however, no correlation between the change in peak ejection velocity or ejection fraction and the development of new wall motion abnormalities. In addition, there was a poor correlation between the number of significantly diseased coronary arteries and the change in peak ejection velocity or change in ejection fraction. An absolute value for the peak velocity of 1.1 m/s and a percentage change from rest to peak exercise of 85% was able to separate subjects with a normal response from those with ischemia induced by left ventricular dysfunction.

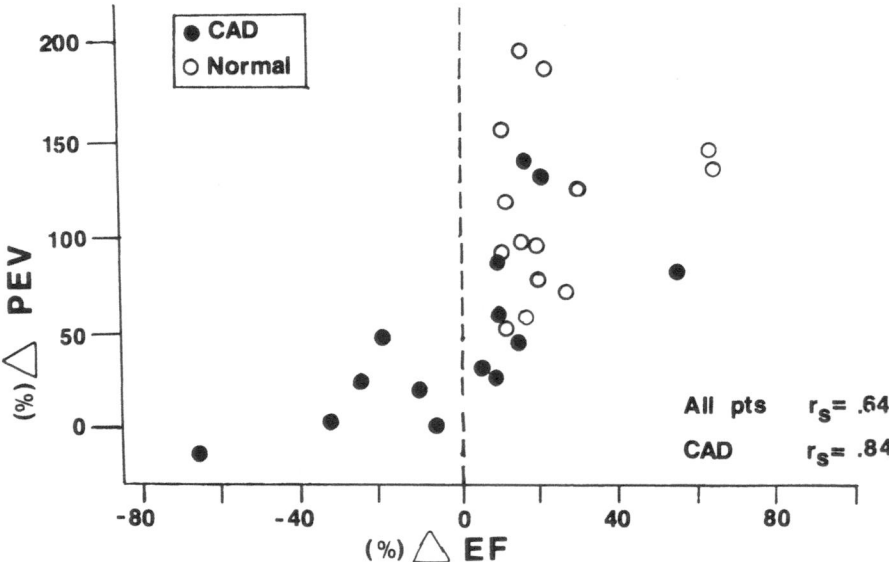

Figure 5. The correlation between the percentage change in ejection fraction (% Δ EF) and the percentage change in peak ejection velocity (% Δ PEV) is shown in normal subjects (open circles) and patients with coronary artery disease (closed circles). (Reprinted with permission of the American Heart Association [15].)

9.5 Other correlative studies

Teague in a study comparing Doppler responses to radionuclide angiography using a continuous wave Doppler device and supine exercise, confirmed the correlation between the change in peak velocity and the change in ejection fraction [17] (Chapter 8). In addition, he showed an even better correlation between the change in ejection fraction and the change in maximal acceleration with exercise. The absolute value of peak velocity was lower in this study than seen by investigators using pulsed Doppler. Daley and his colleagues also demonstrated the relationship between changes in ejection fraction and changes in peak velocity [18, 19]. He showed that patients with a normal ejection fraction who had an increase in this ejection fraction of greater than 5% during exercise (normal response) had an increase in peak velocity from approximately 70 cm/s to 95 cm/s. The mean acceleration similarly increased. In contrast, those with an abnormal resting ejection fraction who did not have an increase in ejection fraction of 5% during exercise, had no increase in peak velocity or mean acceleration.

Mehta studies 165 patients 3 to 4 weeks after an acute myocardial infarction with a continuous wave Doppler probe [20]. Of the original 165 patients, 98 had a negative stress test. In those with a negative stress test, the peak velocity increased slightly from 41 ± 10 to 45 ± 11 cm/sec ($p < 0.01$) and the maximal acceleration increased from 16 ± 3 to 21 ± 5 m/s/s ($p < 0.001$). In contrast, the 67 subjects with a positive stress test had no change in peak velocity at 40 ± 8 cm/s and a smaller rise in maximal acceleration than those with a negative stress test. He then demonstrated that the 32 subjects who had 1 or 2 vessel coronary artery disease had an increase in peak velocity from 44 to 46 cm/s. Likewise, the maximal acceleration was similar to that of those with a negative stress test, increasing from 16 ± 3 to 20 ± 4 m/s/s. Those with three vessel coronary artery disease had a slight fall in the peak velocity and no essential change in the maximal acceleration with exercise. In addition, those who completed only stage 1 or stage 2 of the Bruce protocol had lower maximal acceleration and peak velocity than those who exercised into stage 3.

Harrison, also using a continuous wave Doppler probe, studied 102 subjects and compared the Doppler results to Thallium scintigraphy [22]. In contrast to the other studies, he found significant overlap in the peak velocity and maximal acceleration between patients with normal thallium and those with abnormal thallium responses. Though there was no significant difference in peak ejection velocity in those with documented multivessel coronary artery disease, the maximal acceleration during exercise was lower in those with multivessel coronary artery disease.

9.6 Confounding variables

Recently, there have been several reports demonstrating some of the limitations of the use of Doppler parameters during exercise. Lazarus and Mehta have both demonstrated that age affects the maximal acceleration and peak velocity attained during exercise [12, 13]. Age alone is significantly and inversely related to the immediate postexercise Doppler maximal acceleration and peak velocity. The maximal acceleration in the youngest (Group 1) aged 21 ± 4 was 55 ± 15 m/s/s, in Group 2, aged 36 ± 5, the postexercise maximal acceleration was 46 subjects, Group 3, the acceleration was only 36 ± 9 m/s/s. Similarly, the peak velocity in group 1 was 1.1 ± 0.2 m/s, in group 2, 1.0 ± 0.2 m/s, and in group 3, 0.8 ± 0.2 m/s. There was no effect of gender, heart rate, preconditioning or blood pressure changes in the flow characteristics.

Drug therapy can also affect Doppler parameters during exercise. Both Mehta and Harrison have demonstrated that β blockade, which has a negative inotropic effect, causes a smaller rise in the peak ejection velocity and mean acceleration in normal subjects compared to a drug free state [13, 22]. Interestingly, verapamil did not affect the Doppler parameters during exercise.

9.7 Possible mechanisms for the responses seen

With exercise, several different physiologic responses occur. There is an increase in left ventricular contractility. In addition, there is vasodilation of the arterial bed and a decrease in the systemic vascular resistance. Both of these responses affect the Doppler parameters of aortic flow.

Sabbah and others have demonstrated that peak velocity and maximal acceleration are both directly correlated with global left ventricular function, i.e. ejection fraction [23–25]. It has also been shown that increases in cardiac contractility induced by dobutamine also can produce an increase in the Doppler parameters of aortic flow. Propranolol, conversely, because of its negative inotropic status, produces a decrease in both the peak velocity and maximal acceleration.

Changes in afterload can also affect Doppler parameters of aortic flow. Elkayam demonstrated that vasodilation with either hydralazine or nitrates can produce an increase in peak velocity and mean acceleration [26]. We have also seen an increase in peak velocity and mean acceleration with vasodilation produced by amyl nitrate.

In normal subjects and those with mild coronary artery disease, then, both the increased contractility and decreased afterload contribute to the increased acceleration and peak velocity of blood flow. With significant coronary artery disease, other mechanisms intervene. In patients with severe coronary artery disease, during exercise, the myocardium becomes ischemic, with resultant loss in contractility. There is then a smaller increase in the peak ejection velocity and maximal acceleration (type 2 response). If one has a significant coronary artery stenosis, there would then be an increase in peak velocity until the myocardium becomes ischemic. With the onset of ischemia, there is then a sudden loss of contractility and a resultant decrease in peak velocity and maximal acceleration, producing the type 2 response mentioned above.

In elderly subjects, the aorta becomes stiffer and less compliant. This leads to less vasodilation with exercise, and hence, less of an increase in peak velocity and maximal acceleration. Beta blockade produces its effect during exercise by decreasing contractility. Because of its negative inotropic effect, there is not the same increase in contractility during exercise as is seen in unmedicated normal subjects, and thus the peak velocity and mean acceleration do not increase to the same extent.

9.8 Conclusions

Patients with significant coronary artery disease often have different Doppler aortic velocity parameters with exercise than normal subjects. The peak velocity and maximal acceleration both increase less in those with coronary artery disease, and can be used to determine the severity of their coronary artery disease by reflecting the changes caused by ischemic myocardium. There are several factors including age and the administration of beta blocking agents that can affect this determination.

In addition, the absolute values for peak velocity and acceleration are affected by the instrumentation used for the examination. The continuous wave Doppler velocity probes provide smaller absolute values for peak velocity than obtained with pulsed Doppler. The maximal acceleration provided by these probes is significantly higher than the mean acceleration calculated with pulsed Doppler, however. This technique currently must be validated in one's own laboratory, developing normal values for each individual laboratory and Doppler device to assure diagnostic accuracy for this technique.

References

1. Chandraratna PA, Nanna M, McKay C, Nimalasurilya A, Swinney R, Elkayam U, Rahimtoola SH. Determination of cardiac output by transcutaneous continuous-wave ultrasound Doppler computer. Am J Cardiol 1984; 53:234–237.
2. Rose JS, Nanna M, Rahimtoola SH, Elkayam U, McKay C, Chandraratna PAN. Accuracy of determination of changes in cardiac output by transcutaneous continuous-wave Doppler computer. Am J Cardiol 1984; 54:1099–1101.
3. Gardin JM, Tobis JM, Dabestani A, Smith C, Elkayam U, Castleman E, White D, Allfie A, Henry WL. Superiority of two-dimensional measurement of aortic vessel diameter in Doppler echocardiographic estimates of left ventricular stroke volume. J Am Coll Cardiol 1985; 6:66–74.
4. Labovitz AJ, Buckingham TA, Habermehl K, Nelson J, Kennedy HL, Williams GA. The effect of sampling site on the two-dimensional echo Doppler determination of cardiac output. Am Heart J 1985; 109:327–332.
5. Ihlen H, Endresen K, Golf S, Nitter-Hauge S. Cardiac stroke volume during exercise measured by Doppler echocardiography: Comparison with thermodilution technique and evaluation of reproducibility. Br Heart J 1987; 58:455–459.
6. Christie J, Sheldahl LM, Tristani FE, Sagar KB, Ptacin MJ, Wann LS. Determination of stroke volume and cardiac output during exercise: Comparison of two-dimensional and Doppler echocardiography, Fick oximetry, and thermodilution. Circulation 1987; 76:539–547.

7. Gardin JM, Dabestani A, Matin K, Allfie A, Russell D, Henry WL. Reproducibility of Doppler aortic blood flow measurements: Studies on intraobserver, interobserver and day-to-day variability in normal subjects. Am J Cardiol 1984; 54:1092–1098.
8. Loeppky JA, Greene ER, Hoekenga DE, Caprihan A, Luft UC. Beat-by-beat stroke volume assessment by pulsed Doppler in upright and supine exercise. J Appl Physiol 1981; 50:1173–1182.
9. Shaw JG, Johnson EC, Volyes WF, Greene ER. Noninvasive Doppler determination of cardiac output during submaximal and peak exercise. J Appl Physiol 1985; 59:722–731.
10. Gardin JM, Kozlowski J, Dabestani A, Murphy M, Kusnick C, Allfie A, Russell D, Henry WL. Studies of Doppler aortic flow velocity during supine bicycle exercise. Am J Cardiol 1986; 57:327–332.
11. Daley PJ, Sagar KB, Wann LS. Doppler echocardiographic measurements of flow velocity in the ascending aorta during supine and upright exercise. Br Heart J 1985; 54:562–567.
12. Lazarus M, Dang TY, Gardin JM, Allfie A, Henry WL. Evaluation of age, gender, heart rate, and blood pressure changes and exercise conditioning on Doppler measured aortic blood flow acceleration and velocity during upright treadmill testing. Am J Cardiol 1988; 62:439–443.
13. Mehta N, Boyle G, Bennett D, Gilmour S, Noble MIM, Mills CM, Pugh S. Hemodynamic response to treadmill exercise in normal volunteers: An assessment by Doppler ultrasonic measurement of ascending aortic blood velocity and acceleration. Am Heart J 1988; 116:1298–1307.
14. Bryg RJ, Labovitz AJ, Mehdirad AA, Williams GA, Chaitman BR. Effect of coronary artery disease on Doppler-derived parameters of aortic flow during upright exercise. Am J Cardiol 1986; 58:14–19.
15. Mehdirad AA, Williams GA, Labovitz AJ, Bryg RJ, Chaitman BR. Evaluation of left ventricular function during upright exercise: Correlation of exercise Doppler with postexercise two-dimensional echocardiographic results. Circulation 1987; 75:413–419.
16. Bryg RJ, Labovitz AJ. Exercise pulsed wave Doppler in the evaluation of coronary artery disease: Importance of peak ejection velocity. Am J Cardiac Imaging 1987; 1:207–214.
17. Teague SM, Corn C, Sharma M, Prasad R, Burow R, Voyles WF, Thadani U. A comparison of Doppler and radionuclide ejection dynamics during ischemic exercise. Am J Cardiac Imaging 1987; 1:145–151.
18. Daley PJ, Sagar KB, Collier BD, Kalbfleisch J, Wann LS. Detection of exercise induced changes in left ventricular performance by Doppler echocardiography. Br Heart J 1987; 58:447–454.
19. Mahn T, Sagar KB, Wann LS. Exercise Doppler echocardiography for evaluating coronary artery disease. Am J Cardiac Imaging 1987; 1:97–102.
20. Mehta N, Bennett D, Mannering D, Dawkins K, Ward DE. Usefulness of noninvasive Doppler measurements of ascending aortic blood velocity and acceleration in detecting impairment of the left ventricular functional response to exercise three weeks after acute myocardial infarction. Am J Cardiol 1986; 58:879–884.
21. Harrison MR, Smith MD, Friedman BJ, DeMaria AN. Uses and limitations of exercise Doppler echocardiography in the diagnosis of ischemic heart disease. J Am Coll Cardiol 1987; 10:809–817.
22. Harrison MR, Smith MD, Nissen SE, Grayburn PA, DeMaria AN. Use of exercise Doppler echocardiography to evaluate cardiac drugs: Effects of propranolol and verapamil on aortic blood flow velocity and acceleration. J Am Coll Cardiol 1988; 11:1002–1009.
23. Sabbah HN, Przybylski J, Albert DE, Stein PD. Peak aortic blood acceleration reflects the extent of left ventricular ischemic mass at risk. Am Heart J 1987; 113:885–890.

24. Sabbah HN, Khaja F, Brymer JF, McFarland TM, Albert DE, Snyder JE, Goldstein S, Stein PD. Noninvasive evaluation of left ventricular performance based on peak aortic blood acceleration measured with a continuous-wave Doppler velocity meter. Circulation 1986; 74:323–329.
25. Elkayam U, Gardin JM, Berkley R, Hughes CA, Henry WL. The use of Doppler flow velocity measurement to assess the hemodynamic response to vasodilators in patients with heart failure. Circulation 1983; 67:377–383.
26. Stein PD, Sabbah HN. Rate of change of ventricular power: An indicator of ventricular performance during ejection. Am Heart J 1976; 91:219–227.

10. Uses and limitations of exercise Doppler echocardiography in the clinical evaluation of ischemic heart disease

MICHAEL R. HARRISON and ANTHONY N. DEMARIA

University of Kentucky, College of Medicine, MN 670 Lexington, Kentucky 40536, U.S.A.

10.1 Introduction

Since the early 1930's, clinicians have used exercise to aid in the diagnosis and evaluation of patients with ischemic heart disease [1]. By increasing myocardial oxygen demand, exercise can induce myocardial ischemia when myocardial oxygen delivery is impaired by significant, flow-limiting coronary atherosclerosis [2]. Methods available for noninvasive evaluation of exercise-induced myocardial ischemia include: electrocardiography, radionuclide techniques, two-dimensional echocardiography, and Doppler echocardiography.

Although only recently employed as a method for identifying ischemic heart disease, early experience with exercise Doppler echocardiography has been very encouraging [3–6]. When combined with exercise, the Doppler examination is usually performed with the transducer at the suprasternal notch and measures the velocity of blood flow in the ascending aorta. Thus, in contrast to other techniques, Doppler echocardiography reflects the hemodynamic consequence of left ventricular contraction, rather than depicting perfusion or contraction of the left ventricular myocardium itself.

The use of Doppler echocardiography during exercise to evaluate ischemic heart disease is predicated on two important points: 1) myocardial ischemia results in impairment of contractile performance of the ischemic area [7], and 2) the onset of contractile dysfunction is rapid [8]. Thus, investigators hypothesized that since ischemia can be induced by exercise in patients with significant flow-limiting coronary atherosclerosis and results in impaired left ventricular systolic performance, the presence and extent of exercise-induced myocardial ischemia might be reflected in Doppler recordings obtained during and immediately following exercise.

In normal subjects, upright exercise results in increased heart rate and stroke volume, resulting in a greatly augmented cardiac output. The elevation in stroke volume is due to increased contractility as well as increased venous return and a marked reduction in systemic vascular resistance. Additionally, the tachycardia of exercise contributes to the increased contractility by the force-frequency relationship of Bowditch [9–11]. It must be recalled, however, that the hemodynamic response to exercise is complex and variable between individuals. Furthermore, it is influenced by multiple factors intrinsic and extrinsic to the myocardium.

Steve M. Teague (ed.) Stress Doppler Echocardiography, 121–135.

In addition to myocardial ischemia, intrinsic factors that may alter an individual's cardiac response to exercise include: exercise capacity, age, cardiovascular conditioning, and previous myocardial infarction. Extrinsic factors with potential to alter one's response to exercise include cardiovascular medications, particularly beta adrenergic antagonists.

10.2 Clinical application

The velocity and acceleration (rate of change of velocity) of blood flow in the ascending aorta have been shown to be reliable descriptors of left ventricular systolic performance [12–14]. By virtue of its ability to provide accurate information on blood flow in the ascending aorta, doppler echocardiography offers a convenient method to assess left ventricular systolic function during exercise [15]. Thus, recent investigations in our laboratory [16] have sought to test the hypothesis that myocardial ischemia due to coronary artery disease might be identified by a decrease in Doppler measurements of flow velocity and acceleration during exercise.

We studied a total of 102 individuals (Table 1). Twenty-eight young, healthy volunteers with no evidence of cardiovascular disease served as a reference group (Controls). These subjects provided information regarding the normal response of peak flow velocity, peak acceleration and flow velocity integral to near maximal exercise. The mean age of this reference group was 28.7 years. The remaining 74 subjects were referred for exercise thallium perfusion scintigraphy for the evaluation of chest pain. These patients were subdivided according to the results of their radionuclide study: normal (Group I, mean age 54.9 years), ischemia (Group II, mean age 55.1 years) and prior infarction only (Group III, mean age 53.8 years). The results of coronary angiography were concordant with the thallium testing in those patients in whom catheterization was performed. There was no significant difference in age between the three patient groups, but patients in groups I, II and III were all significantly older than the young control subjects.

Table 1. Age and exercise characteristics of the study population.

	#	Age (mean)	Mean duration of exercise (min)	Maximal HR (average)	# Maximal HR ≥ 85% predicted
Controls	28	28.7	12.7	169.3	28
Group I (normal scans)	25	54.9	8.5 ± 2.9	147.5	19
Group II (ischemia)	37	55.1	7.3 ± 2.7	127.3	16
Group III (infarction only)	12	53.8	7.2	129.6	5
Total	102				

* p = NS
† p ≤ 0.005

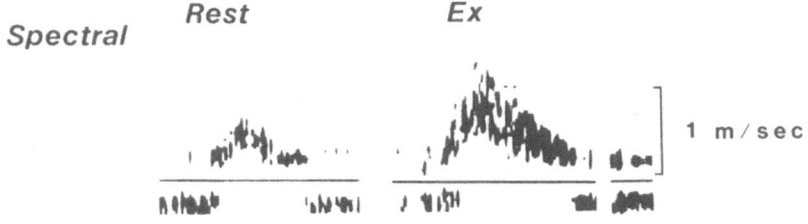

Spectral

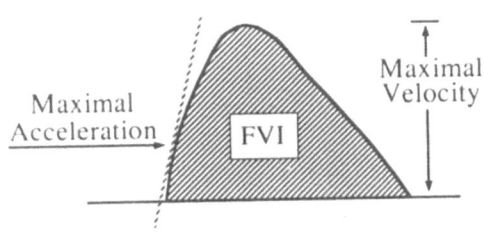

DIGITAL REPORT:	Peak ACCEL (m/sec/sec)	Peak Modal VEL (m/sec)	FVI (cm)	TIME
Rest	15	0.63	7.6	0:00
1	19	0.81	11.0	1:59
2	22	0.90	11.4	4:40
3	30	1.02	10.8	7:36
4	38	1.19	11.4	13:11
Exercise stopped				
5	46	1.11	7.2	0:10

Figure 1. Representative spectral (top) and digital (bottom) printouts from Doppler instruments. The accompanying diagram (middle) illustrates several commonly obtained measurements. ACCEL = acceleration; Ex = exercise; FVI = flow velocity integral; VEL = velocity. (Reprinted with permission from The American College of Cardiology (J Am Coll Cardiol 1987; 10:809–17).)

All subjects were exercised on a standard treadmill using the Bruce protocol [17]. For the 74 patients referred for thallium testing, thallium-201 was administered according to standard procedure [18]. Continuous-wave Doppler examinations were performed from the suprasternal notch, with the subject in the standing position. A nonimaging transducer was positioned to record the maximal flow signal as determined by audio and spectral outputs. Doppler recordings were made at baseline prior to exercise, during the last half of each exercise stage, and immediately after exercise (no warm-down period).

Two nonimaging instruments were employed, and most subjects were studied sequentially with both machines. A full spectral recording was available from one unit (Irex), and enabled measurement of maximal velocity (fastest velocity traveled by RBC's in the Doppler recording) with the aid of a digitizing pad and computer. The second unit (ExerDop, A.H. Robins) is capable of measuring peak modal velocity (peak velocity of the greatest number of RBC's, which is slightly lower than maximal velocity), but lacks the capability of a full spectral tracing. Peak acceleration is derived internally by the instrument at a high sample rate (200 Hz) using a 2 point integrated slope algorithm. Flow velocity integral is also derived internally by this instrument. ExerDop provides Doppler measurements in the form of a digital printout (Figure 1).

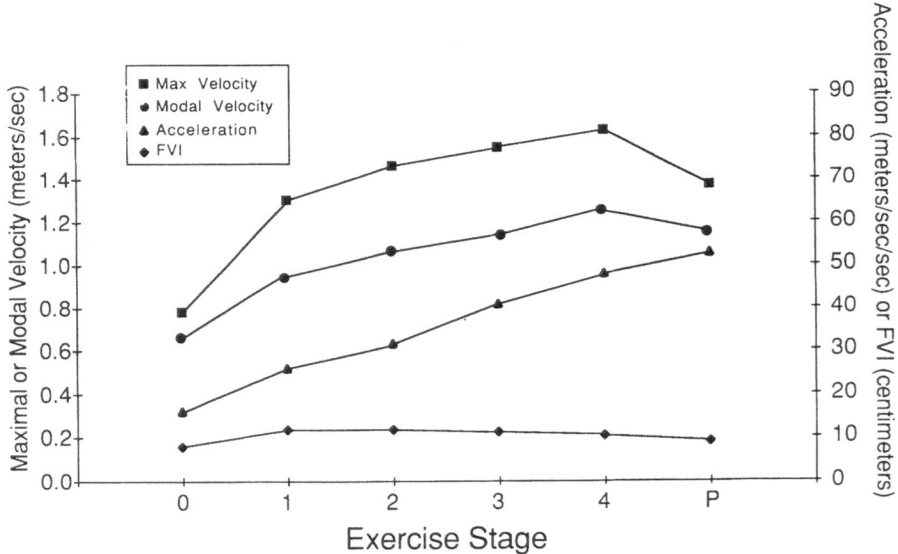

Figure 2. Mean Doppler flow values for young normal subjects. Values are shown for baseline (rest), each stage of exercise, and immediately post-exercise (P). FVI = flow velocity integral; Max = maximal. (Reprinted with permission of The American College of Cardiology (J Am Coll Cardiol 1987; 10:809–17).)

10.3 Results

In all four groups of subjects (young control group and patient Groups I–III), the values for peak velocity and acceleration were significantly higher immediately post-exercise compared to baseline. The young control group exercised an average 12.7 min and achieved an average peak heart rate of 169.3 bpm. As shown in

Figure 2, a progressive increase in maximal velocity, peak modal velocity, and acceleration occurred with advancing levels of exercise. Both maximal and modal velocity decreased slightly in the immediate post-exercise period, while peak acceleration continued to increase. Flow velocity integral increased early in the exercise protocol, then plateaued, and decreased slightly at peak exercise. Qualitatively similar results were obtained for Groups I–III despite lower exercise capacity. Specifically, the nearly universal response of aortic blood flow velocity and acceleration to exercise is to increase, regardless of the presence or absence of ischemia.

There was considerable difference, however, when quantitative changes during exercise were analyzed. The mean value for maximal velocity achieved during exercise by patients examined by thallium scintigraphy was significantly less than that achieved by control subjects (1.36 m/s for Controls vs 1.19 m/s Group I and 1.09 m/s Group II). Despite differing from control values, however, there was no significant difference in response of maximal velocity to exercise for patients in Group I versus Group II (Figure 3). Thus, for this cohort of patients referred for exercise testing, the response of maximal velocity to exercise was no different for patients with ischemia on thallium perfusion scintigraphy vs those with normal myocardial perfusion scans. Similar results were obtained for modal velocity.

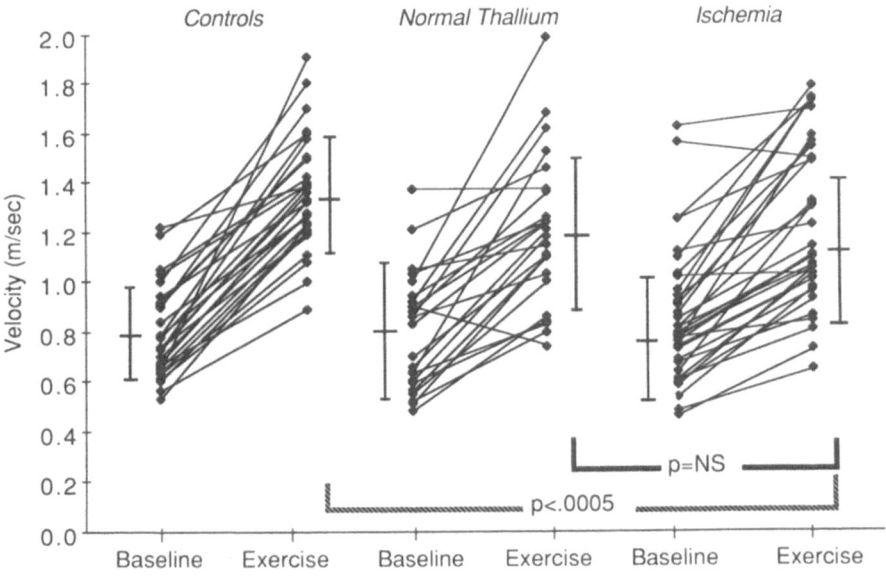

Figure 3. Individual, mean and standard deviation values for maximal aortic flow velocity at baseline and immediately after exercise. The p values refer to the difference between groups for the mean change in flow velocity. (Reprinted with permission from the American College of Cardiology (J Am Coll Cardiol 1987; 10:809–17).)

126

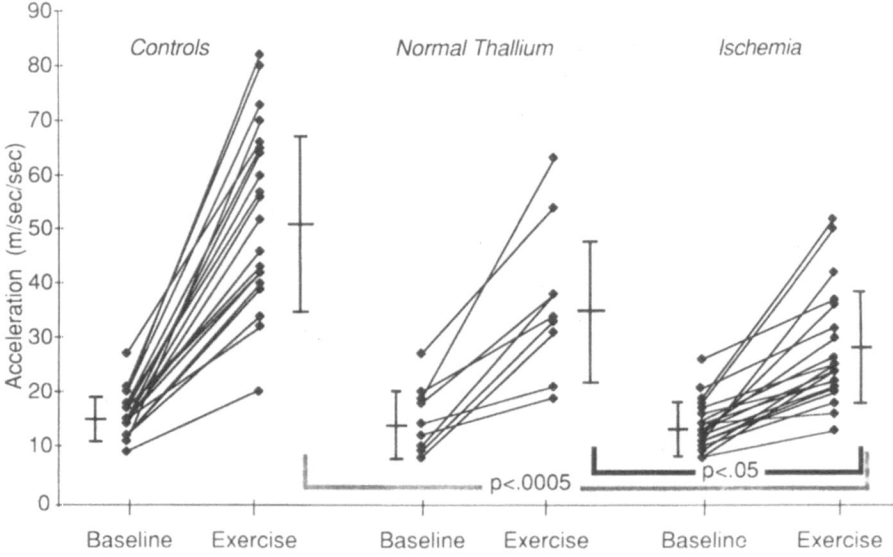

Figure 4. Values for peak acceleration of aortic blood flow at baseline and immediately after exercise. (Reprinted with permission from the American College of Cardiology (J Am Coll Cardiol 1987; 10:800–17).)

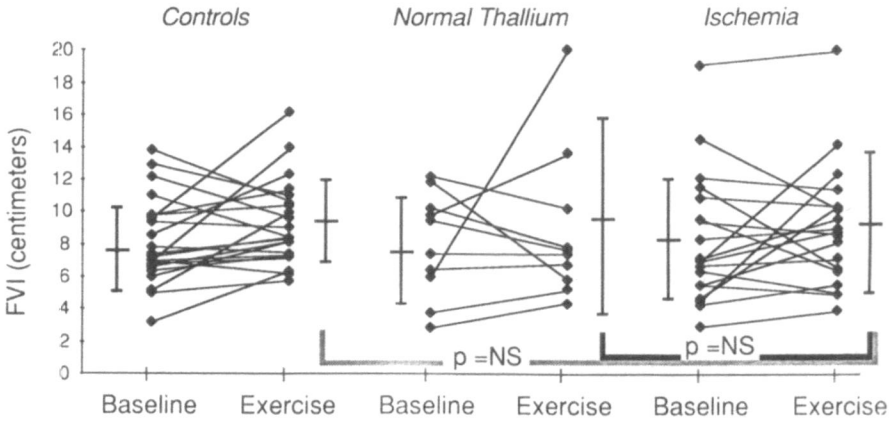

Figure 5. Flow velocity integral (FVI) at baseline and immediately after exercise. (Reprinted with permission from The American College of Cardiology (J Am Coll Cardiol 1987; 10:809–17).)

As was the case for velocity, values for peak acceleration at maximal exercise in the young control group were significantly greater than for either group I or II. In contrast to velocity, however, peak acceleration appeared to distinguish between patients with exercise-induced ischemia and those without ischemia (Figure 4). The mean value achieved by patients with ischemic responses to exercise-thallium imaging was less (27.8 m/s^2) compared to patients with normal perfusion scans (36.8 m/s^2). Thus, measurement of low peak acceleration with exercise by Doppler echocardiography can ostensibly identify patients with a high likelihood of exercise-induced myocardial ischemia.

The response of flow velocity integral to exercise was variable and failed to distinguish controls from patients and abnormal versus normal scans (Figure 5).

10.4 Effect of exercise capacity on Doppler results

It is apparent from Figure 2 that velocity and acceleration of aortic blood flow increase as the level of upright exercise increases. Thus, if peak exercise Doppler values are to be compared between individuals or between groups, equivalent levels of exertion must be performed. Similarly, if an individual is to have serial exercise Doppler studies, Doppler measurements must be evaluated in the context of exercise level at which they are obtained.

10.5 Effect of age on Doppler results

For the older patient group with normal thallium perfusion studies (Group I), average exercise duration was 8.7 min. Values of maximal velocity achieved at that level of exercise for Group I averaged 1.19 m/s. When compared to values of maximal velocity achieved by the young control group for stage 3 of the exercise protocol (comparable exercise level and duration), it is obvious that age plays an important role in determining one's Doppler response to exercise. Indeed, values for maximal velocity for the control group at stage 3 averaged 1.55 m/s, significantly higher ($p < 0.01$) than the velocity achieved by the older subjects in Group I (normal scans) even when the effects of cardiac medication (see below) were accounted for. Similar effects of age were apparent for peak modal velocity.

Peak acceleration at 8.7 min exercise averaged 36.8 m/s^2 for Group I patients. As was the case for velocity, peak acceleration for the young control group (41 m/s^2) was higher at the same level of exertion than peak acceleration in Group I. Thus, for velocity (maximal and modal) and acceleration, age is inversely related to Doppler measurements. Recently, others [19] have reported similar findings with regard to the effects of age on these Doppler parameters, and confirmed our impression that if exercise Doppler values from patients are to be compared to exercise Doppler values from a reference group, age must be considered.

10.6 Effect of previous myocardial infarction

Patients in Group III (thallium evidence of infarction only) were similar in age and exercise duration to patients in Group II (thallium evidence of ischemia) and therefore offered a means by which to evaluate the ability of exercise Doppler to distinguish transient exercise-induced left ventricular dysfunction versus permanent left ventricular dysfunction. Group III patients increased their maximal velocity from 0.76 m/s at baseline to 1.13 m/s immediately post-exercise and increased their peak acceleration from 14.7 m/s^2 at baseline to 24.7 m/s^2 at immediately post-exercise. The response of these Doppler parameters to exercise was not significantly different for patients with prior infarction versus those with thallium evidence of ischemia. Thus, exercise Doppler echocardiography appears to be limited in its ability to distinguish transient from permanent LV dysfunction.

10.7 Effects of beta adrenergic antagonists

From our earliest experience with exercise Doppler echocardiography, patients on beta blocking medication appeared to have a blunted response of velocity and acceleration to exercise. Since previous reports on exercise Doppler have included patients being treated with beta blockers [5], we attempted to address this issue in our study population. Because 36 of the 74 patients referred for thallium study were currently receiving beta blocking medication, we analyzed the results of velocity and acceleration for patients in Group I (normal scans) and Group II (ischemia) who had achieved 85% of their age-predicted maximal heart rate. It is unlikely that beta blockade was significant in this subpopulation. In contrast to the significant decrease in peak acceleration observed between Group II and Group I when all patients were included, when comparison was limited to the subset of patients who reached 85% of age-predicted maximal heart rate there was no difference between peak acceleration during exercise for patients with ischemic versus normal scans (Group II 33.6 versus Group I 36.8 m/s^2, p = NS) (Figure 6). Similarly, velocity (maximal and modal) was unable to distinguish patients with ischemic thallium scans from patients with normal thallium scans in this subpopulation. Thus, use of beta adrenergic antagonists appears to account for much of the lowering of Doppler-measured flow velocity and acceleration since Doppler's ability to predict exercise-induced ischemia was lost when patients receiving beta blockers were eliminated. Presumably, the patients with myocardial ischemia (Group II) were more likely to have been using beta blocking medication, and it was the medication that accounted for the lower values for peak acceleration in Group II compared to patients with normal scans (Group I).

To insure that any change in Doppler values due to exercise-induced ischemia was not missed due to a delay in measurements immediately post-exercise, analysis of velocity and acceleration data was performed for the highest exercise stage achieved while still exercising. As was the case for velocity and acceleration in Groups I and II measured immediately post-exercise, no difference in Doppler parameters could be ascribed to the effects of ischemia when analysis was restricted to patients not receiving beta blockers.

To further assess the possibility of an ischemia-induced difference in Doppler results, the values for maximal velocity and peak acceleration at maximal exercise were compared with baseline values and expressed as a percentage increase from baseline. Results of this analysis, however, were unchanged from those found for absolute values.

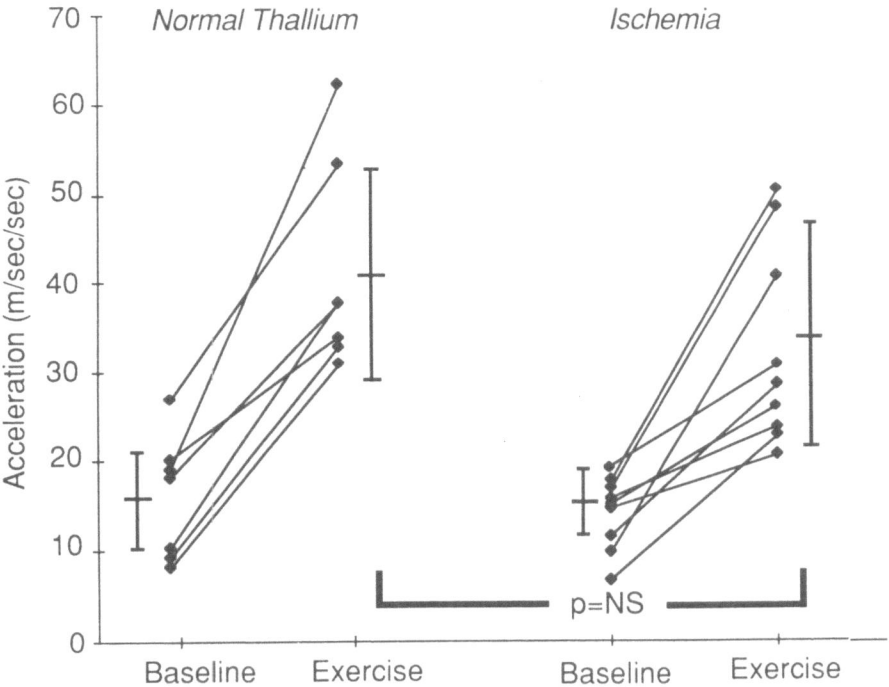

Figure 6. Peak acceleration at baseline and immediately after exercise for patients with normal (Group I) and ischemic (Group II) thallium studies who achieved at least 85% of their age-predicted maximal heart rate. (Reprinted with permission from The American College of Cardiology (J Am Coll Cardiol 1987; 10: 809–17).)

We have since confirmed the impression that beta adrenergic antagonists exert an important influence on Doppler values of velocity and acceleration [20]. Twenty young healthy volunteers were studied with the exercise Doppler protocol as described above. Initially, the test was done in the drug-free (control) state. Immediately following the control test, 1 mg/kg of propranolol was administered orally. Ninety minutes later, these subjects underwent the same exercise Doppler protocol, achieving the same exercise duration as seen in the control test (propranolol test).

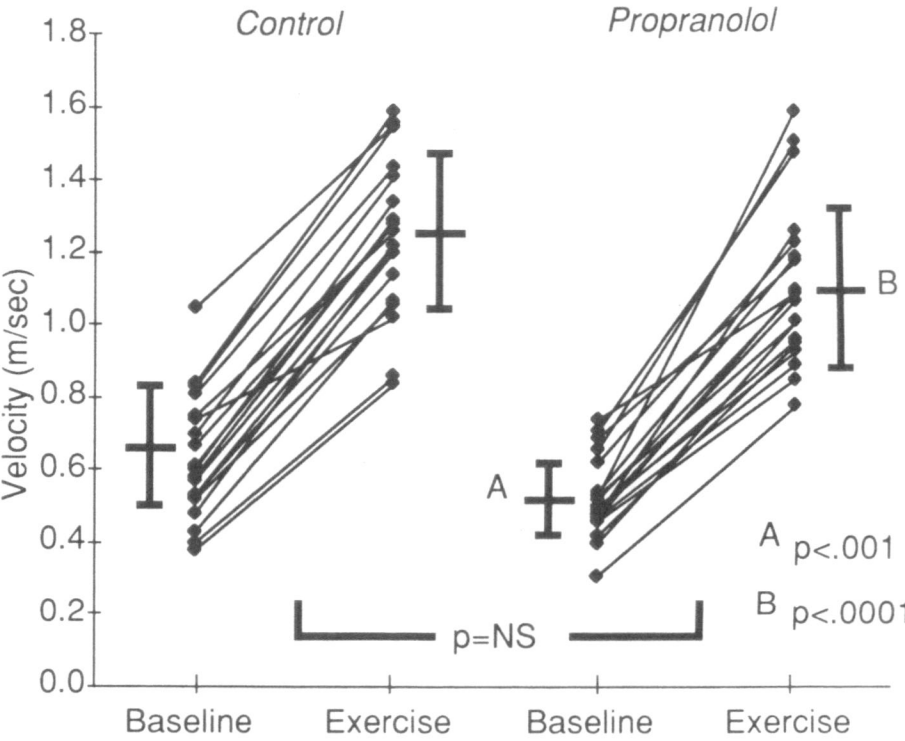

Figure 7. Individual, mean and standard deviations values for peak modal velocity measured at rest and immediately after exercise for the control and propranolol exercise tests. A refers to the difference in Doppler values at rest for drug versus control test, and B refers to the difference in Doppler values during exercise for drug versus control test. The brackets refer to the change in Doppler-derived value from rest to exercise for the drug versus the control test. (Reprinted with permission from The American College of Cardiology (J Am Coll Cardiol 1988; 11:1002–9).)

The results of this study were clear. Propranolol, in clinically useful doses, caused remarkable blunting of both aortic flow velocity and acceleration (Figures 7 and 8). Propranolol lowered values for aortic flow velocity at rest and during exercise, and the extent of propranolol's effect was similar for each situation. Thus, the rise in velocity during exercise was unchanged between the control and propranolol tests (Figure 7). In contrast, the effects of beta blockade on peak acceleration are most profound during exercise. Propranolol caused peak acceleration at rest and maximal exertion to be lowered compared to control, but affected the value of peak acceleration at maximal exercise to a greater extent. Thus, the exercise-induced rise in peak acceleration from baseline to maximal exercise was blunted (Figure 8). The finding of a diminished rise in Doppler values of peak acceleration is similar to the results noted by ourselves (see above) and others for patients with heart disease and suggest that much of what has been attributed to an effect of myocardial ischemia

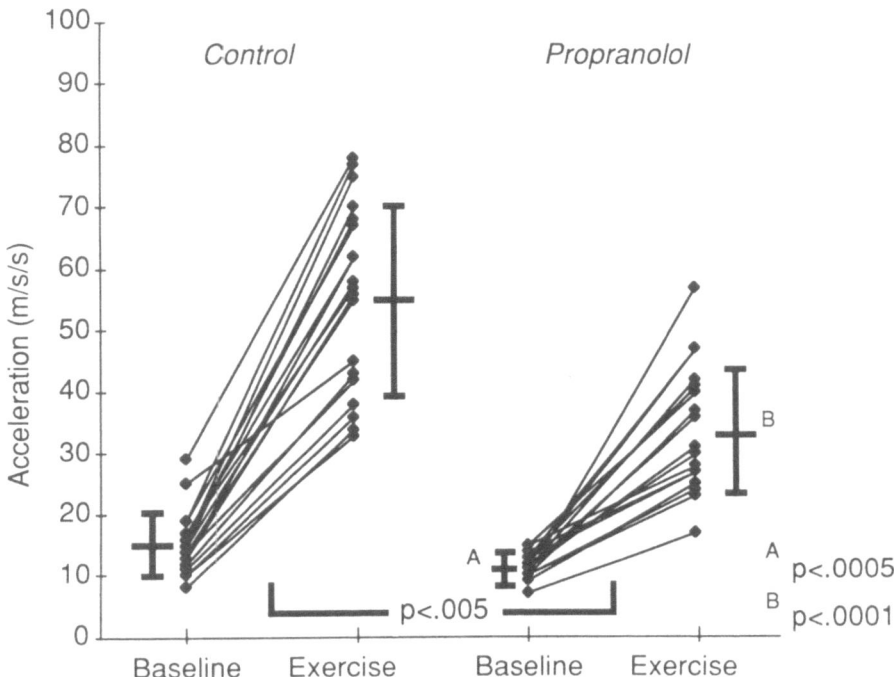

Figure 8. Peak acceleration of aortic blood flow at baseline and immediately after exercise for the control and propranolol tests. Abbreviations as in Figure 7. (Reprinted with permission from The American College of Cardiology (J Am Coll Cardiol 1988; 11:1002–9).)

may actually have been due to the presence of beta receptor antagonists. Similar results of exercise Doppler studies done on patients receiving beta blocking medication [21] have recently been reported by others.

The negative effect of propranolol on Doppler velocity and acceleration appears specific for beta adrenergic antagonists. We conducted the same exercise Doppler protocol on the same subjects, but replaced propranolol with verapamil. Despite its well described negative inotropic properties, verapamil failed to alter either velocity or acceleration at rest or during exercise (Figure 9) [20]. When another calcium channel antagonist, nifedipine, was used in place of verapamil, Doppler values of velocity and acceleration at rest were actually increased relative to control. The augmentation of Doppler values by nifedipine was probably related to reflex sympathetic stimulation due to the potent vasodilatory properties of that drug, but serves as another example of the multiple factors that may influence Doppler measurements [22].

132

Table 2. Age and exercise characteristics for patients achieving at least 85% of their age-predicted maximum heart rate.

	#	Age (mean)	Mean duration of exercise (min)	Maximal HR (average)
Group I (normal scans)	19	55.7	8.7±3.26	157.7±17.4
Group II	16	56.3	7.6 ± 2.9	147.3 ± 15.7
Multivessel CAD	(9)	56.6	6.9 ± 2.2	140.6 ± 10.9
Total	35			

*p=NS; **p≤0.05; †p=NS; ††p≤0.005;

Note: The number of multivessel CAD patients is listed parenthetically because these patients were also counted for Group II.

CAD = coronary artery disease;

* indicates p value for the difference between Group I and Group II;

† indicates p value for the difference between Group I and multivessel CAD.

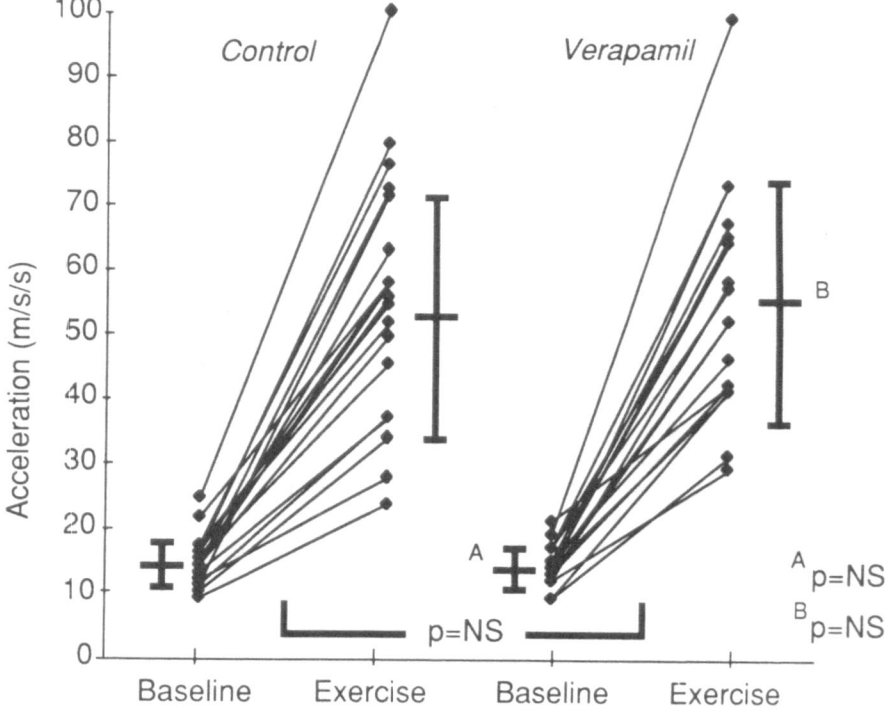

Figure 9. Flow acceleration at baseline and immediately after exercise for the control and verapamil exercise test. Abbreviations as in Figure 7. (Reprinted with permission from The American College of Cardiology (J Am Coll Cardiol 1988; 11:1002–9).)

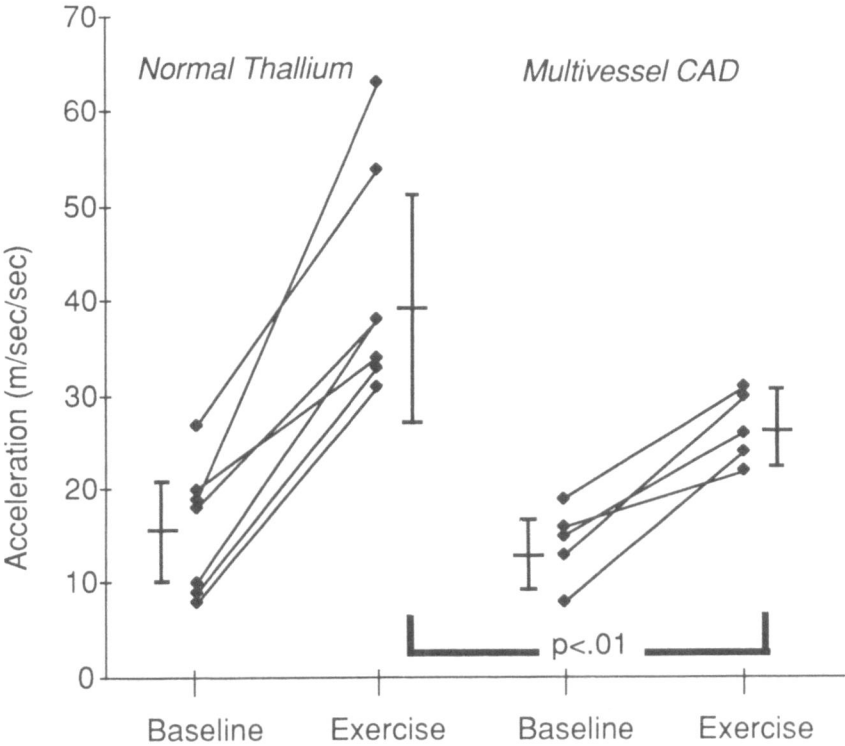

Figure 10. Peak acceleration at baseline and immediately after exercise in patients with normal thallium studies (Group I) and patients with ischemic thallium studies (Group II) who also had angiographically proven multivessel coronary artery disease (CAD). All subjects shown achieved 85% or greater of their age-predicted maximal heart rate. (Reprinted with permission from The American College of Cardiology (J Am Coll Cardiol 1987; 10:809–17).)

10.8 Multivessel coronary disease

We did identify a population in which exercise Doppler techniques may provide clinically useful information [12]. Nine patients in our study (7 with maximal velocity data and 5 with acceleration data) had angiographically documented multivessel coronary artery disease (mean = 2.3 vessels with ≥ 75% stenosis), ischemia on thallium perfusion scintigraphy and an exercise heart rate at least 85% of the age-predicted maximum (Table 2). These patients were compared to patients in Group I (normal scans) who had also achieved at least 85% of their age-predicted maximal heart rate during exercise. In this small but well defined subgroup with multivessel coronary disease and exercise-induced ischemia who were not affected by beta blocking medication, peak acceleration at maximal exercise was significantly lower than that seen for patients of similar age and exercise capacity who were also not affected by beta blockers during the test, but did not have exercise-induced ischemia (Figure 10). This finding is in agreement with the results of Sabbah et al. [23] who used the dog model to demonstrate that of the Doppler parameters measured, peak acceleration correlated most closely with the percentage of myocardial mass rendered ischemic by coronary occlusion. Furthermore, at least 21% or more of the left ventricular mass must be rendered ischemic for significant lowering of peak acceleration to occur. Thus, areas of ischemia large enough to influence results of exercise Doppler echocardiography may be present in patients with multivessel coronary artery disease, and exercise Doppler may provide valuable information regarding the extent of exercise-induced ischemia.

10.9 Conclusions

Initial work from several laboratories [3–6] including our own [16] showed exercise Doppler echocardiography to be very promising for evaluation of patients with ischemic heart disease. Indeed, as a group, patients with coronary artery disease have less of an increase in aortic flow velocity and acceleration with exercise than do individuals without evidence of heart disease. As work in this field continues, however, limitations regarding clinical application of this technique to individual patients are becoming apparent. Exercise capacity, age, previous myocardial infarction, and beta blocking medication all exert important influence on the hemodynamic response to exercise as reflected in the Doppler-measured values of velocity and acceleration. Nonetheless, with appropriate patient selection, exercise Doppler echocardiography may prove to be useful in the evaluation of patients with ischemic heart disease. Future studies must carefully consider the known limitations to this method and be aware that other, as yet unknown, limitations may exist.

References

1. Goldhammer S, Scherf D. Electrokardiographische Untersuchungen bei Kranker mit Angina Pectoris ("ambulatorischer Typus"). Z Klin Med 1933; 122:134.
2. Sheffield LT. Exercise stress testing. In: Braunwald E (ed.). Heart Disease: A Textbook of Cardiovascular Medicine. Philadelphia. W.B. Saunders. 1988:223–41.
3. Teague, SM, Mark DB, Radford M, et al. Doppler velocity profiles reveal ischemic exercise responses. Circulation 1984; 70(suppl II):II–185. (abstract).
4. Bryg RJ, Labovitz AJ, Mehdirad AA, Williams GA, Chaitman BR. Effect of coronary artery disease on Doppler-derived parameters of aortic flow during upright exercise. Am J Cariol 1986; 58:14–19.
5. Mehta N, Bennett D, Mannering D, Dawkins K, Ward DE. Usefulness of noninvasive Doppler measurement of ascending aortic blood velocity and acceleration in detecting impairment of the left ventricular functional response to exercise three weeks after acute myocardial infarction. Am J Cardiol 1986; 58:879–84.
6. Mehdirad AA, Williams GH, Labovitz AJ, Bryg RJ, Chaitman BR. Evaluation of left ventricular function during upright exercise: Correlation of exercise Doppler with post

exercise two-dimensional echocardiographic results. Circulation 1987; 75:413–19.

7. Osakada G, Hess OM, Gallather KP, Kemper WS, Ross J, Jr. End-systolic dimension-wall thickness relations during myocardial ischemia in conscious dogs. Am J Cardiol 1985; 51:1750–58.

8. Amano J, Thomas JX Jr, Lavalle M, Mirsky I, Glover D, Manders WT, Randall WC, Vatner SF. Effects of myocardial ischemia on regional function and stiffness in conscious dogs. Am J Physiol 1987; 252:H110–17.

9. Bowditch HP. Uber die Eigenthumlichkeiten der Reizarbeit, welche die Muskelfasern des Herzens zeigen. Ber Verh der kongiglich sachischen ges Wissenschaften zu Leipzig. 1871: 23:652.

10. Grossman W. Evaluation of systolic and diastolic function of the myocardium. In: Cardiac Catheterization and Angiography (3rd Ed.), Philadelphia, Lea and Febiger, 1986:302.

11. Mahler F, Yoran C, Ross J Jr. Inotropic effect of tachycardia and poststimulation potentiation in the conscious dog. Am J Physiol 1974; 227:569–75.

12. Bennett ED, Barclay SA, Davis AL, Mannering D, Mehta N. Ascending aortic blood velocity and acceleration using Doppler ultrasound in the assessment of left ventricular function. Cardiovasc Res 1984; 18:632–38.

13. Sabbah HN, Khaja F, Brymer JF, et al. Noninvasive evaluation of left ventricular performance based on peak aortic blood acceleration measured with a continuous wave Doppler velocity meter. Circulation 1986; 74:323–29.

14. Noble MIM, Trenchard D, Guz A. Left ventricular ejection in conscious dogs: Measurement and significance of the maximum acceleration of blood from the left ventricle. Circ Res 1966; 19:139–47.

15. Stein PD, Sabbah HN, Albert DE, Snyder JE. Continuous wave Doppler for the noninvasive evaluation of aortic blood velocity and rate of change of velocity: Evaluation in dogs. Med Instrum 1987; 21:177–82.

16. Harrison MR, Smith MD, Friedman BJ, DeMaria AN. Uses and limitations of exercise Doppler echocardiography in the diagnosis of ischemic heart disease. J Am Coll Cardiol 1987; 10:809–17.

17. Doan AE, Peterson DR, Blackmon JR, Bruce RA. Myocardial ischemia after maximal exercise in healthy men. Am Heart J 1965; 69:11–22.

18. Okada RD, Boucher CA, Strauss HW, Pohost GM. Exercise radionuclide imaging approaches to coronary artery disease. Am J Cardiol 1980; 46:1188–1204.

19. Lazarus M, Danz TU, Gardin JM, Allfie A, Henry WL. Evaluation of age, gender, heart rate and blood pressure and exercise conditioning on Doppler measured aortic blood flow acceleration and velocity during upright treadmill testing. Am J Cardiol 1988; 62:439–43.

20. Harrison MR, Smith MD, Nissen SE, Grayburn PA, DeMaria AN. Use of exercise Doppler echocardiography to evaluate cardiac drugs: Effects of propranolol and verapamil on aortic blood flow velocity and acceleration. J Am Coll Cardiol 1988; 11:1002–9.

21. Mehta N, Boyle G, Bennett D, Gilmour S, Noble MIM, Mills CM, Pugh S. Hemodynamic response to treadmill exercise in normal volunteers: An assessment by Doppler ultrasonic measurement of ascending aortic blood velocity and acceleration. Am Heart J 1988; 116:1298–1307.

22. Harrison M, Grayburn P, Smith M, DeMaria AN. Evaluation of the hemodynamic effects of calcium channel antagonists by exercise Doppler: Comparison of verapamil and nifedipine. J Am Coll Cardiol 1989; 11:122A (abstract).

11. Assessment of the effect of coronary artery bypass grafting on left ventricular function by stress Doppler cardiography

ABDUL-MAJEED SALMASI

Irvine Laboratory for Cardiovascular Investigation and Research, St Mary's Hospital, London W2 1NY, U.K.

11.1 Introduction

Coronary artery bypass graft surgery (CABG) is a widely used method of treating patients with coronary artery disease. It is associated with improvement in postsurgical lifestyle. It relieves angina pectoris in over 85% of patients [1, 2] and prolongs life especially in patients with disease in the three main coronary arteries or the left main coronary artery [1–3]. One of the major anticipated goals of CABG is correction of left ventricular function as the status of left ventricular function is an important factor in the survival of patients with coronary artery disease [4–6]. However the effect of CABG on left ventricular function has been the subject of much debate. This is due to conflicting reports with results suggesting improvement [7, 8] or no improvement or even deterioration [9, 10]. Some of the factors which have led to such mixed reports are the techniques used in the evaluation, the timing of te postoperative assessment and finally whether the assessment was carried out at rest or during exercise.

Studying resting ventricular function too early following CABG did not show any improvement by various investigators [11, 12]. Using systolic time intervals as measures of left ventricular performance it has been suggested that in the early postoperative period there is an increased adrenergic activity which may influence left ventricular function after the operation of CABG for two weeks or more [12]. Such a phenomenon therefore may mask any left ventricular dysfunction in the early postoperative periods. The results obtained from studying left ventricular function at rest following CABG varied widely between different investigators with some showing improvement [13–17] while others showed failure of improvement or even deterioration [10, 18–22].

Both from the research and the clinical points of view it would be beneficial to study left ventricular function sequentially, not only at rest but also with exercise, following CABG in order to allow for better understanding of the natural history. This will not be possible unless a rather simple cheap and safe technique is applied with high reproducibility and which can be carried out at frequent intervals without any side effects or biological danger. The usefulness of Doppler ultrasound during exercise in various clinical situations and its use to study and evaluate various

Steve M. Teague (ed.) Stress Doppler Echocardiography, 137–153.
© 1990 *Kluwer Academic Publishers.*

cardiac conditions have been discussed in the previous chapters. One of the important uses of this approach is to evaluate the effect of CABG on left ventricular function.

11.2 Doppler technique and the original experience

The technique used was the transcutaneous aortovelograph (TAV) introduced originally by Light and Cross (1972) [23]. Various investigators reported on the value of the TAV at rest both qualitatively and quantitatively in studying and assessing various cardiac conditions including myocardial infarction, cardiomyopathy, aortic valve disease and others beside its value in general medical conditions such as shock [23–31]. Its value in assessing the effect of different therapeutic agents has also been reported [32]. The method is based on measuring mainstream blood velocity in the aortic arch using a 2MHz transducer via the suprasternal notch and in between the neck blood vessels. This is carried out at rest and at maximal-tolerated supine exercise.

The transcutaneous aortovelograph (TAV, type 1006, manufactured by Murihead Medicals, Beckenham, Kent, England) which was based on the original machine developed by Cross and Light [33] was used.

Pre-exercise recordings are obtained after at least 5 minutes of supine rest, with the subject's shoulder and head slightly elevated and the legs horizontal. The transducer is placed on the suprasternal notch and directed downwards and laterally in a direction tangential to the distal part of the aortic arch. Its position is adjusted until the highest pitched sound is heard on the loudspeaker and signals with maximum peak frequency are recorded.

11.3 Exercise studies

Supine exercise is carried out on a bicycle ergometer which is attached to the end of a couch. A standard protocol with step-wise increase in work load [34] is used. The ECG is monitored continuously, and blood pressure is recorded at minute intervals during exercise, at peak exercise and during the recovery phase until they returned to pre-exercise levels.

The distance travelled by the blood in each cycle is given by the area of each systolic complex (systolic velocity integral) and termed the 'stroke distance' (Sd). This is an index of stroke volume [25]. The distance travelled per minute (stroke distance x heart rate) is the 'minute distance' and is an index of cardiac output in the subject. Five consecutive complexes from each recording are measured, and analysed on a digitiser-microprocessor programmed to average and derive peak velocity (Vp), stroke distance (Sd), minute distance (Md) and flow time (Tf), and early systolic acceleration.

The technique is highly reproducible with a coefficient of variation for the stroke distance of 5.2% at rest and 5.9% at maximal exercise [35]. The coefficient of variation for the percentage change in the stroke distance with exercise (%ΔSd) was 10.7% [36].

Our experience with Doppler stress testing goes back to 1982 and 1983 when the first reports came out of St Mary's Hospital, London [37, 38]. These preliminary studies indicated the usefulness of using Doppler ultrasound evaluating left ventricular function with exercise in normal subjects and in patients with coronary artery disease. Subsequent study [39] has confirmed that the $\%\Delta Sd$ was linearly related to invasively derived (by left ventriculography) ejection fraction (r = 0.8). The $\%\Delta Sd$ was also found to be robust against variation in exercise time and age [35]. For these reasons the percentage change in the stroke distance with exercise ($\%\Delta Sd$) is the most appropriate TAV index of left ventricular performance and its response to exercise.

In normal subjects the stroke distance increases with exercise by 9–48% [35]. In patients with coronary artery disease on the other hand, the stroke distance decreases with exercise when there is left ventricular dysfunction (as evidenced by left ventriculography [39]. The $\%\Delta Sd$ with exercise in patients with coronary disease was found to be a function of the number of coronary arteries with significant stenoses; it also decreases linearly with increasing number of diseased coronary arteries and the presence of history of previous myocardial infarction [39].

11.4 The coronary artery bypass grafting (CABG) study

Because the status of left ventricular performance is a good predictor of survival in patients with coronary artery disease [3–5], the effects of coronary artery bypass surgery on left ventricular function may have important implications on the prognosis. Various studies have been carried out and in all of them assessment of left ventricular performance was carried out either invasively or noninvasively. Some of the noninvasive studies involved the use of radio-labelled substances injected into the circulation; a reason which renders the repetition of these tests for follow up purposes rather difficult.

Exercise ECG testing has its own limitations in assessing the effect of coronary artery bypass grating. The disappearance of chest pain following CABG does not always imply improved coronary blood flow, as intra-operative infarcts or even placebo effect may be responsible for the relief of pain [40]. Despite the improvement in exercise tolerance and disappearance of symptoms following CABG, reversal of ischaemic ST segment response to exercise following CABG was noted in only 50% of patients [41]. Another mechanism which may influence the result of exercise testing is the training programma which may produce improvement in exercise tolerance following CABG [12].

Because of the above reasons a study has been carried out at St Mary's Hospital, London to evaluate the effect of CABG on left ventricular function using the continuous-wave Doppler ultrasound technique of TAV with exercise [42]. Thirty consecutive patients (all male) in the age range 39–70 years (mean 55.4, SD 7.9) with coronary artery disease confirmed by coronary arteriography, and who were due to undergo CABG were studied. None of the patients had previous cardiac surgery or myocardial infarction within the six months prior to the study. All the

140

patients were free from valvular or myocardial heart disease and none of them was receiving digoxin or antiarrhythmic therapy.

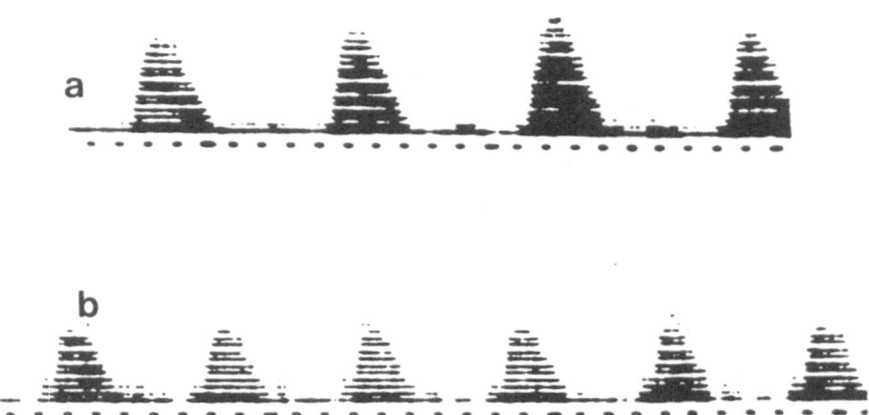

Figure 1. Continuous-wave Doppler ultrasound recordings using transcutaneous aortovelo-graphy from a patient with 3-vessel coronary disease and ejection fraction of 38%. Note that the area of the triangle (systolic velocity integral or stroke distance) has decreased at maximal (3 minute) exercise (b) as compared to the pre-exercise recording (a), thus suggesting a decrease in the stroke volume with exercise. Tf: flow time; Vp: peak velocity.

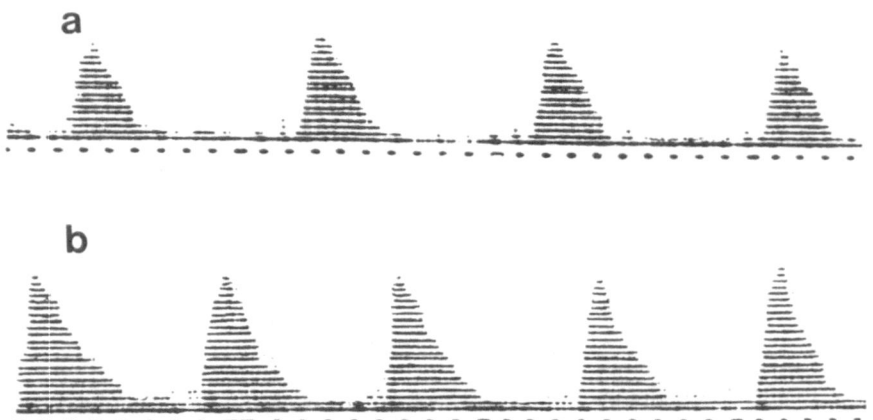

Figure 2. Aortic blood velocity recording by TAV of the same patient in Figure 1 following coronary artery bypass grafting. The stroke distance indicated by the area of the triangle at maximal (4.5 minute) exercise (b) increases as compared to the pre-exercise recording (a), thus suggesting an increase in the stroke volume. The response of the stroke distance to exercise is in contrast to that observed in Figure 1.

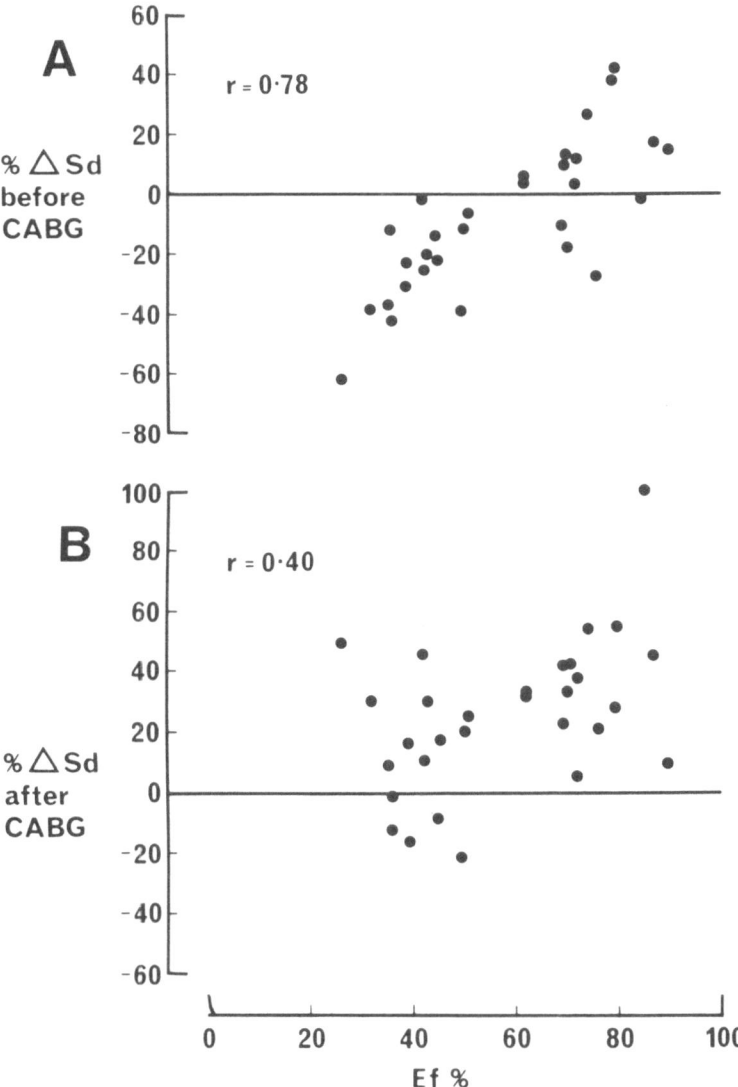

Figure 3. The correlation between pre-operative resting ejection fraction (EF) assessed invasively by left ventriculography and the percentage change in the stroke distance (%△Sd) before coronary artery bypass grafting (A) and after the operation (B). The correlation is weaker after CABG than before the operation, thus demonstrating an improvement in the left ventricular function following the operation.

142

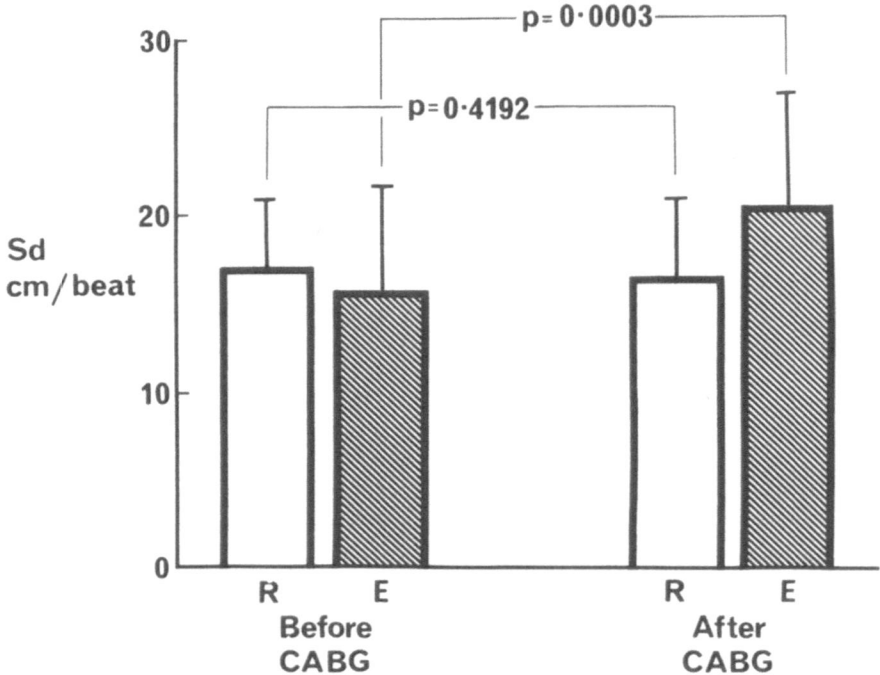

Figure 4. Stroke distance (Sd) as mean and standard deviation before and after coronary artery bypass grafting (CABG) at rest and at maximal tolerated supine exercise. No significant change in the resting Sd is noted after CABG while a significant increase took place following the operation.

Prior to surgery, 21 patients were receiving beta-adrenergic blockade and 13 patients had history of myocardial infarction more than 6 months prior to the study. However, other anti-anginal medication like calcium-antagonists or nitrates were discontinued a week before the studies. All these patients had TAV studies at rest and at maximal-tolerated supine exercise during the week before and six weeks after operation. None of the patients developed peri-operative myocardial infarction. Before surgery exercise was terminated in four patients due to knee or thigh pain and exhaustion. None of the patients developed arrhythmia. After CABG, exercise was terminated due to exhaustion in all patients, none developed ST segment depression and/or chest pain.

Coronary artery bypass grafting was carried out and the patients had an average of 3.57 grafts. Two patients had 2 grafts, 13 patients had 3 grafts, 11 patients had 4 and 4 patients received 5 grafts. Figures 1 and 2 are typical examples of TAV recordings before and after CABG.

11.5 Preoperative data

Prior to surgery the average exercise time was 3.9 (SD 1.1). Resting heart rate was 63 (SD 10) which rose to 103 (SD 17) beats per minute at maximal exercise. The stroke distance decreased with exercise in 19 patients hence resulting in a negative percentage change in stroke distance (%ΔSd), ten of whom had a history of myocardial infarction. In 16 of these 19 patients, the resting ejection fraction (EF) was below 60%. The %ΔSd showed a good correlation with the resting ejection fraction (r = 0.78, p = 0.001), (Figure 3a), thus confirming our previous findings [39]; thus the stroke distance decreased with exercise in patients with ejection fraction below 60%.

11.6 Postoperative data

Six weeks after the operation, when the TAV study was repeated, none of the patients was receiving any medication apart from aspirin and persantin. Digoxin, which was used routinely in the postoperative period, was discontinued 4 weeks after the operation. Exercise time was 4.9 minutes (SD 1.3) which was a significant

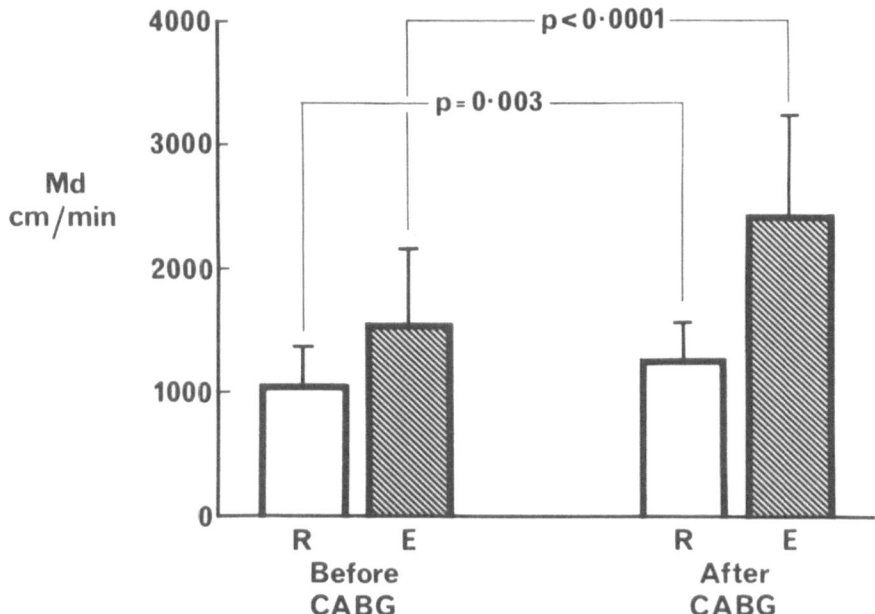

Figure 5. Minute distance (Md) as mean and standard deviation before and after coronary artery bypass grafting (CABG) prior to and at maximal tolerated supine exercise. Both the resting and maximal exercise values for the Md did increase following CABG. The reason for the increase in the resting Md is mainly due to stopping the beta-adrenergic blocking agents after the operation.

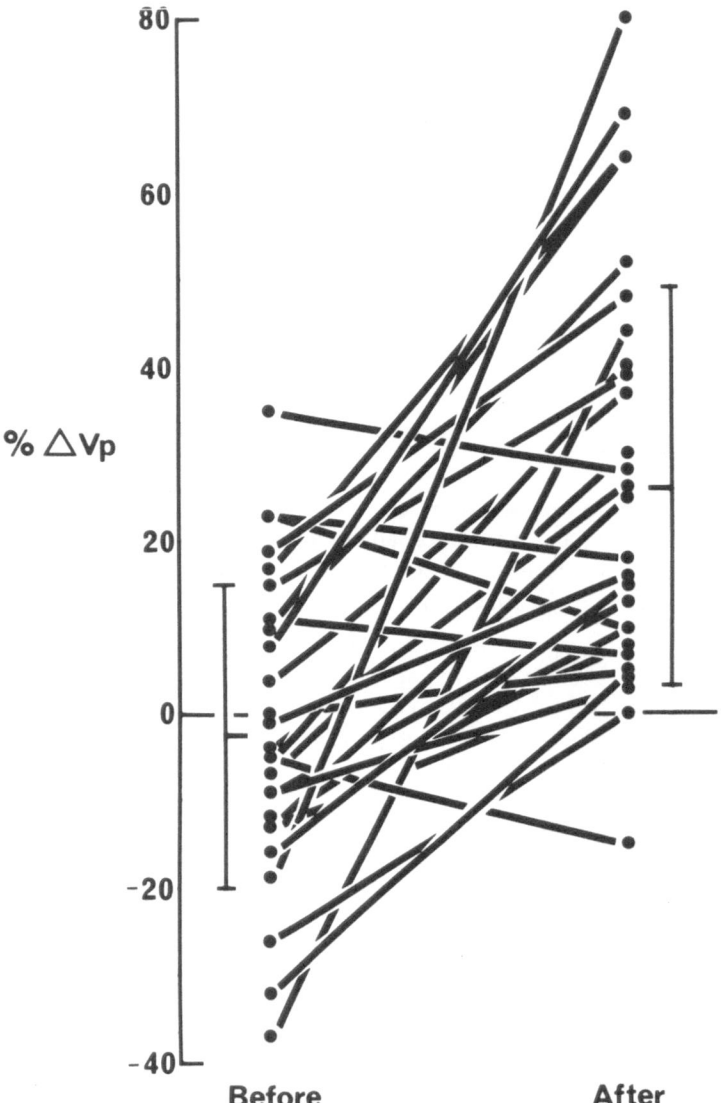

%△Vp

Before   After

Figure 6. Comparison of the percentage change in the peak velocity (%△Vp) in individual patients who underwent coronary artery bypass grafting (CABG) before and after the operation and the mean and its 95% confidence limits.

improvement over the pre-exercise value (p = 0.002). However, this improvement was not a function of number of grafts (r = 0.19). The heart rate at rest was 80 (SD 14) which rose to 120 (SD 19) at maximal exercise. The significant improvement in heart rate both at rest (p < 0.001) and with exercise (p < 0.001) postoperatively was mainly due to the withdrawal of beta-adrenergic blockade.

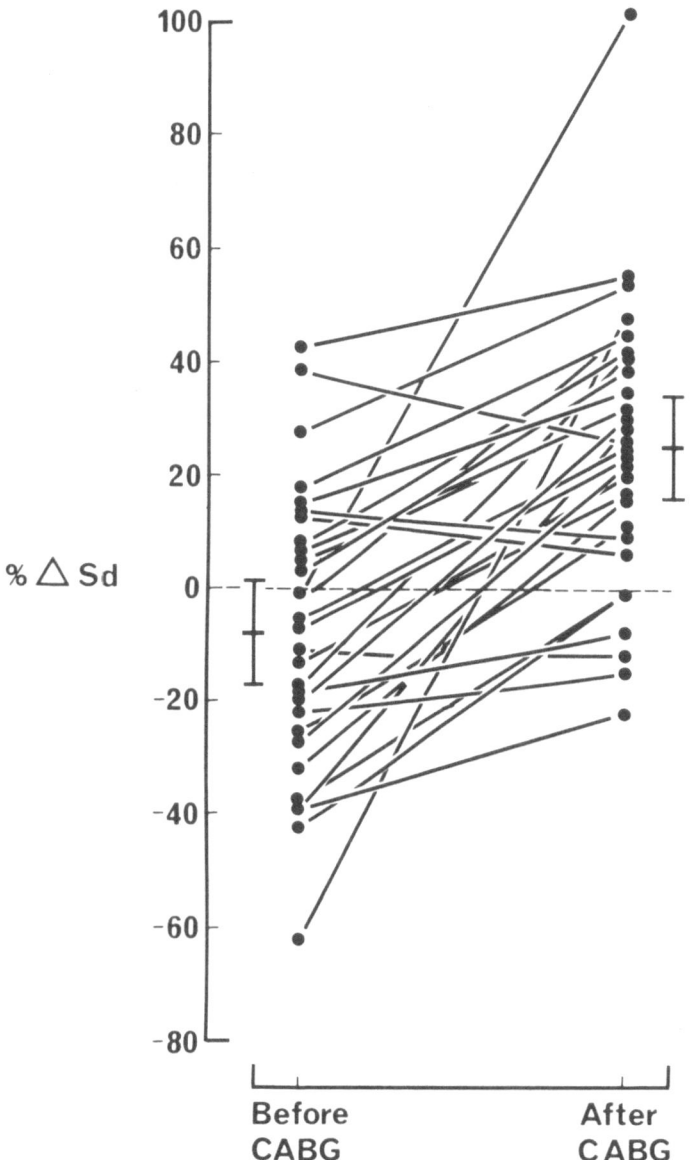

Figure 7. Comparison of the percentage change in the stroke distance (%△Sd) in individual patients and the mean (and its 95% confidence limits) before and after the operation of coronary artery bypass grafting (CABG). Mean change = 33.6%, SE of the change = 5.1, p < 0.001. (Salmasi A-M, in AM Salmasi & AN Nicolaides (Eds.) Cardiovascular applications of Doppler ultrasound. Churchill-Livingstone. 1989. pp. 127–144). Reproduced with permission.

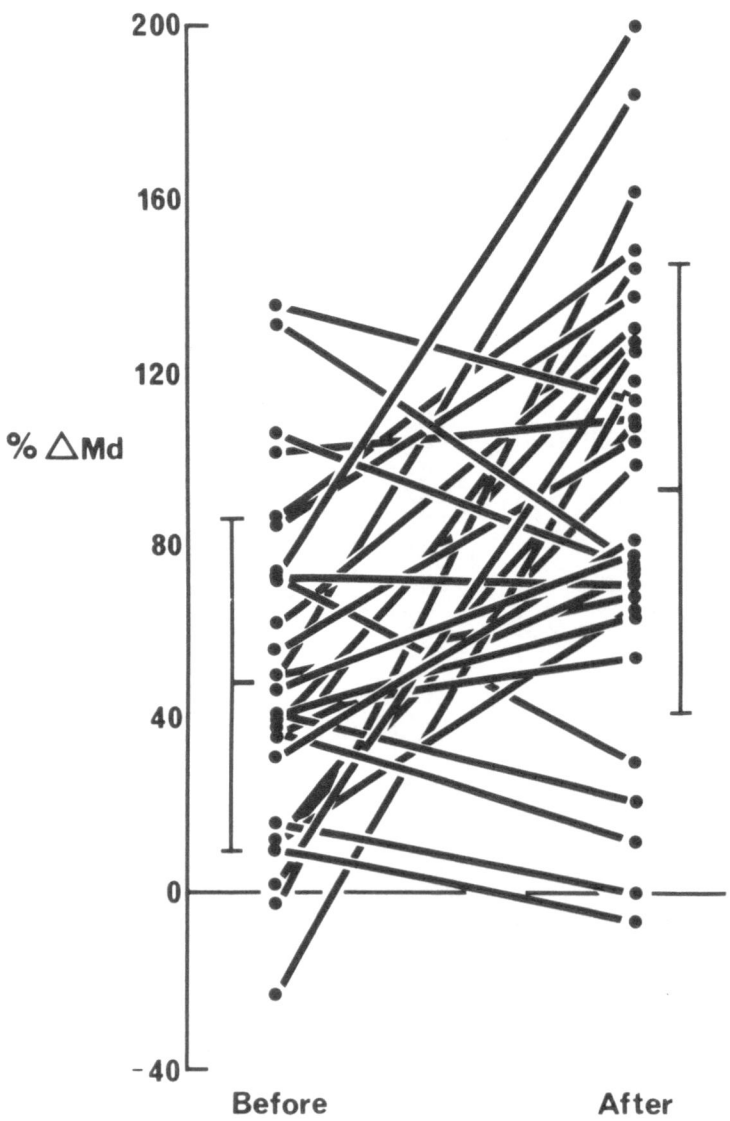

Figure 8. Comparison of the percentage change in the minute distance (%ΔMd) before and after coronary artery bypass grafting (CABG) in 30 patients and its mean (and 95% confidence limits). A significant increase in the %ΔMd is noted (p < 0.001). (Salmasi A-M. In AM Salmasi & AN Nicolaides (Eds.) Cardiovascular applications of Doppler ultrasound. Churchill-Livingstone. 1989. pp. 127–144). Reproduced with permission.

Whereas a significant increase in the peak exercise values for the Sd, and Md, occurred after surgery (Figures 4 and 5), no significant changes were noticed in the resting values except for the Md which increased significantly by an average of 28% following CABG. This is mainly due to the disappearance of the effects of beta-adrenergic blockade postoperatively. However, the percentage changes with exercise in peak velocity, stroke distance and minute distance increased significantly following CABG (Figures 6, 7 and 8). A weaker relation between postoperative %ΔSd and pre-operative ejection fraction was noted (Figure 3b); thus suggesting improvement in %ΔSd following CABG.

The increase in the exercise TAV values suggests that CABG has improved LV function possibly by reversing the myocardial ischaemic process.

11.7 Significance of the early systolic acceleration

Early invasive studies both in animals and in humans have demonstrated the usefulness of the maximum acceleration in assessing left ventricular function. In 1966, Noble and associates [43] using catheter tip velocity probe invasively in dogs showed that maximum acceleration was highly responsive to changes in left ventricular inotropic state. Using the same invasive technique Jewitt and associates in 1974) [44] reported that maximum acceleration was a good predictor of subsequent mortality in patients with acute myocardial infarction. Bennett and colleagues (1974 [45] using this invasive approach measured the maximum acceleration of the aortic blood by continuously differentiating the velocity signal, in twelve patients undergoing diagnostic coronary arteriography. The authors [45] found a close relationship between maximum acceleration and ejection fraction and reported that the maximum acceleration was inversely related to the severity of coronary artery disease. The maximum acceleration recorded in patients with definite coronary artery disease was below 1100 cm/sec^2, while in patients with chest pain but no definite coronary artery disease it was higher than 1500 cm/sec^2 [45].

Recently through non-invasive approach, Mehta and Bennett [46] measured maximum acceleration via application of a continuous-wave Doppler probe in the suprasternal notch, reported a significantly lower maximum acceleration (37%) in patients with acute myocardial infarction than in normal subjects. Also they found that the maximum acceleration was significantly lower in the non-survivors than in the survivors in their patients studied [46].

In this study of the evaluation of the effect of CABG on left ventricular function using Doppler ultrasound measurement of aortic blood velocity during physical exercise, the maximum early systolic acceleration was measured (Figure 9). The acceleration prior to exercise has not changed significantly following the operation. However, the acceleration at maximal exercise has increased significantly following CABG. This is mainly due to increasing peak velocity and, to a lesser extent, to a reduction in the time from beginning of the systolic signal till the peak velocity (time to peak velocity = t-Vp).

148

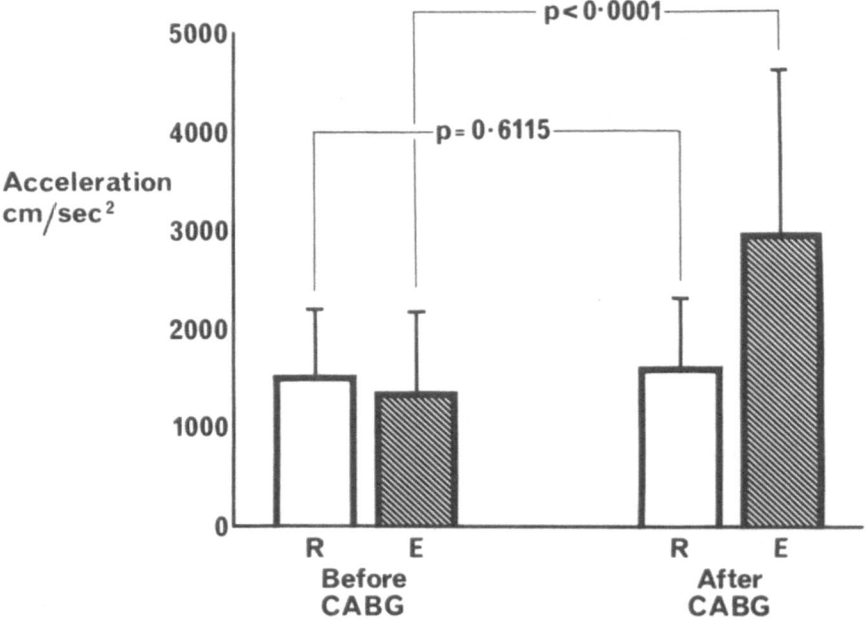

Figure 9. Comparison of the early systolic acceleration (mean and SE) in the 30 patients who underwent coronary artery bypass grafting (CABG) at rest and at maximal tolerated supine exercise both before and after CABG. While no change was observed in the resting value a highly significant increase in the maximal exercise acceleration is observed.

In keeping with other investigators [7], by carrying out the post-operative studies 6 weeks after CABG, rather than much earlier, factors which may have influenced left ventricular performance such as increased adrenergic activity [12] have thus been avoided.

11.8 Effect of beta-adrenergic blockade

It has been reported that beta-adrenergic blockade may improve myocardial contractility and hence ejection fraction, even when the ejection fraction is below 40%. Using radionuclide techniques, Marshall and associates (1981) [47] reported that following clinically effective anti-anginal doses of propranolol, patients with coronary artery disease who had positive exercise results, showed an improvement in the global as well as regional left ventricular performance. Improvement in the exercise response of the ejection fraction following oral propranolol therapy in coronary artery disease was reported by Battler and associates (1979) [48]. In the study reported here, therefore, the beta-blockades prior to CABG either improved or did not have significant effect on the left ventricular function. Also if they were to be stopped prior to TAV testing this would have been risky and a lower workload would have thus been achieved.

11.9 Effect of previous myocardial infarction

Before CABG the ejection fraction measured by left ventriculography in patients with previous history of myocardial infarction (44.8%, SD 14.5%) was lower (p = 0.001) than in patients without such a history (67.2% ± 15.7%). Prior to CABG the stroke distance in eleven out of thirteen patients with such a history was reduced during exercise (i.e. negative % Sd). The five patients with % Sd below zero following CABG had a history of an old myocardial infarction also (Figure 7).

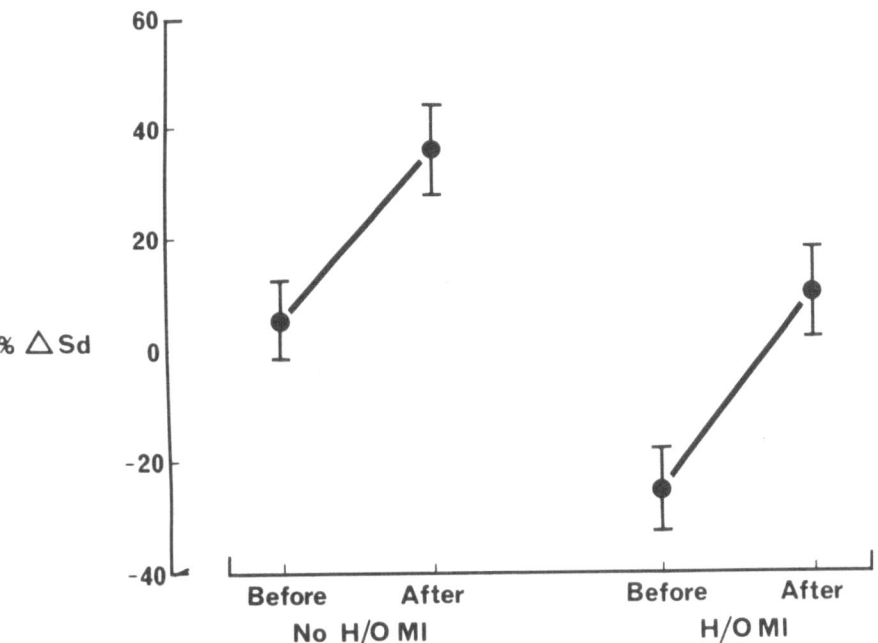

Figure 10. Comparison of the (mean + SD) percentage change in the stroke distance (%ΔSd) before and after coronary artery bypass grafting (CABG) in patients with and without history of myocardial infarction (H/O MI). There is no significant (p = 0.7) difference in the degree of improvement in %ΔSd following CABG between patients with H/O MI (mean 36.0, SE 6.0) and those without H/O MI (mean 32.0, SE 4.6). Patients with H/O MI had a lower %ΔSd than patients without H/O MI both before and after CABG.

There was no significant difference ($p = 0.7$) in the mean change (post CABG – pre CABG) for %ΔSd between patients with a history of myocardial infarction (mean 36.0, SE 6.0) and those without such a history (mean 32.0, SE 4.6). However, although no significant differences were observed in the amount of improvement of the %ΔSd (Figure 7), after operation, the %ΔSd in patients with a history of myocardial infarction was lower than those without such a history (Figure 10).

The results suggest that a history of myocardial infarction prior to CABG has a depressant effect on the overall myocardial function during exercise. This is in agreement with a previous report [39]. However, the degree of improvement in left ventricular performance in the myocardial infarct patients after revascularisation as a result of CABG, was similar to that in patients without infarction indicating that the effect of the degree of revascularisation was similar in the two groups. This is further supported by the lack of difference in the number of coronary bypass grafts between the two groups. However, the existence of a myocardial infarct scar tended to exert a similar degree of reduction in overall left ventricular function before and after CABG. This suggests that patients with a previous history of myocardial infarction do benefit from CABG to the same extent as do patients without such a history. The explanation for this finding may be that revascularisation has only improved the function (or led to a reversal in the dysfunction) in the ischaemic area, while the dead (infarcted) myocardium remained non-functioning.

In a study by Taylor and associates [7], on 56 patients with exertional angina using multiple gated ventricular scintigraphy at rest and during dynamic exercise, before and six weeks after CABG, they showed that resting ejection fraction did not change following CABG. However, during exercise it increased significantly in the 52 patients who were asymptomatic following CABG. Taylor and colleagues [7] also showed that exercise-induced regional wall motion abnormalities prior to CABG disappear after the operation. The presence of previous myocardial infarction did not have any influence on these results. On the other hand, in patients who continued to experience exertional angina following CABG, Taylor and colleagues [7] reported a fall in both resting and exercise ejection fraction. However, in the study reported here, none of the patients were symptomatic following CABG.

11.10 Conclusion

Left ventricular dysfunction in patient with coronary artery disease improves following revascularisation of the ischaemic myocardium as a result of the operation of coronary artery bypass grafting. This is only evident if left ventricular function is assessed during exercise. Exercise myocardial function improves by the sixth weeks following CABG, equally in patients with and without previous myocardial infarction, but those who have lower left ventricular function before CABG tend to have a lower function following CABG.

The use of a suptrasternally approachable continuous-wave Doppler ultrasound with exercise to assess the effect of CABG on left ventricular function proves, therefore, to be of value as a simple non-invasive test. It is free of risks and can be repeated as frequently as necessary. These facts render this technique to be of value in the follow-up of patients and in studying their natural history following such operative procedures.

References

1. Rahimtoola SH. Coronary bypasss surgery for chronic angina – 1981: A perspective. Circulation 1982; 65:225–241.
2. Ross RS. Ischaemic heart disease – an overview. Am J Cardiol 1975; 36:496–505.
3. Keogh BE, Taylor KM. Coronary artery surgery and angioplasty. Cardiovascular Update. 1987; 9:3–11 (Second series).
4. Bourassa MG, Lesperance J, Campeau L, Saltiel J. Fate of left ventricular contraction following aortocoronary venous grafts. Circulation 1972; 46:724–730.
5. Cohn PF, Gorlin R, Cohn LH, Collins JJ. Left ventricular ejection fraction as a prognostic guide in surgical treatment of coronary and vascular heart disease. Am J Cardiol 1974; 34:136–141.
6. Nelson GR, Cohn PF, Gorlin R. Prognosis in medically treated coronary artery disease. Influence of ejection fraction compared to other parameters. Circulation 1975; 52:408–412.
7. Taylor NC, Barber RW, Crossland P, English TAH, Wraight EP, Petch MC. Effects of coronary artery bypass grafting on left ventricular function assessed by multiple gated ventricular scintigraphy. Br Heart J 1983; 50:149–156.
8. Roberts AJ, Lichtenhal PR, Spies SM, Kaplan KJ. Periperative myocardial damage in coronary artery bypass graft surgery: Analysis of multifunctional aetiology and evaluation of diagnostic techniques. In: Moran JM, Michaelis LL (eds.). Surgery for the complications of myocardial infarction. 1980; Grune and Stratton Inc., pp. 79–80.
9. Wolf NM, Kreulen TH, Bove AA, McDonough MT, Kessler KM, Strong M, LeMole G, Spann JF. Left ventricular function following coronary bypass surgery. Circulation 1978; 58:63–70.
10. Hammermeister KE, Kennedy JW, Hamilton GW, Stewart DK, Gould KL, Lipscomb K, Murray JA. Aorto-coronary saphenous vein bypass. Failure of successful grafting to improve resting left ventricular function in chronic angina. N Engl J Med 1974; 290:186–192.
11. Mintz LJ, Ingels NB Jr, Daughters GT, Stinson EB, Alderman EL. Sequential studies of left ventricular function and wall motion after coronary arterial bypass surgery. Am J Cardiol 1980; 45:210–216.
12. Boudoulas H, Lewis RP, Vasko JS, Karayannacos PE, Beaver BM. Left ventricular function and adrenergic hyperactivity before and after saphenous vein bypass. Circulation 1976; 53:802–806.
13. Hamby RI, Tabrah F, Aintablian A, Hartstein ML, Wisoff BG. Left ventricular haemodynamics and contractile pattern after aortocoronary bypass surgery. Am Heart J 1974; 88:149–159.
14. Chatterjee K, Swan HJC, Parmley WW, Sustaita H, Marcus HS. Ventricular asynergy and function in patients with coronary heart disease. Circulation 1973; 47:276–286.
15. Ress G, Bristow JD, Kremkau EL, et al. Influence of aortocoronary bypass surgery on left ventricular performance. N Engl J Med 1971; 284:1116–1120.
16. Levine JA, Bechtel DJ, Cohn PF, et al. Ventricular function before and after direct revascularization surgery. Circulation 1975; 51:1071–1078.
17. Chatterjee K, Matloff JM, Swan HJC, et al. Abnormal regional metabolism and mechanical function in patients with ischaemic heart disease: Improvement after suc-

cessful regional revascularization by aortocoronary bypass. Circulation 1975; 52:390–399.

18. Bussman WD, Mayer V, Kober G, Kaltenbach M. Ventricular function at rest, during leg raising and physical exercise before and after aorto-coronary bypass surgery. Am J Cardiol 1979; 43:488–501.

19. Kent KM, Borer JS, Green MV, et al. Effects of coronary artery bypass on global and regional left ventricular function during exercise. N Engl J Med 1978; 298:1434–1439.

20. Shepherd RL, Itscoitz SB, Glancy DL, et al. Deterioration of myocardial function following aortocoronary bypass operation. Circulation 1974; 49:467–475.

21. Kennedy JW, Hammermeister KE, Hamilton GW, Gould KL. Failure of successful myocardial revascularization to alter left ventricular function. Am J Cardiol 1974; 33:74 (abstract).

22. Arbogast R, Solignac A, Bourassa MG. Influence of aortocoronary saphenous vein bypass surgery on left ventricular volumes and ejection fraction. Am J Med 1973; 54: 290–296.

23. Light LH, Cross G. Cardiovascular data by transcutaneous aortovelography. In: Roberts C (ed.). Blood Flow Measurement. London: Sector Publishing 1972: 60–63.

24. Light LH. Transcutaneous aortovelography. A new window on the circulation. Br Heart J 1976; 38:433–442.

25. Sequeira RF, Light LH, Cross G, Raftery EB. Transcutaneous aortovelography. A quantitative evaluation. Br Heart J 1976; 38:443–450.

26. Bilton AH, Brotherhood J, Cross G, Hanson GC, Light LH, Sequeira RF. Transcutaneous aortovelography as a measure of central blood flow. J Physiol 1978; 281:4–9.

27. Distante A, Moscarelli E, Rovai D, L'Abbate A. Monitoring changes in cardiac output by transcutaneous aortovelography, a non-invasive Doppler technique: Comparison with thermodilution. J Nucl Med All Sci 1980; 24:171–175.

28. Arnim Th v, Holte H-d, Light LH. Transcutane aortale Velographie – Eine neue Method zur nichtinvasive Doppler-sonographischen Bestimmung eines Schlag-volumenindex. Zeitschr Kardiol 1982; 71:596 (abstract).

29. Light LH, Sequeria RF, Cross, G, Bilton A, Hanson GC. Floworientated circulatory patient assessment and management using transcutaneous aortovelography, a non-invasive Doppler technique. J Nucl Med All Sci 1979; 23:137–144.

30. Light LH, Cross G. Convenient monitoring of cardiac output and global left ventricular function by transcutaneous aortovelography – an effective alternative to cardiac output measurements. In: Spencer M (Ed.). Cardiac Doppler Diagnosis. Boston: Martinus Nijhoff 1983: 69–80.

31. Buchtal A, Hanson GC, Peisach AR. Transcutaneous aortovelography, potentially useful techniques in management of critically ill patients. Br Heart J 1976; 38:451–456.

32. Salmasi A-M. Doppler stress testing. In: Salmasi A-M, Nicolaides AN (eds.). Cardiovascular Applications of Doppler Ultrasound. Churchill-Livingstone, Edinburgh, in press.

33. Cross G, Light LH. Non-invasive intrathoracic blood velocity measurement in the assessment of cardiovascular function. Biomed Eng 1974; 9:464–471.

34. Salmasi AM, Nicolaides AN, Vecht RJ, Hendry WG, Salmasi SN, Nicolaides EP, Kidner PH, Besterman EMM. Electrocardiographic chest wall mapping in the diagnosis of coronary artery disease. Br Med J 1983; 287:9–12.

35. Salmasi A-M, Salmasi S, Dore C, Nicolaides AN. Non-invasive assessment of changes in aortic blood velocity and its derivatives with exercise in normal subjects by Doppler ultrasound. J Cardiovasc Surgery 1987; 28:321–327.

36. Salmasi SN. Electrocardiographic chest wall mapping and transcutaneous aortovelography. Ph.D Thesis, London University, 1989.

37. Salmasi SN, Salmasi AM, Hendry WG, et al. Exercise-induced changes in stroke volume measured non-invasively in coronary artery disease. Ultrasound Med Biol

1982; 8(A):170 (abstract).

38. Salmasi SN, Salmasi AM, Hendry WG, *et al.* Exercise-induced changes in stroke volume measured non-invasively in coronary artery disease. Acta Cardiologica 1983; 6:337–339.

39. Salmasi A-M, Salmasi S, Nicolaides AN, Dore C, Hendry WG, Kidner PH. Noninvasive assessment of left ventricular function in coronary artery disease by Doppler stress testing. J Cardiovasc Surgery 1987; 28:313–320.

40. Hossack KF, Bruce RA, Ivey TD, Kusumi F. Changes in cardiac functional capacity after coronary bypass surgery in relation to adequacy of revascularisation. J Amer Coll Cardiol 1984; 3:47–54.

41. Laptin ES, Murray JA, Bruce RA, Winterscheid L. Changes in maximal exercise performance in the evaluation of saphenous vein bypass surgery. Circulation 1973; 47:1164–1173.

42. Salmasi AM, Salmasi SN, Nicolaides AN, Dore C, Kidner PH. Assessment of the effect of coronary artery bypass grafting on left ventricular performance by Doppler measurement of the aortic blood velocity during exercise. J Cardiovasc Surg 1988; 29:89–94.

43. Noble MIM, Trenchard D, Guz A. Left ventricular ejection in conscious dogs. 1. Measurements and significance of the maximum acceleration of blood from the left ventricle. Circ Res 1966; 19:139–147.

44. Jewitt D, Gabe I, Mills C, Maurer B, Thomas M, Shilingford J. Aortic velocity and acceleration measurements in the assessment of coronary heart disease. Europ J Cardiol 1974; 1:299–305.

45. Bennett ED, Else W, Miller GAH, Sutton GC, Miller HC, Nobel MIM. Maximum acceleration of blood from left ventricle in patients with ischaemic heart disease. Clin Sci Mol Med 1974; 46:49–59.

46. Mehta N, Bennett ED. Impaired left ventricular function in acute myocardial infarction assessed by Doppler measurement of ascending aortic blood velocity and maximum acceleration. Am J Cardiol 1986; 57:1052–1058.

47. Marshall RC, Wisenberg G, Schelbert HR, Henze E. Effect of oral propranolol on rest, exercise and post-exercise left ventricular performance in normal subjects and patients with coronary artery disease. Circulation 1981; 63:572–583.

48. Battler A, Ross J Jr., Slutsky R, Pfisterer M, Ashurn W, Froelicher V. Improvement by oral propranolol of exercise-induced left ventricular dysfunction in patients with coronary artery disease. Am J Cardiol 1979; 44:318.

12. Doppler assessment of stress induced ischemic diastolic dysfunction

GEORGE D. MITCHELL

University of Connecticut, School of Medicine, Saint Francis Hospital and Medical Center, 114 Woodland St., Hartford, CT, 06105, U.S.A.

12.1 Introduction

Considerable interest has recently been focused on the importance of diastolic left ventricular (LV) dysfunction in the production of signs and symptoms in acquired heart disease. Studies in patients presenting with symptoms of congestive heart failure, for example, have estimated that 34% to 42% will have normal left ventricular ejection fractions, implying a major role for abnormalities of left ventricular compliance and/or relaxation [1, 2, 3]. Pulsed Doppler echocardiography has emerged as a clinically useful tool in the noninvasive evaluation of abnormalities of LV filling, by virtue of its beat to beat analysis of the velocity of transmitral blood flow. Abnormal left ventricular diastolic function has been studied using this technique in patients with hypertension [4, 5, 6], hypertrophic cardiomyopathy [7, 8, 9, 10], and dilated cardiomyopathy [11], with a prevalent pattern being identified of a shift in ventricular filling from early to late diastole. Reduced flow velocity in early diastole has been attributed to impaired relaxation with consequent compromise of early diastolic filling. Increased transmitral flow velocity in late diastole is felt to reflect a compensatory increase in the atrial contribution to left ventricular filling. The effects of myocardial ischemia on diastolic ventricular function are more complex. It is the intention of this review to briefly outline what is known on an experimental level of the effects of ischemia on ventricular diastolic function, to briefly summarize the validation of the Doppler method of assessment of LV filling in comparison with previous techniques, to describe what has been ascertained of the effects of ischemic heart disease on Doppler parameters of diastolic function, and to attempt to delineate the utility of Doppler assessment of transmitral flow with exercise in the detection of stress induced myocardial ischemia.

12.2 Experimental studies

During the past 10–15 years, many investigators have attempted to analyze the effects of myocardial ischemia on diastolic ventricular function in animal preparations, predominantly by studying myocardial compliance changes as reflected by

Steve M. Teague (ed.) Stress Doppler Echocardiography, 155–171.
© 1990 *Kluwer Academic Publishers*.

alterations in the LV pressure-volume relationship at end-diastole [12]. Experimental coronary artery ligation has been shown to acutely increase LV compliance, whereas pacing induced ischemia has been noted to produce the opposite effect of a decrease in compliance (i.e. increased myocardial stiffness) [13, 14, 15, 16]. The underlying mechanisms thought to explain these contradictory effects of 'supply' and 'demand' ischemia are multifactorial. Supply ischemia results in a collapse of the coronary vasculature (the so-called 'garden hose effect'), which is felt to lead to a reduction in its contribution to chamber stiffness. Segmental dyskinesis (stretching and elongation of the ischemic region) which occurs during coronary occlusion, may lead to an increase in ventricular volume at a given pressure, thereby increasing chamber compliance [12, 17, 18]. Tissue metabolic factors leading to increased levels of cytostolic calcium are felt to play a role in the observed decreased compliance during demand ischemia [12, 19]. The duration of ischemia also appears to be an important factor as variable degrees of 'ischemic contracture' may occur with more prolonged ischemia, leading to further decreases in myocardial compliance [12].

12.3 Ischemia and diastolic dysfunction in humans

The effects of myocardial ischemia on diastolic left ventricular function in humans has been studied extensively using invasive hemodynamic techniques [20, 21, 22, 23, 24, 25, 26, 27], radionuclide techniques [28, 29, 30], or a combination of the two [31]. Simultaneous measurement of intraventricular pressure and contrast ventriculographic volume during angina at rest [26] and during pacing induced ischemia [20, 21, 22, 26] has demonstrated a shift in the pressure/volume relationship consistent with decreased LV compliance (increased stiffness). Pressure measurements during pacing induced ischemia [23] and during supine bicycle exercise induced ischemia [25] have shown abnormal decay in LV pressure in early diastole suggesting a primary effect of ischemia on myocardial relaxation. A landmark study by Mann, et al. [23], studying pacing induced ischemia, showed a decrease in the rate and increase in the time constant of pressure decay, confirming the effect of ischemia on relaxation. Strong arguments were also made against a contribution of extrinsic compression of the LV by the pericardium and right ventricle, or by changes in the 'erectile effect' of the coronary vasculature. Radionuclide studies at rest in patients with coronary disease [29], and during exercise induced ischemia [28, 30], have shown a decrease in the peak rate of diastolic filling and a reduction in the proportion of filling in early diastole. Sharma, et al. [26] also provided invasive evidence of a shift in filling from early to late diastole during spontaneous angina in the cath lab. Thus a primary effect of ischemia on diastolic LV function in humans has been clearly shown. A more easily obtained, less expensive, noninvasive technique would facilitate the study of these phenomena in larger numbers of patients and serially in individual patients.

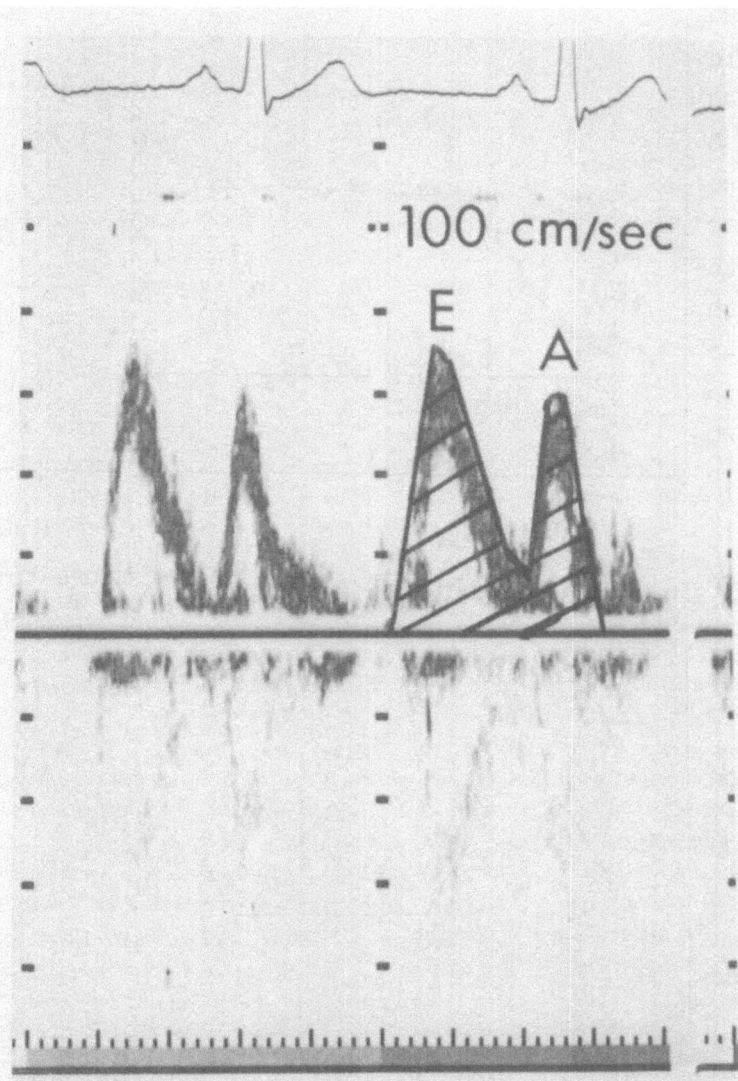

Figure 1. Sample spectral display of Doppler transmitral flow velocity. E = peak velocity in early diastole; A = peak velocity during atrial systole; integrated area under the darkest outline of the spectral display = mean flow velocity.

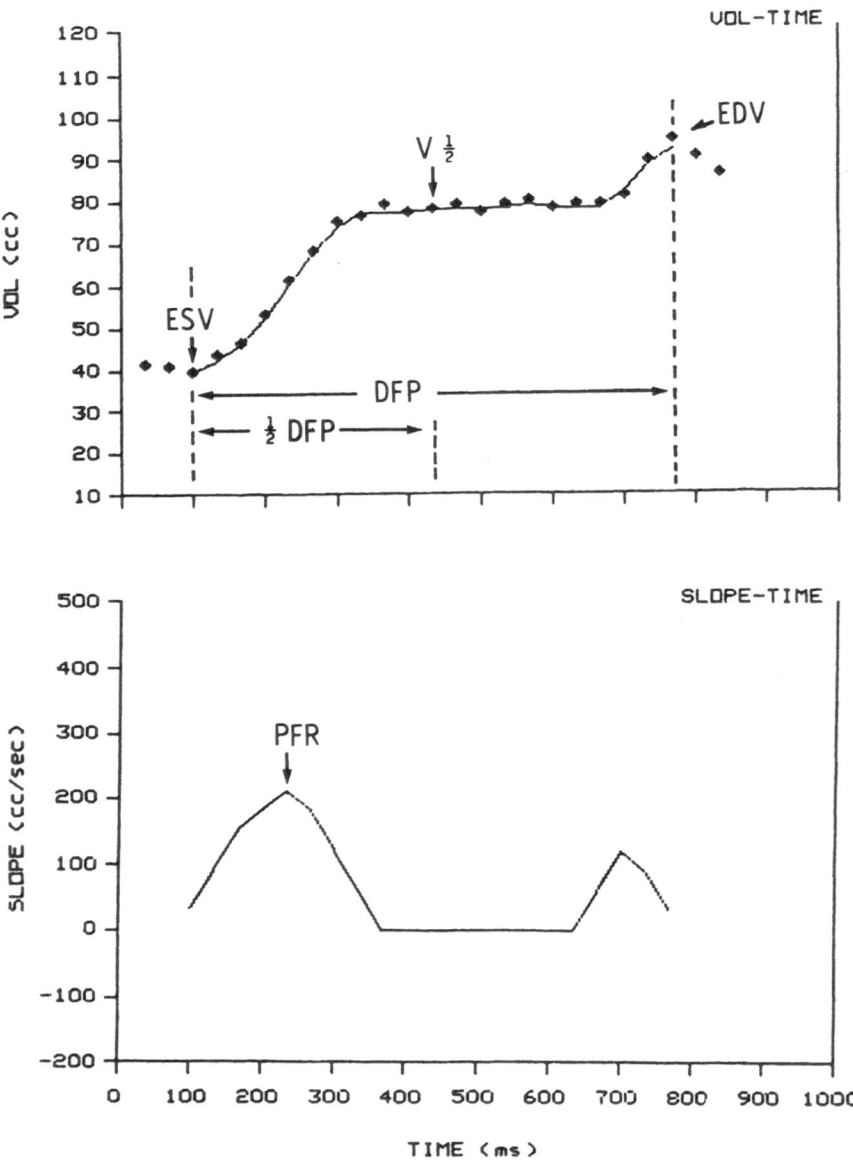

Figure 2. Top) Computer-generated graphic display of an angiographic frame-by-frame left ventricular volume curve during diastole. The diastolic filling period (DFP) is determined as the time between the end-systolic volume (ESV) and end-diastolic volume (EDV). V 1/2 is the abolute volume of the left ventricle at one half DFP. Bottom) Instantaneous slope or derivative of the volume curve. Peak filling rate (PFR) represents the largest derivative within the first half of diastole. Reproduced with permission from Rokey *et al.* [33].

12.4 Pulsed Doppler assessment of left ventricular filling

Prior to the use of Doppler echocardiography in the analysis of left ventricular filling, the clinical assessment of diastolic function was made by obtaining filling rates and filling fractions from frame-by-frame analysis of contrast ventriculgrams or time-activity curves by gated blood pool scintigraphy. Doppler assessment of LV filling is accomplished by measuring the velocities of transmitral flow in diastole. The heart is imaged in the apical 4-chamber view, and the pulsed Doppler sample voume is placed on the ventricular side of the mitral annulus near the tips of the mitral leaflets [32]. The spectral display thus obtained has a characteristic biphasic apeparance as illustrated in Figure 1. Two peak velocities are recorded, representing flow in early diastole (E) and during atrial contraction (A).

Rokey, *et al.* [33] compared peak filling rates obtained using the product of peak early diastolic Doppler flow velocity and mitral annular cross sectional area, with those obtained from frame by frame analysis of contrast ventriculograms. The derivative of the contrast volume curve (bottom panel of Figure 2) was found to morphologically resemble the Doppler-derived velocity profile. Mean values for peak filling rates and for first one-half of diastole filling fractions, obtained by the two methods, were nearly identical. A significant correlation was found between peak flow velocity alone and angiographic peak filling rate. Patients with low angiographic filling rates tended to have an early diastolic peak velocity of less than 45 cm/sec. Patients with low filling rates also tended to have a relative increase in flow velocity during atrial contraction. An E/A ratio (ratio of early to late peak flow velocity) less than 1.0 correlated with low angiographic filling rate. A cutoff value of 1.0 allowed separation of normal from reduced one-half filling fraction angiographically in 93% of patients studied.

Spirito, *et al.* [34] evaluated variables obtained directly from the Doppler diastolic flow velocity waveform alone, and compared them with volumetric measurements of diastolic filling using time-activity curves obtained by radionuclide angiography. The timing of flow velocities by Doppler appeared to coincide exactly with changes in relative volume by radionuclide angiography (Figure 3). The slope of the descent of the early diastolic peak flow velocity correlated well with the radionuclide angiographic peak filling rate (R = 0.79). E/A ratios taken directly from the Doppler spectral display correlated well witht he ratio of percent of LV filling occurring during rapid filling and that occurring during atrial systole. The two techniques showed agreement in classifying patients as having normal or abnormal diastolic function in 84% of the patients studied. In a similar study, Friedman, *et al.* [35] digitized the Doppler flow velocity waveform and assessed the fraction of left ventricular filling during early diastole and atrial systole by calculating the ratios of the integrated component velocities to the integration of the total diastolic spectral display. The fraction of diastolic filling during early diastole and atrial systole correlated well with the corresponding parameters obtained by analysis of radionuclide time-activity curves (R values of 0.84 and 0.85 respectively).

160

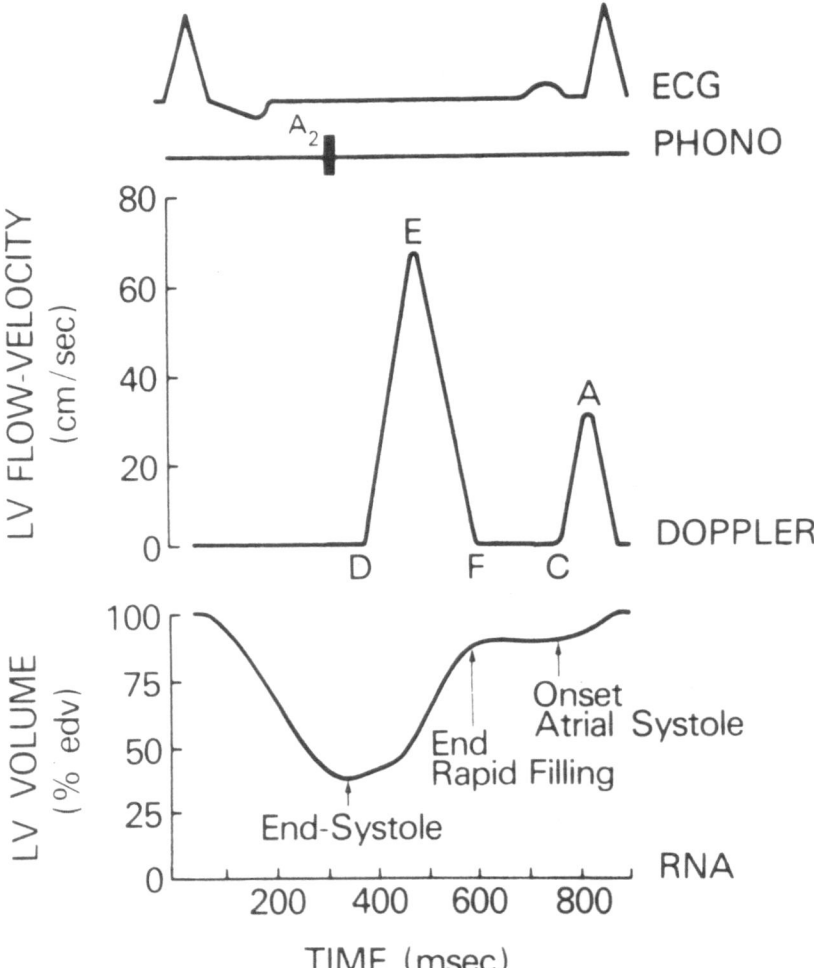

Figure 3. Superimposed Doppler left ventricular (LV) diastolic flow velocity waveform (middle) and radionuclide angiographic (RNA) time-activity curve (bottom), obtained in a normal subject. Cycle length (878 ms) was identical in the two studies. Changes in flow velocity appear to occur at the same time as changes in relative volume. The early diastolic flow velocity peak occurs during the period of left ventricular (LV) rapid filling. At the end of rapid filling, flow velocity begins to decrease and reaches zero baseline at the beginning of diastasis. At the end of diastasis and after atrial systole (A), both flow velocity and filling rate increase again. A2 = aortic component of the second heart sound in the phonocardiogram (PHONO); ECG = electrocardiogram; edv = end-diastolic volume. Reproduced with permission from Spirito *et al.* [34].

These landmark studies demonstrate that indexes derived from the Doppler transmitral flow velocity waveform provide a reliable assessment of diastolic function in patients with cardiac disease. The Doppler technique provides a useful noninvasive, beat to beat analysis of diastolic function, comparing favorably with previous invasive, time consuming, and expensive methods.

12.5 Supply ischemia and the Doppler technique

The effects of myocardial ischemia on the Doppler parameters of left ventricular filling have been studied in patients with acute myocardial infarction (MI) [36, 37], during the balloon inflation phase of percutaneous transluminal coronary angioplasty (PTCA) [38,39], and in patients with coronary artery disease before and after successful PTCA [40,41]. Significant decreases in the E/A ratio compared with controls were seen in patients with acue MI, with the degree of decrease in E/A ratio correlating with both Killip class and hospital mortality. Supply ischemia induced by balloon inflation during PTCA resulted in a lowering of the early diastolic filling velocity and a greater contribution of atrial systole to ventricular filling, within 15–30 seconds of coronary occlusion. Although Wind, *et al.* [40] documented lower peak E velocities and lower E/A ratios and E/A integral ratios in patients with coronary artery disease, no improvement toward normal values was seen in the first 24 hours following successful PTCA. Masuyama, *et al.* [41] however, found that depressed early diastolic filling velocities increased significantly by 9 days post-PTCA. At the time of late follow-up, recurrent decrease in the E velocity was a reliable marker of restenosis. Thus, supply ischemia in humans is associated with the typical abnormalities of the Doppler derived transmitral flow waveform consistent with decreased left ventricular compliance.

12.6 Stress induced ischemia and the Doppler technique

As can be seen from the above discussion, the assessment of ischemic diastolic dysfunction using pulsed Doppler analysis of transmitral flow, has focused on abnormalities of the peak velocity in early diastole (E), the peak velocity during atrial contraction (A), the ratio of the two (E/A ratio), and the integration of the total waveform as well as its two major components (see Figure 1) to yield total and partial velocity integrals. The time-velocity integral represents the mean velocity obtained by digitization of the spectral envelope of the transmitral flow velocity waveform, normalized for the diastolic filling period. The time-velocity integral bears a closer relationship to flow than peak velocities alone, as the product of the time velocity integral and the cross-sectional area of the mitral annulus has correlated well with thermodilution measurement of stroke volume, with an R value by linear regression as high as 0.96 [42]. With increased heart rates (as would occur with exercise or atrial pacing), a phenomenon has been observed in which the E and A velocities tend to merge, preventing analysis of individual integrated

162

velocities [43]. Thus, partial integrals (E and A integrals) cannot be assessed accurately with the increased heart rates to be expected with exercise.

The effect of exercise induced tachycardia on the pulsed Doppler transmitral flow velocity waveform has only very recently been investigated. Iwase *et al.* [44] studied patients with hypertrophic cardiomyopathy treated with diltiazem, undergoing supine bicycle exercise. The response seen in healthy controls was for the E and A velocities to increase dramatically, while maintaining an unchanged E/A ratio. Rassi, *et al.* [45,46] studied normal subjects undergoing supine bicycle exercise, and found that mean mitral flow velocity increased greater than two-fold (41.9 cm/sec to 109.7 cm/sec) from baseline to peak exercise. The mitral time-velocity integral, however, did not change significantly due to a greater than two-fold decrease in the diastolic filling period. Figure 4 illustrates the dramatic increase in transmitral flow velocities with exercise in a normal subject. Again, the degree of fusion of the E and A velocities at increased heart rates prevents separate analysis of E and A velocity integrals. Clearly, it can be seen that distinguishing abnormalities of the distribution of diastolic filling induced by ischemia, in the setting of increased heart rates, is complicated by the above technical problems in waveform analysis. In addition, decreases in the E velocity and integral, and increases in A velocity and integral, seen in models of supply ischemia, may be masked by the normal physiologic response of both parameters to exercise, when investigating demand ischemia.

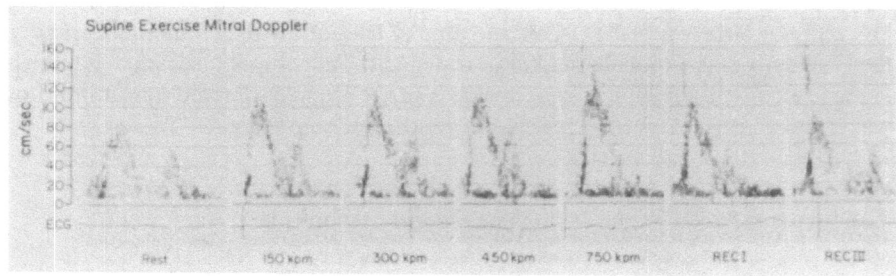

Figure 4. Representative single-beat Doppler velocity recordings at rest, during exercise, and recovery. ECG = electrocardiogram; REC = recovery. Reproduced with permission from Rassi *et al.* [46].

In an attempt to overcome these technical difficulties, Iliceto, *et al.* [47] studied patients with coronary artery disease using pacing induced ischemia, but assessed the transmitral flow velocity waveform during post-atrial pacing recovery, thus analyzing changes in the E and A velocities and integrals in the presence of demand ischemia, but at heart rates no different than baseline. A significant rearrangement of left ventricular filling was found with a decrease in E velocity, a compensatory increase in A velocity, and an increase in the ratio of atrial time-velocity integral to total time velocity integral. The Doppler waveform returned to baseline, however, by one minute of recovery from pacing.

Given the inherent difficulties in assessing Doppler parameters of left ventricular filling at increased heart rates, we attempted to prospectivley assess whether useful information could be obtained using this technique in patients undergoing treadmill stress testing in the evaluation of coronary artery disease. Realizing that separate E and A integrals and deceleration time of the E velocity would not be measurable at increased heart rates due to the fusion of E and A velocities, the only remaining parameters that could be practically assessed would be the peak E and A velocities, their ration (E/A ratio), the mean velocity for the total waveform, and the time-velocity integral for the total waveform.

12.7 Doppler technique during stress testing

A total of 28 consecutive patients, over a 4 month period at the UCLA Noninvasive Laboratories, underwent simultaneous digital stress echocardiography and stress thallium imaging using standard upright treadmill exercise protocols [48]. The 'ischemic' group (Group I) included 18 patients; 12 with evidence of reversible perfusion defects by SPECT thallium imaging (Group IA), and 6 with negative thallium scans but with exercise induced wall motion abnormalities by stress echocardiography (Group IB). The 'non-ischemic' group (Group 2) included 10 patients with known or suspected coronary artery disease, with normal stress thallium imaging, normal stress echocardiography, and normal ECG stress testing. During this same time period 10 'controls' (Group 3) were identified as age matched patients undergoing stress echocardiography for evaluation of atypical chest pain but without evidence of coronary artery disease.

Resting and immediate post-exercise 2-dimensional (2-D) and Doppler echocardiographic imaging was performed on supine subjects with a Hewlett-Packard 77020A echocardiograph with a 2.5 MHz transducer and pulsed Doppler capability. Optimal windows for obtaining parasternal and apical views at rest were clearly marked on each patient's chest wall. Immediate post-exercise images were obtained in all cases within 30–60 seconds of termination of upright treadmill exercise. Digitized cine loops of 2-D images obtained using the apical 4-chamber, 2-chamber and long axis, as well as the parasternal short-axis veiws were made on a Microsonics digitizing system. The grading system used for wall motion analysis has been described previously [48]. The profile of transmitral flow by pulsed Doppler was obtained with the sample volume placed on the ventricular side of the mitral annulus near the tips of the mitral leaflets in the apical 4-chamber view. Pulsed Doppler measurements were obtained immediately after 2-D imaging. Beats used for analysis were those that showed the greatest peak flow velocities regardless of the phase of respiration. Four parameters of LV filling were obtained from analysis of the Doppler spectral display: (1) peak E, (2) peak A, (3) E/A ratio (4) mean mitral flow velocity-obtained by digitizing the contour of the darkest outline of the spectral display (see Figure 1). The time-velocity integral is the mean velocity normalized for the diastolic filling period (see above). Digitization was performed using a standard, commercially available digitizing pad from Trinity Systems. Statistical methods used were described previously [48].

A summary of the overall results of simultaneous digital stress echocardiography and stress thallium imaging is shown in Figure 5. Of note is the fact that of the 10 patients with known or suspected coronary artery disease with 'non-ischemic' studies, 7 had resting wall motion abnormalities consistent with previous infarction (Group 2A). The mean ages, baseline heart rates, post exercise heart rates, percentages of maximum predicted heart rate at peak exercise, and double-products achieved were comparable in all groups. There was a trend toward greater use of calcium antagonists and beta-blocking drugs in Groups 1 and 2, compared with Group 3. Table 1 lists the data for the response of the mean mitral flow velocity to exercise in all groups.

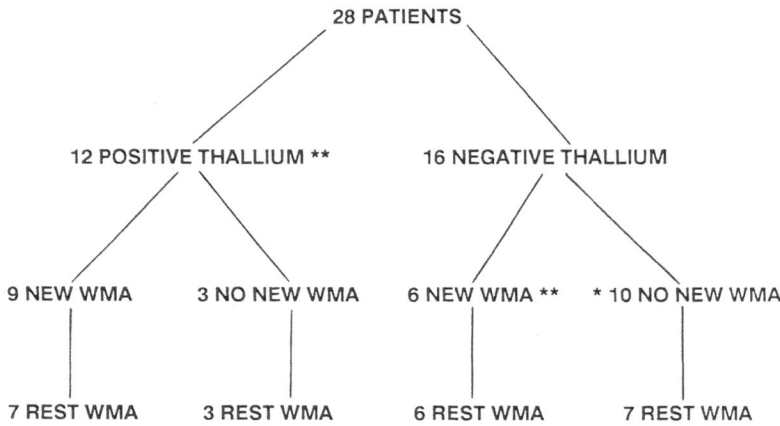

** Constitute ischemic group

* Constitute non-ischemic group

WMA = wall motion abnormality

Figure 5. Overall results of simultaneous digital stress echocardiography and stress thallium imaging in 28 consecutive patients with known or suspected coronary artery disease. * = non-ischemic group; ** = ischemic group. WMA = wall-motion abnormality.

In controls the mean mitral flow velocity doubled, from baseline to post-exercise, whereas in patients with evidence of exercise induced ischemia by stress echo and stress thallium, the mean mitral flow velocity increased by only 33%. Sample Doppler tracings in a control and an ischemic patient are shown in Figure 6. There was no difference in the response of mean mitral flow velocity with exercise if one compares patients with ischemia demonstrated by reversible thallium perfusion

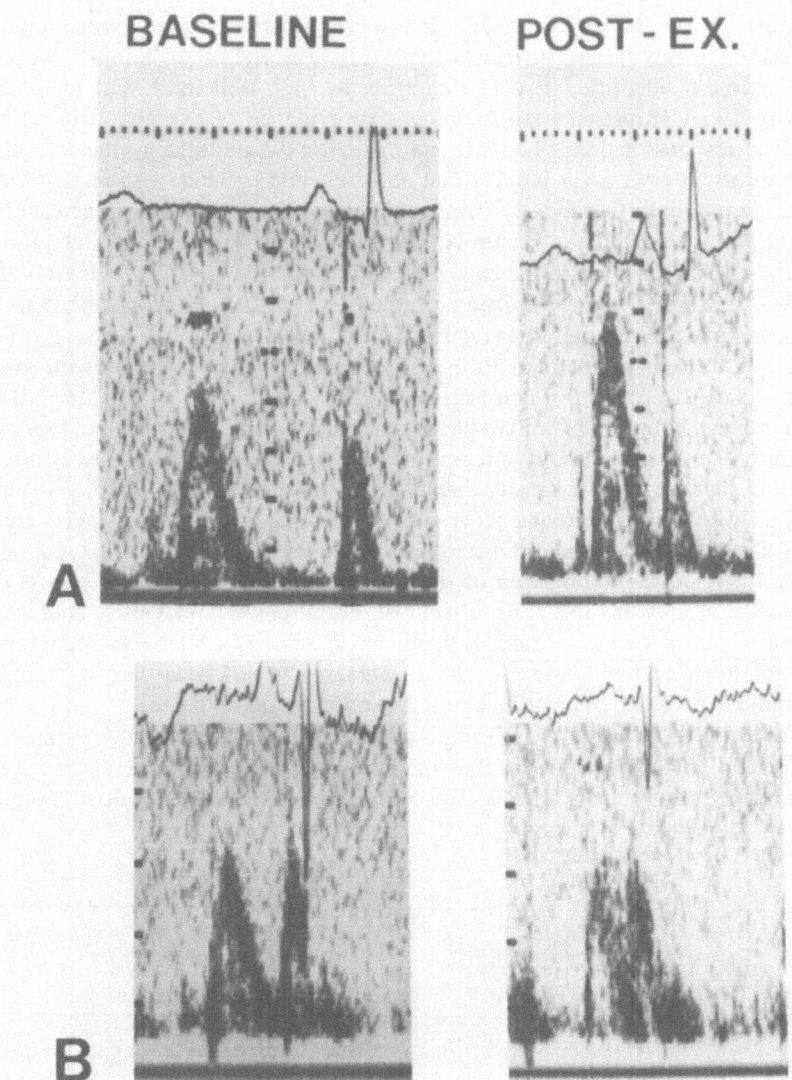

BASELINE   POST-EX.

A

B

Figure 6. Pre-exercise and post-exercise spectral display of Doppler transmitral flow velocity in 2 representative patients. A) control: a 61 year old female, 13 minute total exercise time on Bruce protocol, reached 88% maximal predicted heart rate, double product = 23,800, baseline mean mitral flow velocity = 33 cm/s, post-exercise mean mitral flow velocity = 67 cm/s (103% increase). B) thallium redistribution and exercise induced wall-motion abnormality developed in this 58 year old male, 11.5 minute total exercise time on Bruce protocol, reached 100% maximal predicted heart rate, double product = 27,200, baseline mean mitral flow velocity = 42 cm/s, post-exercise mean mitral flow velocity = 53 cm/s (26% increase). Each division = 20 cm/s.

defects versus those with ischemia demonstrated by exercise induced wall motion abnormalities (Group 1A vs. Group 1B). If one uses a cut-off for the normal degree of increase in mean mitral flow velocity with exercise of 50%, the Doppler response correctly identified 9 of 10 controls as 'non-ischemic', and predicted ischemia in 15 of 18 patients with noninvasive evidence of exercise induced ischemia. The response among 'non-ischemic patients' was similar to the response among controls. It is of great interest that non-ischemic patients with resting wall motion abnormalities (Group 2A) demonstrated the same degree of increase in mean mitral flow velocity as controls, suggesting that the proposed abnormal response to exercise (failure to increase mean mitral flow velocity by at least 50%) is a marker of exercise induced ischemia, rather than merely a non-specific marker of resting compliance abnormalities related to prior ischemic injury.

The failure in ischemic patients to increase transmitral flow velocity with exercise to the same extent seen in non-ischemics and controls, may be a reflection of ischemia induced compromise of stroke volume, LV filling or both. If one looks at the response of the time-velocity integral to exercise in all groups (Table 2) it can be seen that there is no significant change from baseline to post-exercise in any group. This would suggest that changes in stroke volume were not significantly different. The smaller decrease in diastolic filling period seen in ischemic patients may reflect a relative prolongation of diastolic filling due to ischemic effects on compliance and/or relaxation. The effects of drugs on the responses noted are interesting in that patients with an 'ischemic' response in the Doppler parameter had a trend toward greater use of calcium antagonists and beta blocking drugs, which should exert a beneficial effect on left ventricular compliance.

In terms of the response of the E/A ratio to exercise, the values for this parameter at baseline and post-exercise, as well as the percent change with exercise, were no different among all groups (Table 3). The overall response of mean velocity, there-

Table 1. Mitral flow velocity data.

Pt Group	Baseline Mitral Flow Velocity (cm/s)	Postexercise Mitral Flow Velocity (cm/s)	Percent Change in Mitral Flow Velocity* (cm/s)	Patients with >50% Increase in Mitral Flow Velocity* (cm/s)
1	39 ± 13	51 ± 18	33 ± 24	3/18
1A	42 ± 15	56 ± 20	31 ± 29	2/12
1B	32 ± 6	41 ± 9	34 ± 24	1/6
2	33 ± 7	59 ± 12	86 ± 53	8/10
2A	35 ± 7	63 ± 10	90 ± 64	5/7
3	31 ± 7	60 ± 12	101 ± 59	9/10

All values are mean ± standard deviation.
* $p = <0.005$ between groups.

Table 2. Diastolic filling period and time-velocity integral data.

Pt Group	Baseline DFP	Postexercise DFP	Percent Change in DFP	Baseline TVI	Postexercise TVI	Percent Change in TVI
1	0.48 ± 0.16	0.37 ± 0.15	23 ± 16	18 ± 5	17 ± 4	−1 ± 18
2	0.48 ± 0.11	0.29 ± 0.06	37 ± 14	16 ± 4	17 ± 4	13 ± 23
3	0.59 ± 0.13	0.34 ± 0.09	40 ± 18	17 ± 4	20 ± 4	11 ± 17
	NS	NS	$p = 0.02$	NS	NS	NS

All values are in mean ± standard deviation.
DFP = diastolic filling period (in seconds of diastole/beat); NS = not significant; TVI = time-velocity integral.

fore, would appear to be a more reliable measure of the effects of exercise induced ischemia on Doppler assessment of LV filling, overcoming the technical drawback of the effect of increased heart rate on the Doppler peak velocities, as previously described.

The above study is the first to assess the response of transmitral flow, as measured by pulsed Doppler echocardiography, to exercise in the evaluation of patients with known or suspected coronary artery disease. The major limitation, besides small numbers of patients, is the absence of angiographic confirmation of the presence of significant coronary artery obstruction. In terms of future directions in the study of this technique, we plan to evaluate a more straightforward model, namely the patient with single vessel coronary artery disease and normal LV systolic function, undergoing PTCA. The evaluation of the response of LV filling to exercise in the presence, and then in the same patient, the absence of exercise induced ischemia, should help to establish the reliability and usefulness of this technique as an adjunct to routine stress echocardiography.

Table 3. E/A ratios.

Pt group	Baseline E/A ratio	Postexercise E/A ratio	Percent change in E/A ratio
1	1.2 ± 0.3	1.3 ± 0.5	10 ± 48
2	1.6 ± 1.7	1.4 ± 0.7	7 ± 32
3	1.2 ± 0.4	1.0 ± 0.2	16 ± 27
	NS	NS	NS

All values are in mean ± standard deviation.

12.8 Summary

Stress echocardiography is continually evolving as a useful adjunct to ECG treadmill stress testing. The role of Doppler echocardiography as an adjunct to stress echocardiography is only recently beginning to be defined. The majority of clinical studies have focused on Doppler parameters of systolic LV function and LV ejection dynamics. The assessment of diastolic function during stress testing has thus far been the least studied aspect of stress Doppler. This review has attempted to demonstrate that pulsed-Doppler provides clinically useful and physiologically meaningful information about abnormalities of LV filling by comparison with other techniques. The effects of ischemia (occurring at rest or produced by atrial pacing, exercise, and coronary occlusion) on diastolic LV function, and the use of pulsed-Doppler to assess abnormalities of transmitral flow induced by ischemia, have been summarized. This should serve as a background to understanding (and formulating ways of studying) the effects of ischemia produced by treadmill stress testing on LV diastolic function.

This review has also concentrated on the technical difficulties and pitfalls in analyzing the Doppler waveform of transmitral flow at the increased heart rates encountered with exercise. The response of transmitral flow to exercise in normals has been described. The experience of one laboratory in the use of Doppler assessment of diastolic function with treadmill exercise in patients with known or suspected coronary artery disease has been described in detail.

Changes in peak E velocity, peak A velocity, and their ratio, with exercise induced myocardial ischemia, are influenced by the normal physiologic response during exercise to increase all velocities as a reflection of increased cardiac output, as elegantly reported by Rassi et al. [46]. Evaluation of the separate integral velocities is technically limited by the fusion of E and A waveforms at the increased heart rates attained with exercise. It is proposed that analysis of the total waveform integral at baseline and post-exercise be compared with the response in normals, in assessing abnormalities of LV filling produced by exercise induced ischemia. Clearly, the clinical role of Doppler assessment of LV filling with exercise, in evaluating patients with coronary artery disease, has yet to be defined. Further studies are needed to validate the use of this technique in treadmill stress testing.

References

1. Dougherty AH, Naccarelli GV, Gray EL, Hicks CH, Goldstein RA. Congestive heart failure with normal systolic function. Am J Cardiol 1984; 54:778–782.
2. Soufer R, Wohlgelernter D, Vita NA, Amuchestegui M, Sostman D, Berger HJ, Zaret BL. Intact systolic left ventricular function in clinical congestive heart failure. Am J Cardiol 1985; 55:1032–1036.
3. Marantz PR, Tobin JN, Wassertheil-Smoller S, Steingart RM, Wexler JP, Budner N, Lense L, Wachspress J. The relationship between left ventricular systolic function and congestive heart failure diagnosed by clinical criteria. Circulation 1988; 77:607–612.
4. Snider AR, Sidding SS, Rocchini AP, Rosenthal A, Dick M, Crowley DC, Peters J. Doppler evaluation of left ventricular diastolic filling in children with systemic hypertension. Am J Cardiol 1985; 56:921–926.
5. Dianzumba SB, Di Pette DJ, Cornman C, Weber E, Joyner CR. Left ventricular filling characteristics in mild untreated hypertension. Hypertension 1986; 8(Suppl I):I–156–160.

6. Phillips RA, Coplan NL, Krakoff LR, Yeager K, Ross RS, Gorlin R, Goldman ME. Doppler echocardiographic analysis of left ventricular filling in treated hypertensive patients. J Am Coll Cardiol 1987; 9:317–322.

7. Kitabatake A, Inoue M, Asao M, Tanouchi J, Masuyama T, Abe H, Morita H, Senda S, Matsuo H. Transmitral blood flow reflecting diastolic behavior of the left ventricle in health and disease. A study by pulsed Doppler technique. Jpn Circ J 1982; 46:92–102.

8. Takenaka K, Dabestani A, Gardin JM, Russell D, Clark S, Allfie A, Henry WL. Left ventricular filling in hypertrophic cardiomyopathy: A pulsed Doppler echocardiographic study. J Am Coll Cardiol 1986; 7:1263–1271.

9. Iwase M, Sotobata I, Takagi S, Miyaguchi K, Jing HX, Yokota M. Effects of diltiazem on left ventricular diastolic behavior in patients with hypertrophic cardiomyopathy: evaluation with exercise pulsed Doppler echocardiography. J Am Coll Cardiol 1987; 9:1099–1105.

10. Maron BJ, Spirito P, Green KJ, Wesley YE, Bonow RO, Arce J. Noninvasive assessment of left ventricular diastolic function by pulsed Doppler echocardiography in patients with hypertrophic cardiomyopathy. J Am Coll Cardiol 1987; 10:733–742.

11. Takenaka K, Dabestani A, Gardin JM, Russell D, Clark S, Allfie A, Henry WL. Pulsed Doppler echocardiographic study of left ventricular filling in dilated cardiomyopathy. Am J Cardiol 1986; 58:143–147.

12. Apstein CS, Grossman W. Opposite initial effects of supply and demand ischemia on left ventricular diastolic compliance: the ischemia-diastolic paradox. J Mol Cell Cardiol 1987; 19:119–128.

13. Pirzada FA, Ekong EA, Vokonas PS, Apstein CS, Hood WB. Experimental myocardial infarction. XIII. Sequential changes in left ventricular pressure-length relationships in the acute phase. Circulation 1974; 53:970–975.

14. Serizawa T, Vogel WM, Apstein CS, Grossman W. Comparison of acute alterations in left ventricular relaxation and diastolic chamber stiffness induced by hypoxia and ischemia. J Clin Invest 1981; 68:91–102.

15. Serizawa T, Carabello BA, Grossman W. Effect of pacing-induced ischemia on left ventricular diastolic pressure-volume relations in dogs with coronary stenoses. Circ Res 1980; 46:430–439.

16. Momomura S, Bradley AB, Grossman W. Left ventricular diastolic pressure-segment length relations and end-diastolic distensibility in dogs with coronary stenoses. Circ Res 1984; 55:203–214.

17. Edwards CH, Rankin JS, McHale PA, Ling D, Anderson RW. Effects of ischemia on left ventricular regional function in the conscious dog. Am J Physiol 1981; 9:H413–H420.

18. Tyberg JV, Forrester JS, Wyatt HL, Goldner SJ, Parmley WW, Swan HJC. An analysis of segmental ischemic dysfunction utilizing the pressure-length loop. Circulation 1974; 49:748–754.

19. Momomura S, Ingwall JS, Parker JA, Sahagian P, Ferguson JJ, Grossman W. The relationships of high energy phosphates, tissue pH, and regional blood flow to diastolic distensibility in the ischemic dog myocardium. Circ Res 1985; 57:822–835.

20. Dwyer EM. Left ventricular pressure-volume alterations and regional disorders of contraction during myocardial ischemia induced by atrial pacing. Circulation 1970; 42:1111–1122.

21. Barry WH, Brooker JZ, Alderman EL, Harrison DC. Changes in diastolic stiffness and tone of the left ventricle during angina pectoris. Circulation 1974; 49:255–263.

22. Mann T, Brodie BR, Grossman W, McLaurin LP. Effect of angina on the left ventricular diastolic pressure-volume relationship. Circulation 1977; 55:761–766.

23. Mann T, Goldberg S, Mudge GH, Grossman W. Factors contributing to altered left ventricular diastolic properties during angina pectoris. Circulation 1979; 59:14–20.

24. Bourdillon PD, Lorell BH, Mirsky I, Paulus WJ, Wynne J, Grossman W. Increased regional myocardial stiffness of the left ventricle during pacing-induced angina in man.

Circulation 1983; 67:316–323.

25. Caroll JD, Hess OM, Hirzel HO, Krayenbuehl HP. Exercise-induced ischemia: The influence of altered relaxation on early diastolic pressures. Circulation 1983; 67:521–528.

26. Sharma B, Behrens TW, Erlein D, Hodges M, Asinger RW, Francis GS. Left ventricular diastolic properties and filling characteristics during spontaneous angina pectoris at rest. Am J Cardiol 1983; 52:704–709.

27. Sasayama S, Nonogi H, Miyazaki S, Sakurai T, Kawai C, Eiho S, Kuwahara M. Changes in diastolic properties of the regional myocardium during pacing-induced ischemia in human subjects. J Amer Coll Cardiol 1985; 5:599–606.

28. Reduto LA, Wickemeyer WJ, Young JB, Del Ventura LA, Reid JW, Glaeser DH, Quinones MA, Miller RR. Left ventricular diastolic performance at rest and during exericse in patients with coronary artery disease. Assessment with first-pass radionuclide angiography. Circulation 1981; 6:1228–1237.

29. Bonow RO, Bacharach SL, Green MV, Kent KM, Rosing DR, Lipson LC, Leon MB, Epstein SE. Impaired left ventricular diastolic filling in patients with coronary artery disease: assessment with radionuclide angiography. Circulation 1981; 64:315–323.

30. Poliner LR, Farber SH, Glaeser DH, Nylaan L, Verani MS, Roberts R. Alteration of diastolic filling rate during exercise radionuclide angiography: A highly sensitive technique for detection of coronary artery disease. Circulation 1984; 70:942–950.

31. Aroesty JM, McKay RG, Heller GV, Royal HD, Als AV, Grossman W. Simultaneous assessment of left ventricular systolic and diastolic dysfunction during pacing-induced ischemia. Circulation 1985; 71:889–900.

32. Gardin JM, Dabestani Ali, Takenaka K, Rohan MK, Knoll M, Russell D, Henry WL. Effect of imaging view and sample volume location on evaluation of mitral flow velocity by pulsed Doppler echocardiography. Am J Cardiol 1986; 57:1335–1339.

33. Rokey R, Kuo LC, Zoghbi WA, Limacher MC, Quinones MA. Determination of parameters of left ventricular diastolic filling with pulsed Doppler echocardography: comparison with cineangiography. Circulation 1985; 71:543–550.

34. Spirito P, Maron BJ, Bonow RO. Noninvasive assessment of left ventricular diastolic function: comparative analysis of Doppler echocardiographic and radionuclide angiographic techniques. J Am Coll Cardiol 1986; 7:518–526.

35. Friedman BJ, Drinkovic N, Miles H, Shih W, Mazzoleni A, DeMaria AN. Assessment of left ventricular diastolic function: comparison of Doppler echocardiography and gated blood pool scintigraphy. J Am Coll Cardiol 1986; 8:1348–1354.

36. Fujii J, Yazaki Y, Sawada H, Aizawa T, Watanabe H, Kato K. Noninvasive assessment of left and right ventricular filling in myocardial infarction with a two-dimensional Doppler echocardiographic method. J Amer Coll Cardiol 1985; 5:1155–1160.

37. Visser CA, deKoning H, Delemarre B, Koolen JJ, Dunning AJ. Pulsed Doppler-derived mitral inflow velocity in acute myocardial infarction: An early prognostic indicator. J Amer Coll Cardiol 1986; 7:136A.

38. Labovitz AJ, Lewen MK, Kern M, Vandormael M, Deligonal U, Kennedy HL. Evaluation of left ventricular systolic and diastolic dysfunction during transient myocardial ischemia produced by angioplasty. J Amer Coll Cardiol 1987; 10:748–755.

39. Henderson M, Schwartz L, Aldridge HE, Prieur T, Rakowski H. Doppler quantitation of diastolic function during PTCA induced ischemia. Circulation 1986; 74:11–357.

40. Wind BE, Snider R, Buda AJ, O'Neill WW, Topol EJ, Dilworth LR. Pulsed Doppler assessment of left ventricular diastolic filling in coronary artery disease before and immediately after coronary angioplasty. Am J Cardiol 1987; 59:1041–1046.

41. Masuyama T, Kodama K, Nakatani S, Nanto S, Kitabatake A, Kamada T. Effects of changes in coronary stenosis on left ventricular diastolic filling assessed with pulsed Doppler echocardiography. J Amer Coll Cardiol 1988; 11:744–751.

42. Lewis JF, Kuo LC, Nelson JG, Limacher MC, Quinones MA. Pulsed Doppler echocardiographic determination of stroke volume and cardiac output: clinical validation of

two new methods using the apical window. Circulation 1984; 70:425–431.

43. Herzog CA, Elsperger KJ, Manoles M, Murakami M, Asinger R. Effect of atrial pacing on left ventricular diastolic filling measured by pulsed Doppler echocardiography. J Amer Coll Cardiol 1987; 9:197A.

44. Iwase M, Sotobata I, Takagi S, Miyaguchi K, Jing HX, Yokota M. Effects of diltiazem on left ventricular diastolic behavior in patients with hypertrophic cardiomyopathy: evaluation with exercise pulsed Doppler echocardiography. J Amer Coll Cardiol 1987; 9:1099–1105.

45. Rassi A, Richards K, Miller J, Crawford M. Echo/Doppler assessment of mitral blood flow during supine exercise. Circulation 1986; 74:II-47.

46. Rassi A, Crawford MH, Richards KL, Miller JF. Differing mechanisms of exercise flow augmentation at the mitral and aortic valves. Circulation 1988; 77:543–551.

47. Iliceto S, Amico A, Marangelli V, D'Ambrosio G, Rizzon P. Doppler echocardiographic evaluation of the effect of atrial pacing-induced ischemia on left ventricular filling in patients with coronary artery disease. J Amer Coll Cardiol 1988; 11;953–961.

48. Mitchell GD, Brunken RC, Schwaiger M, Donohue BC, Krivokapich J, Child JS. Assessment of mitral flow velocity with exercise by an index of stress-induced ischemia in coronary artery disease. Am J Cardiol 1988; 61:536–540.

13. Pharmacologic Doppler stress testing in coronary artery disease

ARTHUR J. LABOVITZ
Division of Cardiology, Department of Internal Medicine,
St. Louis University School of Medicine, St. Louis, Missouri, U.S.A.

It has been over a decade since the initial studies confirming that transcutaneous Doppler ultrasound could be used to accurately assess ascending aortic blood flow velocities [1–3]. As described in detail elsewhere in this book, a number of parameters derived from the aortic velocity profile accurately reflect global left ventricular systolic function (Figure 1). In fact, Doppler evaluation of aortic blood flow velocities provides one of the few non-invasive methods by which beat-to-beat changes in left ventricular function may be assessed.

13.1 Doppler and left ventricular function

A number of studies both from the experimental model as well as in the clinical setting have confirmed the accuracy by which Doppler velocimetry may be applied in determining stroke volume and cardiac output compared with invasive measurements of the same [4–7]. These volume measurements require the integration of the mean velocity over an entire cardiac cycle (flow velocity integral) and the cross sectional area of the aortic valve anulus. In addition, several investigators have shown that the simple measurement of the peak aortic velocity also reflects and is dependent upon to a large extent, left ventricular systolic function. Gardin demonstrated that peak aortic flow velocity was significantly higher in normal individuals than in patients with cardiomyopathy [8]. Other investigators have reported that peak aortic acceleration as well as mean acceleration as measured by Doppler ultrasound also shows a good correlation with left ventricular systolic performance and left ventricular ejection fraction [9,10]. Having the ability therefore, to evaluate parameters of left ventricular systolic function on a beat-to-beat basis, Doppler provides a technique by which one may assess dynamic changes in left ventricular function that may occur secondary to an intervention.

13.2 Using Doppler to assess drug effects

Several chapters in this book are devoted to the use of Doppler in evaluating left ventricular function during exercise. The purpose of this chapter will be to review

Steve M. Teague (ed.) Stress Doppler Echocardiography, 173–182.
© 1990 *Kluwer Academic Publishers.*

174

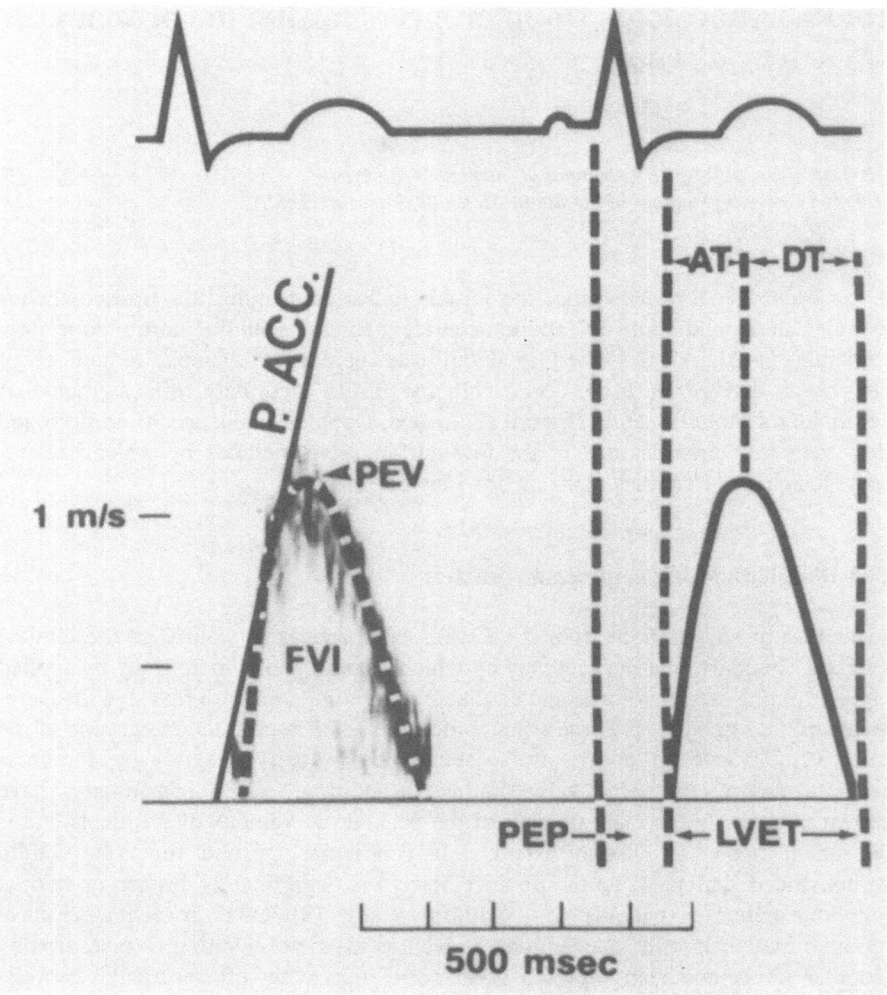

Figure 1. Parameters of left ventricular systolic function measured from a Doppler tracing of ascending aortic blood flow. PEV = peak ejection velocity; PACC = peak acceleration; FVI = flow velocity integral; PEP = pre-ejection period; LVET = left ventricular ejection time; AT = acceleration time; DT = deceleration time.

the effects of various pharmacologic maneuvers on Doppler aortic blood flow velocities and explore the potential for this technique in the evaluation of patients with coronary artery disease (Figure 2). Elkayam and co-workers examined a group of 13 patients with left ventricular dysfunction and congestive heart failure by Doppler echocardiography [11]. Eighteen drug interventions with vasodilators were

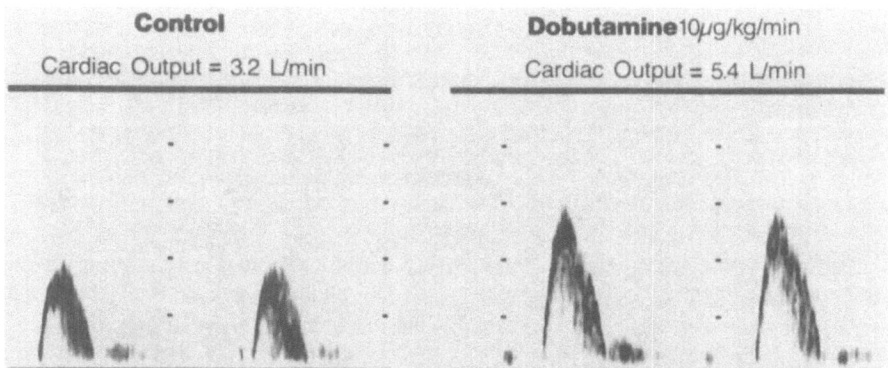

Figure 2. Aortic blood flow velocities at baseline (left) and following equilibration on 10 micrograms/kilogram/minute of dobutamine (right). Note the marked increase in stroke volume and cardiac output.

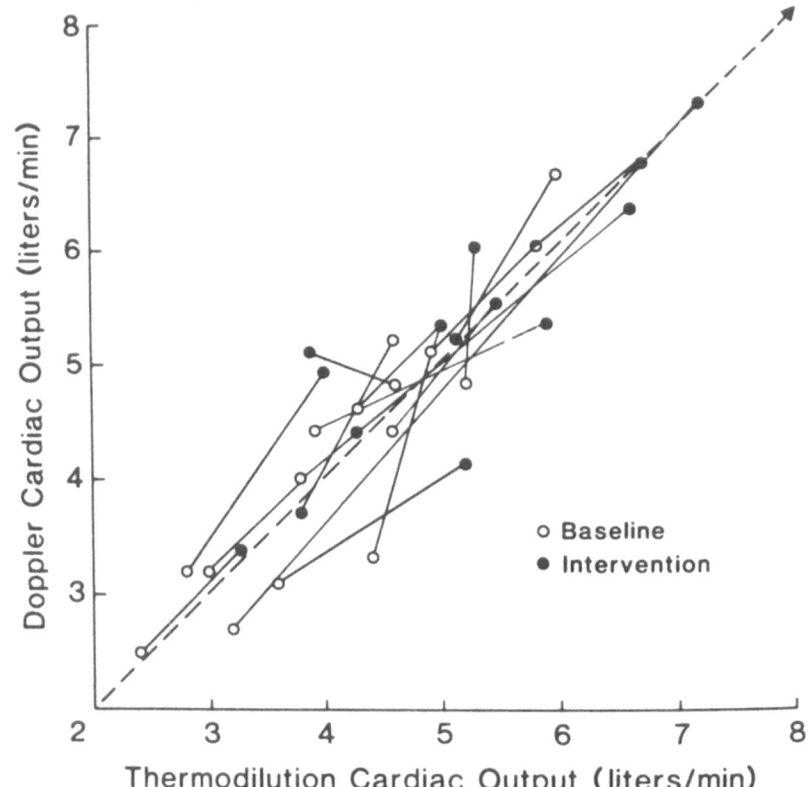

Figure 3. Baseline and interventional (following drug administration) cardiac output data in individual patients as measured by Doppler versus thermodilution. The dashed line is the line of identity. From Reference 12 with permission.

176

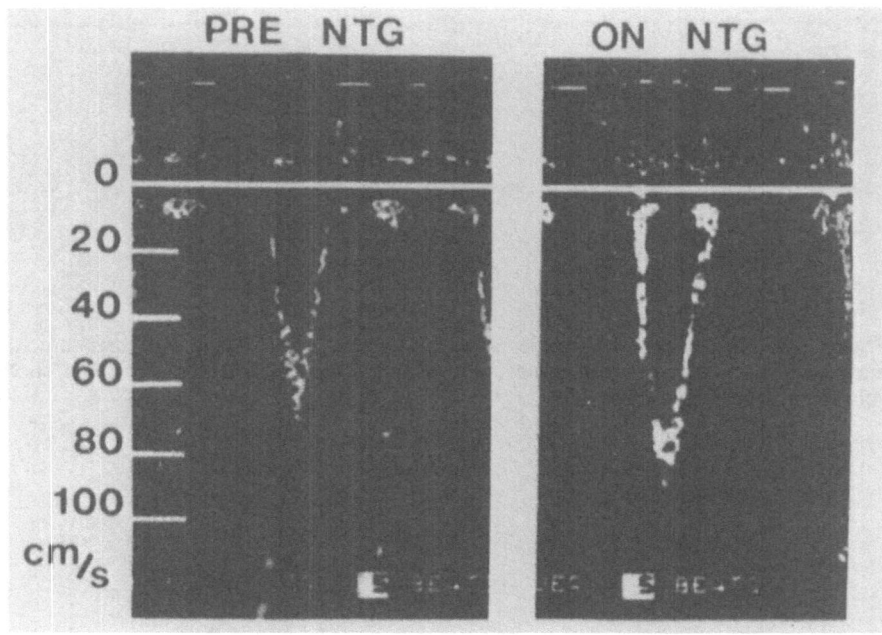

Figure 4. Increase in peak velocity of aortic flow from the left ventricular outflow tract in a patient with mitral regurgitation during nitroglycerin infusion. NTG = nitroglycerin. From Reference [13] with permission.

performed in which aortic blood flow velocity parameters were measured prior to and following administration of nitroprusside, hydralazine, or nitroglycerin. Improvement in stroke volume with vasodilator therapy correlated well with both changes in Doppler flow velocity integral (r = 0.65) as well as changes in the peak flow velocity (r = 0.75). Likewise, Rose reported on excellent correlation between Doppler and thermodilution derived cardiac output (r = 0.88) following drug intervention in a group of 16 patients [12] (Figure 3). Keren and co-workers demonstrated significant increases in cardiac output measured by Doppler in a group of patients with chronic heart failure and functional mitral regurgitation following administration of intravenous nitroglycerin [13] (Figure 4).

Wallmeyer demonstrated in the dog model that the pharmacologic manipulation can have profound influence on Doppler measured blood flow velocities [14]. Infusions of Dobutamine and propranolol induced significant increases and decreases respectively in peak aortic velocity and mean acceleration. These measurements correlated very well with invasive measurements of aortic flow, maximal acceleration of aortic flow and maximum dP/dt. Pharmacologic influence of aortic flow was further demonstrated when Harrison examined 20 young health volunteers by Doppler following the administration of propranolol and verapamil by Doppler echocardiography and found significant decreases in both peak velocity and peak acceleration following administration of the drug (see chapter 10 (ed.)) [15]. Studies examining the effects of pharmacologic interventions in the diagnosis of coronary artery disease, however, in large series of patients have been limited.

13.3 Dipyridamole stress testing

Intravenous Dipyridamole is a potent coronary vasodilator which has been demonstrated to be useful in the evaluation of the functional significance of coronary artery disease. Thallium perfusion imaging following dipyridamole induced vasodilatation can demonstrate perfusion defects in regions supplied by stenosed coronary arteries. Recognizing the potential application of Doppler echocardiography in this setting, we undertook a study to compare the echocardiographic and Doppler parameters of left ventricular systolic function with thallium perfusion imaging following intravenous dipyridamole and the diagnosis of coronary artery disease.

The study population consisted of 100 patients undergoing dipyridamole thallium imaging for standard indications including pre-operative assessment of cardiac risk and functional assessment of suspected coronary artery disease in patients unable to perform standard exercise testing. There were 58 men and 42 women with a mean age of 62 years (range 38 to 82 years). Following a baseline Doppler and echocardiographic studies, Dipyridamole was infused intravenously in the standard fashion at a rate of 0.14 mg/kg/min over four minutes for a total dose of 0.56 mg/kg. At peak dipyridamole effect (approximately four minutes following the infusion), two mCi of Thallium[201] were injected and a repeat Doppler and two-dimensional echocardiographic examination was performed.

Myocardial perfusion imaging was performed 5–10 minutes following the thallium injection and repeated four hours later. Ascending aortic blood flow velocity was evaluated using continuous wave Doppler for peak modal velocity, peak acceleration and flow velocity integral. Two-dimensional echocardiographic images were recorded both in the parasternal and apical views and were analyzed for segmental wall motion and bi-plane left ventricular ejection fraction.

Table 1. Baseline parameters

	Thallium negative	Thallium positive	p value
Number	41	53	–
Age (years)	59 ± 12	65 ± 10	< 0.01
Base heart rate (beats/min.)	77 ± 13	74 ± 12	NS
Base acceleration (m/s^2)	25 ± 16	26 ± 14	NS
Base velocity (m/s)	0.9 ± 0.4	0.9 ± 0.4	NS
Base ejection fraction (%)	53 ± 7	50 ± 10	NS

NS = not significant.

178

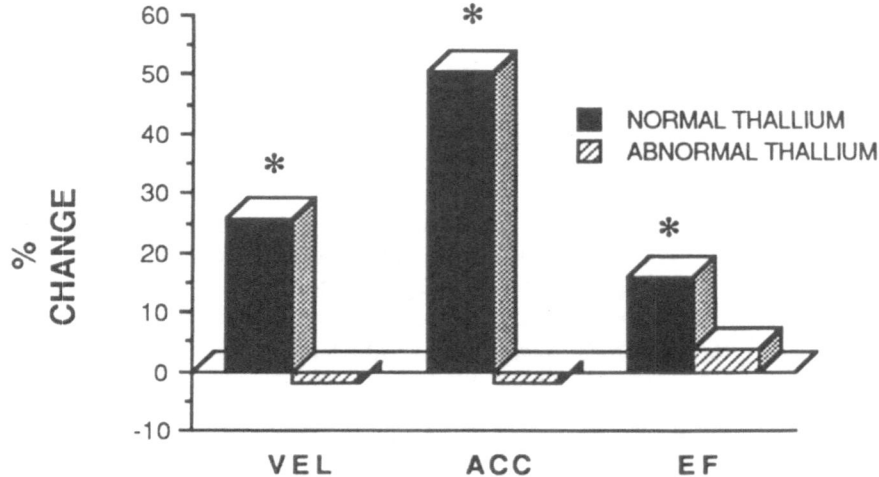

Figure 5. Percent change from baseline to peak dipyridamole effect in velocity (Vel), acceleration (Acc), and LV ejection fraction (EF) in patients with normal and abnormal thallium images following intravenous dipyridamole. (*p < 0.05.)

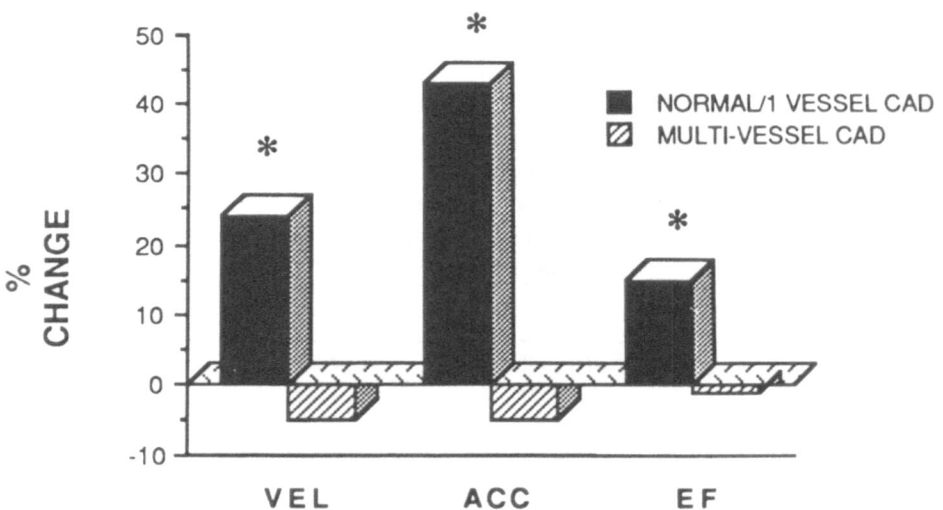

Figure 6. Percent change from baseline to peak dipyridamole effect in velocity (Vel), acceleration (Acc), and LV ejection fraction (EF) in patients with and without multi-vessel disease.

CORONARY ARTERY DISEASE

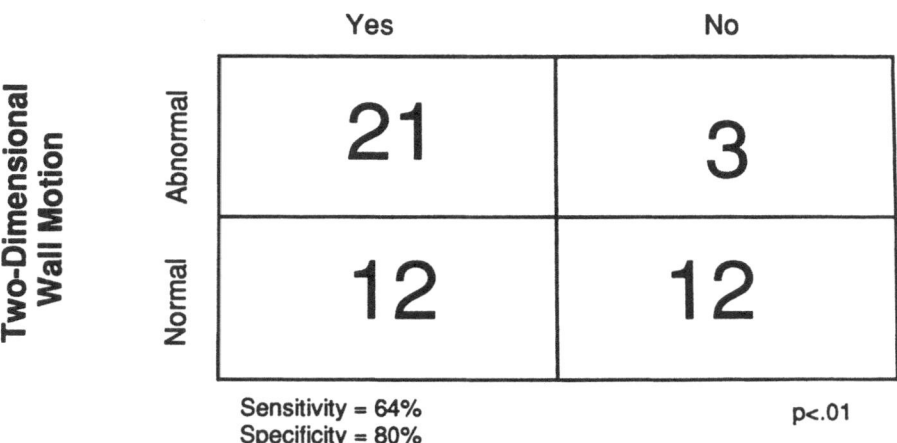

Figure 7. Comparison of the results of coronary arteriography and 2-dimensional wall motion analysis. There were 12 patients with significant CAD in whom 2-dimensional wall motion was judged to be normal. Only 3 individuals without significant CAD were found to have wall motion abnormalities on 2-dimensional echocardiography.

CORONARY ARTERY DISEASE

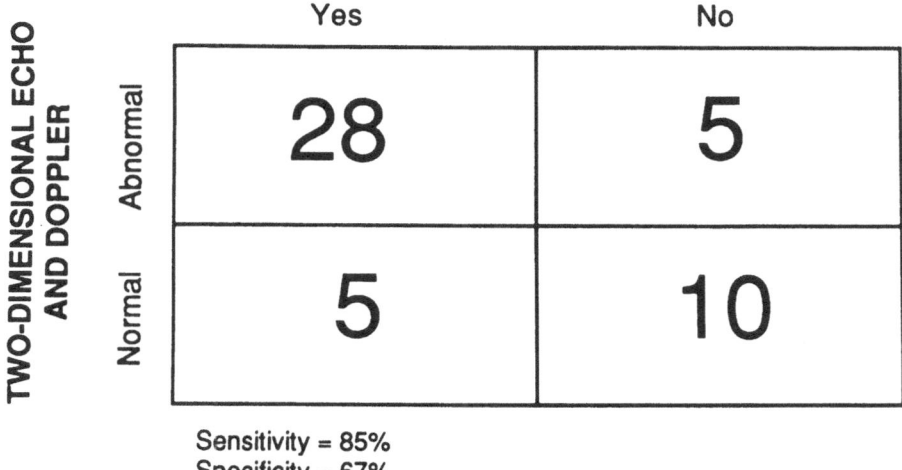

Figure 8. When either 2-dimensional wall motion abnormality by echocardiography or an abnormal Doppler response was found, the presence of CAD was likely. Sensitivity with a combination of these parameters was 85%.

Fifty-five of the patients in the study group underwent cardiac catheterization. Three patients had technically inadequate thallium scans and three had technically inadequate Doppler echocardiographic studies. Correlative data was therefore available in the remaining 94 patients.

Table 1 summarizes the baseline parameters in patients with negative and positive thallium scans. Although those with abnormal thallium scans were significantly older, there was no difference in the Doppler echocardiographic parameters of acceleration, velocity and ejection fraction prior to dipyridamole infusion. Following IV dipyridamole, however, there was a marked difference in these parameters between the two groups. Those with thallium evidence of ischemia showed a blunted response in each of these three parameters while those with normal thallium scans demonstrated increases in velocity, acceleration and ejection fraction of 26, 51 and 16% respectively (all $p < 0.05$) (Figure 5).

In the 55 patients who underwent cardiac catheterization, 15 were found to have normal coronary arteries, 14 single and 26 multivessel disease. Only the percent change in acceleration (57 versus 7, $p < 0.01$) was significantly different in patients with normal or abnormal coronary anatomy. This was due to a large extent to the individual variability among patients. Many patients with single vessel coronary disease had changes in their Doppler echocardiographic parameters similar to patients with normal coronary arteries. Thallium perfusion imaging, likewise, showed a decreased sensitivity in patients with single vessel coronary artery disease.

13.4 Multivessel coronary disease

The differences in the Doppler echocardiographic parameters were much greater when patients were stratified according to the presence of multivessel disease (Figure 6). Two-dimensional segmental wall motion analysis revealed that in the 33 patients with significant coronary artery disease, 12 had normal wall motion (Figure 7). Of the 15 patients without significant coronary artery disease, three had abnormal segmental wall motion. However, when either abnormal Doppler results (a decrease in peak velocity or acceleration following dipyridamole), or abnormal two-dimensional echocardiographic results were combined, the sensitivity of cardiac ultrasound in the detection of significant coronary artery disease increased to 85% (Figure 8).

Previous studies examining the use of two-dimensional echocardiography alone following intravenous dipyridamole have shown the technique to be relatively insensitive but highly specific for the detection of coronary artery disease. Not surprisingly, the sensitivity of this technique increases proportionately with the degree of stenosed coronary arteries and has been reported to be in the range of 37, 71 and 100% for single, double and triple vessel coronary artery disease respectively.

The present study demonstrates significant differences in aortic flow velocities following intravenous dipyridamole in patients with normal versus abnormal thallium perfusion. These differences are most marked in patients with multivessel coronary artery disease. The combination of Doppler and two-dimensional echocardiographic results appear to increase the sensitivity of cardiac ultrasound in the detection of coronary artery disease following intravenous dipyridamole. Importantly, the technique appears to be widely applicable in that technically adequate images can be obtained in the vast majority of patients studied in contrast to exercise studies in which technically difficult post exercise image acquisition remains a significant problem.

13.5 Summary

Few data are available examining the use of 'pharmacologic' stress testing in patients with suspected coronary artery disease utilizing Doppler echocardiography. This remains a promising area in which Doppler echocardiography may be applied in the detection and assessment of coronary artery disease, particularly in patients unable to exercise and in laboratories or offices in which radionuclide capabilities are not present. Further studies are needed to assess the effects of a variety of other pharmacologic agents including beta blockers and inotropic drugs in this patient population.

References

1. Light H. Transcutaneous aortovelography. British Heart Journal 1976; 38:433–442.
2. Huntsman LL, Gams E, Johnson CC, Fairbanks E. Transcutaneous determination of aortic blood flow velocities in man. Am Heart J 1975; 89:605–612.
3. Angelsen BAJ, Brubakk AO. Transcutaneous measurement of blood flow velocity in the human aorta. Cardiovasc Res 1976; 10:368–379.
4. Steiningart RM, Meller J, Barovick J, Patterson R, Herman MV, Teichholz LE. Pulsed Doppler echocardiographic measurement of beat-to-beat changes in stroke volume in dogs. Circulation 1980; 62:542–548.
5. Magnin PA, Stewart JA, Myers S, VonRamm O, Kisslo JA. Combined Doppler and phased array echocardiographic estimation of cardiac output. Circulation 1981; 63:388–392.
6. Goldberg SJ, Sahn DJ, Allen HD, Valdes-Cruz LM, Hoenecke H, Carnahan Y. Evaluation of pulmonary and systemic blood flow by 2-dimensional Doppler echocardiography using fast fourier transform spectral analysis. Am J Cardiol 1982; 50:1394–1400.
7. Labovitz AJ, Buckingham TA, Habermehl K, Nelson J, Kennedy HL, Williams GA. The effects of sampling site on two-dimensional Echo-Doppler determination of cardiac output. Am Heart J 1985; 109:327–332.
8. Gardin JM, Iseri LT, Elkayam U, Tobis J, Childs W, Burn CS, Henry WL. Evaluation of dilated cardiomyopathy by pulsed Doppler echocardiography. Am Heart J 1983; 106:1057–1065.
9. Sabbah HN, Khaja F, Brymer JF, McFarland TM, Albert DE, Snyder JE, Goldstein S, Stein PD. Noninvasive evaluation of left ventricular performance based on peak aortic blood acceleration measured with a continuous-wave Doppler velocity meter. Circulation 1986; 74:323–329.
10. Mehta N, Bennett DE. Impaired left ventricular function in acute myocardial infarction

assessed by Doppler measurement of ascending aortic blood velocity and maximum acceleration. Am J Cardiol 1986; 57:1052–1058.

11. Elkayam U, Gardin JM, Berkley R, Hughes CA, Henry WL. The use of Doppler flow velocity measurement to assess the hemodynamic response to vasodilators in patients with heart failure. Circulation 1983; 67:377–383.

12. Rose JS, Nanna M, Rahimtoola SH, Elkayam U, McKay C, Chandraratna PA. Accuracy of determination of changes in cardiac output by transcutaneous continuous-wave Doppler computer. Am J Cardiol 1984; 54:1099–1101.

13. Keren G, Bier A, Strom AJ, Laniado S, Sonnenblick EH, LeJemtel TH. Dynamics of mitral regurgitation during nitroglycerin therapy: A Doppler echocardiographic study. Am Heart J 1986; 112:517–525.

14. Wallmeyer K, Wann LS, Sagar KB, Kalbfleisch J, Klopfenstein HS. The influence of preload and heart rate on Doppler echocardiographic indexes of left ventricular performance: comparison with invasive indexes in an experimental preparation. Circulation 1986; 74:181–186.

15. Harrison MR, Smith MD, Nissen SE, Grayburn PA, DeMaria AN. Use of exercise Doppler echocardiography to evaluate cardiac drugs: effects of Propranolol and Verapamil on aortic blood flow velocity and acceleration. J Am Coll Cardiol 1988; 11:1002–1009.

14. Effects of abrupt coronary occlusion on Doppler ejection dynamics in man

FAREED KHAJA, HANI N. SABBAH, JAMES F. BRYMER, and
PAUL D. STEIN

*Henry Ford Heart and Vascular Institute, 2799 West Grand Boulevard,
Detroit, Michigan 48202, U.S.A.*

In experimental animals, brief periods of acute coronary artery occlusion can result in a marked impairment of regional left ventricular wall function [1–3]. The magnitude of global impairment of left ventricular function that accompanies regional wall motion abnormalities is dependent upon the extent of left ventricular ischemic mass [4]. Recently, with the advent of percutaneous transluminal coronary angioplasty (PTCA), transient occlusion of a coronary artery with the angioplasty balloon provided a model through which regional and global left ventricular function can be assessed in patients during brief periods of myocardial ischemia.

Studies intended for the evaluation of global or regional left ventricular performance during transient ischemia in patients undergoing PTCA must take into account the possible existence of a well developed collateral circulation to the coronary vessel undergoing PTCA. Patients undergoing PTCA are by definition patients with significant coronary artery disease. In such a patient cohort, a considerable number may have well developed collaterals providing sufficient blood supply such that a complete occlusion of a proximal coronary artery will not result in ischemia accompanied by regional myocardial dysfunction. In a recent echocardiographic study, Alam *et al.* reported a lack of regional wall motion abnormalities during coronary occlusion in two of three patients undergoing PTCA in whom coronary collateral filling was present to the coronary artery being dilated [5]. For this very reason, other studies which evaluated regional left ventricular function during angioplasty excluded patients with angiographic evidence of collateral vessels [6, 7].

With this in mind, we examined the effects of abrupt coronary artery occlusion, produced by balloon inflation during PTCA, on Doppler ejection indices of global left ventricular performance [8]. Peak velocity and peak acceleration of blood in the ascending aorta were measured noninvasively with a continuous-wave Doppler velocimeter (ExerDop, Quinton Instruments Co., Seattle, WA) using the suprasternal notch approach. The Doppler velocimeter and its use in patients has been described in detail [9]. Whereas these Doppler indices of global systolic left ventricular function have been shown to be sensitive to regional ischemia in experimental animals [8, 9], their sensitivity to regional ischemia, as it pertains to global left ventricular function in a patient population with coronary artery disease was, until recently, not fully elucidated [8].

Steve M. Teague (ed.) Stress Doppler Echocardiography, 183–190.
© 1990 *Kluwer Academic Publishers.*

14.1 Patient population and study methods

A total of 37 patients undergoing PTCA were entered into the study. Approximately 20% of all eligible patients were excluded because of a poor Doppler signal almost always related to obesity. Among the 37 patients studied, 19 underwent PTCA of the proximal left anterior descending coronary artery, 15 of the right coronary artery and 3 of the proximal circumflex coronary artery. All patients had a subtotal coronary stenosis of the vessel undergoing PTCA. In all patients, the luminal diameter at the stenosis was ≥70%.

Table 1. Hemodynamics, medications, diagnosis and clinical history in patients included in the study. (Modified from Khaja *et al.*, Ref. [8] with permission).

	Patients with collaterals n = 14	Patients without collaterals n = 23
Age (years)	57 ± 10	56 ± 10
Sex		
Male	10	15
Female	4	8
Heart Rate (beats/min)	71 ± 11	69 ± 10
Systolic pressure (mm Hg)	126 ± 21	137 ± 20
Diastolic pressure (mm Hg)	72 ± 10	75 ± 10
History of infarction	7 (50%)	8 (35%)
Diagnosis		
Angina pectoris	5 (36%)	9 (39%)
Unstable angina	5 (36%)	10 (43%)
Post infarction angina	4 (29%)	4 (17%)
Beta blockers or calcium channel blockers	12 (86%)	23 (100%)
Chest pain during occlusion	5 (36%)	17 (74%)
ECG changes during occlusion	4 (29%)	18 (78%)
Number of diseased vessels		
1 vessel	7 (50%)	13 (67%)
2 vessels	5 (30%)	8 (35%)
3 vessels	2 (14%)	2 (9%)
Vessel dilated		
LAD	4 (29%)	15 (65%)
CIRC	1 (7%)	2 (9%)
RCA	9 (64%)	6 (26%)

LAD = left anterior descending coronary artery; CIRC = circumflex coronary artery; RCA = right coronary artery.

In each patient selective coronary arteriography was performed prior to PTCA and was used to assess the presence or absence of existing collateral vessels supplying the coronary artery to undergo PTCA. Coronary collaterals, when present, were graded as follows: 0 = none, 1 = filling of side branches without visualization of the epicardial segment, 2 = partial filling of the epicardial segment, 3 = complete filling of the epicardial segment by collateral flow [10]. Patients were divided into two groups based on the presence or absence of existing collateral vessels. Group I consisted of 23 patients without collaterals. Group II consisted of 14 patients with collaterals. In this group, 6 patients had grade 1 collaterals, 4 had grade 2, and 4 patients had grade 3 collaterals.

In each patient, coronary occlusion was maintained for a period of at least 40 sec (range 40–57 sec). Lead II of the electrocardiogram was recorded continuously and was used to identify ischemic changes during coronary occlusion. Each patient was also queried as to whether he or she experienced chest pain during the period when the balloon was inflated. The hemodynamics, medications and clinical history in the two groups of patients are shown in Table 1. Doppler measurements were made continuously in each patient beginning 10 to 30 seconds before balloon inflation and ending approximately one minute after balloon deflation. Because of beat-to-beat variability of the Doppler parameters [11], and for statistical purposes, data in each patient were averaged over a period of 10 sec during the preocclusion period (baseline), the occlusion period and the reperfusion period. During the occlusion and reperfusion periods, the 30 to 40 sec time period was selected for averaging.

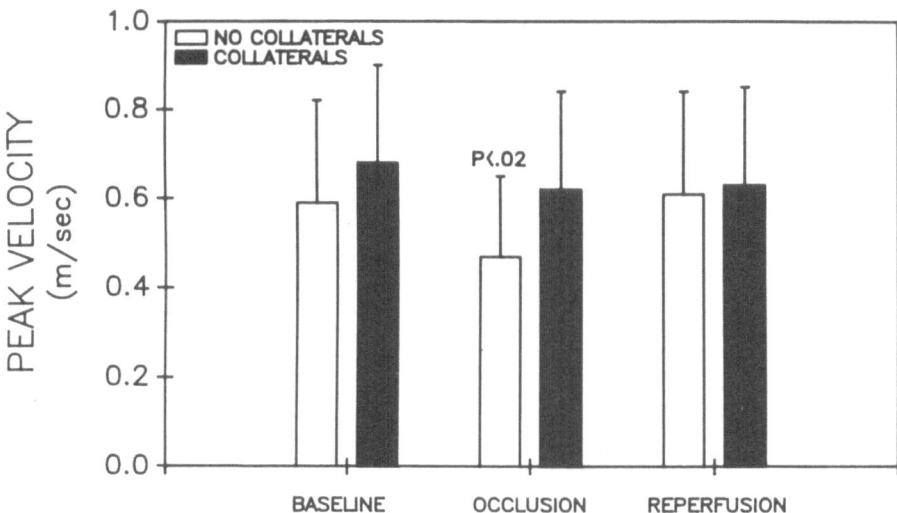

Figure 1. Bar graph denoting mean ± STD of peak velocity prior to coronary occlusion (Baseline), 30 to 40 seconds after balloon inflation (Occlusion) and 30 to 40 seconds after balloon deflation (Reperfusion). The changes of peak velocity are shown for patients without collateral vessels (open bars) and patients with pre-existing collateral vessels (solid bars) which supply the coronary artery undergoing angioplasty.

186

14.2 Observations in patients without collaterals (Group I)

In this group of patients, peak velocity was 0.59 ± 0.23 m/sec at baseline, decreased to 0.47 ± 0.18 m/sec during coronary occlusion ($P < 0.02$) and returned to preocclusion levels (0.61 ± 0.23 m/sec) 30 to 40 seconds after reperfusion (balloon deflation) (Figure 1). An example of the time course of change of phasic blood velocity during coronary occlusion and reperfusion in a patient without collaterals is shown

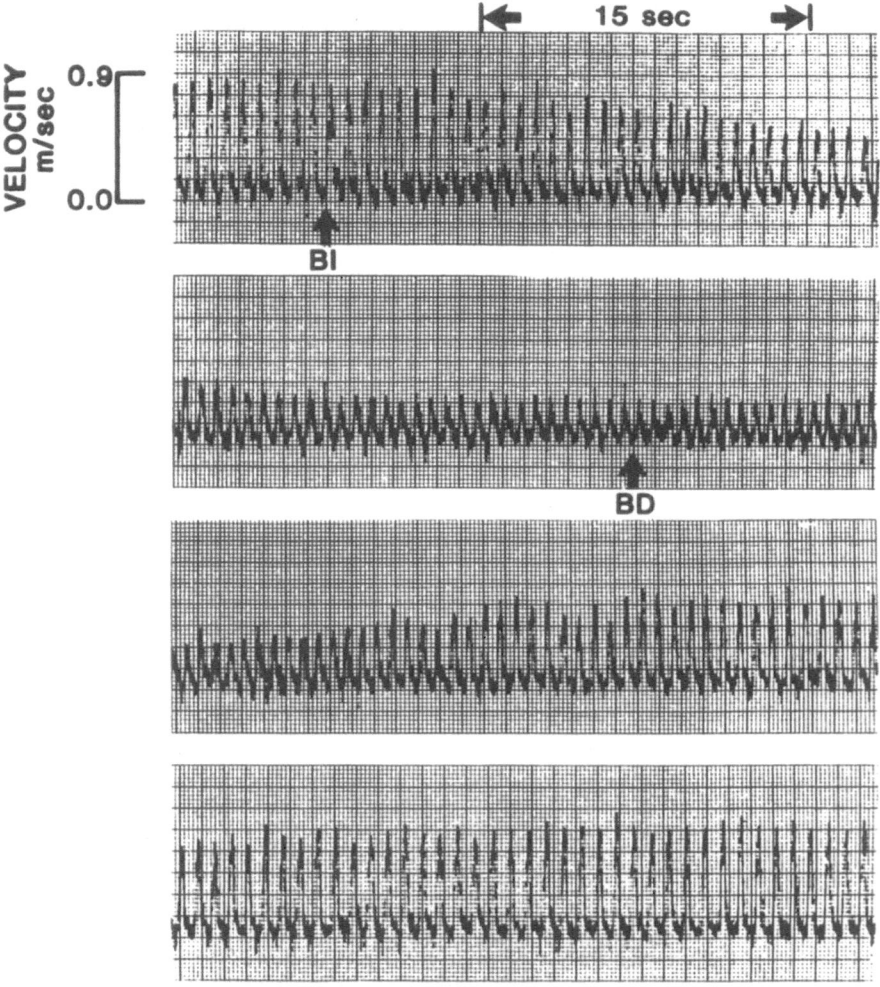

Figure 2. Continuous recording of phasic aortic blood velocity in a patient without collaterals supplying the coronary artery undergoing angioplasty. First arrow (top panel) indicated onset of balloon inflation (BI). Second arrow indicates onset of balloon deflation (BD). Note reduction of peak velocity during coronary occlusion and its recovery during reperfusion. (Reproduced from Khaja *et al.*, Ref. [8], with permission).

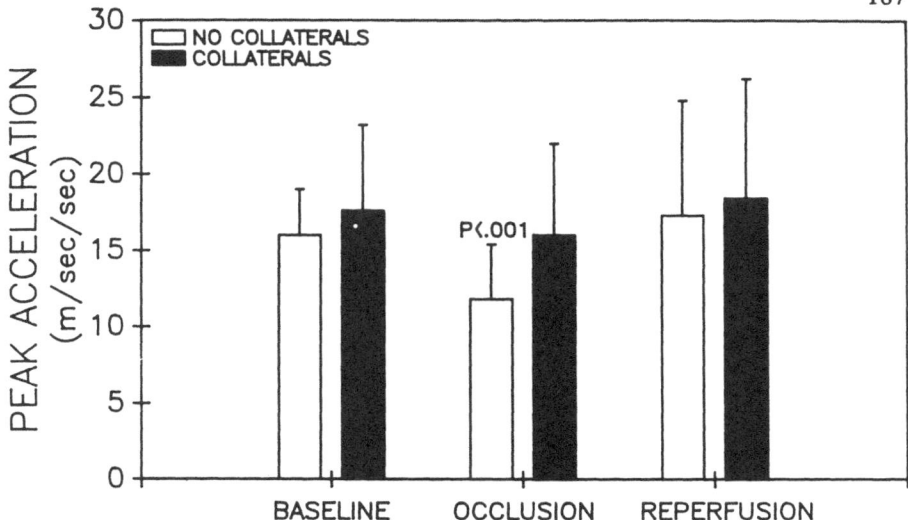

Figure 3. Bar graph denoting mean ± STD of peak acceleration prior to coronary occlusion (Baseline), 30 to 40 seconds after balloon inflation (Occlusion) and 30 to 40 seconds after balloon deflation (Reperfusion). The changes of peak acceleration are shown for patients without collateral vessels (open bars) and patients with collateral vessels (solid bars).

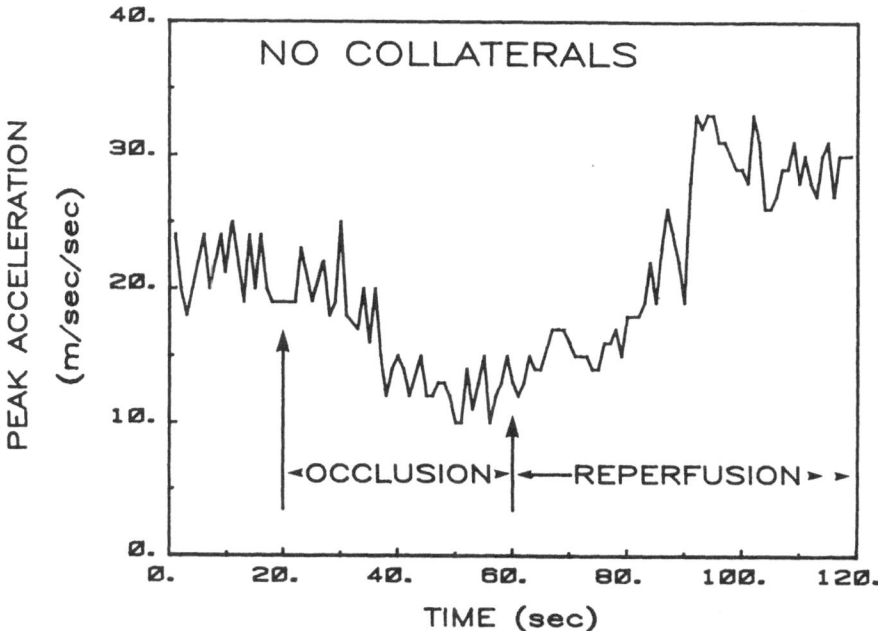

Figure 4. Time course of change of peak acceleration during coronary occlusion and reperfusion in a patient without collaterals supplying the coronary artery undergoing angioplasty. Note the reduction of peak acceleration during coronary occlusion and overshoot of peak acceleration during reperfusion. (Reproduced from Khaja *et al.*, Ref. [8], with permission).

in Figure 2. Peak acceleration in this group was 16.0 ± 3.0 m/sec/sec at baseline, decreased to 11.8 ± 3.6 m/sec/sec during coronary occlusion ($P < 0.001$) and returned to near preocclusion levels (17.3 ± 7.5 m/sec/sec) 30 to 40 seconds after reperfusion (Figure 3). An example of the time course of change of peak acceleration during coronary occlusion and reperfusion is shown in Figure 4. In this group of patients, reductions of peak velocity and peak acceleration during coronary occlusion were accompanied, in general, by electrocardiographic (ECG) changes compatible with ischemia. Among the 23 patients without collaterals, 18 (78%) had ischemic ECG changes and 17 (74%) had chest pain of varying severity during coronary occlusion.

Among the 23 patients without collaterals, 8 had a previous history of a myocardial infarction. In these patients, peak acceleration at baseline was significantly lower than in patients without a history of infarction (14.3 ± 2.0 vs. 17.0 ± 3.2 m/sec/sec) ($P < 0.05$). During coronary occlusion, peak acceleration decreased to 10.7 ± 2.9 m/sec/sec in patients with infarction in comparison to 12.5 ± 3.9 m/sec/sec in patients without infarction. Even though the percent reduction of peak acceleration during coronary occlusion relative to baseline was the same in these two subgroups, on an absolute scale, peak acceleration declined to lower levels in the infarction group. This suggests a greater reduction of global left ventricular function during abrupt coronary occlusion if underlying segmental wall dysfunction is present.

14.3 Observations in patients with collaterals (Group II)

In this group of 14 patients, peak velocity was 0.68 ± 0.22 m/sec at baseline. Peak velocity remained relatively unchanged during coronary occlusion (0.62 ± 0.22 m/sec) and reperfusion (0.63 ± 0.22 m/sec) (Figure 1). Peak acceleration was 17.6 ± 5.6 m/sec/sec at baseline and also remained relatively unchanged during coronary occlusion (16.0 ± 6.0 m/sec/sec) and reperfusion (18.4 ± 7.8 m/sec/sec) (Figure 3). An example of the time course of change of peak acceleration during coronary occlusion and reperfusion in a patient without collaterals is shown in Figure 5.

14.4 Discussion of findings

The above observations clearly indicate that in patients with coronary artery disease without pre-existing collateral vessels, abrupt coronary occlusion can lead to a profound compromise of global left ventricular performance. In contradistinction, in patients with collateral vessels to the coronary artery undergoing angioplasty, left ventricular function is preserved during transient coronary occlusion. Preservation of global left ventricular function in the presence of collateral vessels appeared, in our study, to be independent of the degree of collateral filling. This unexpected observation can be explained on the basis of the work of Rentrop *et al.* who demonstrated improved collateral channel filling during coronary occlusion

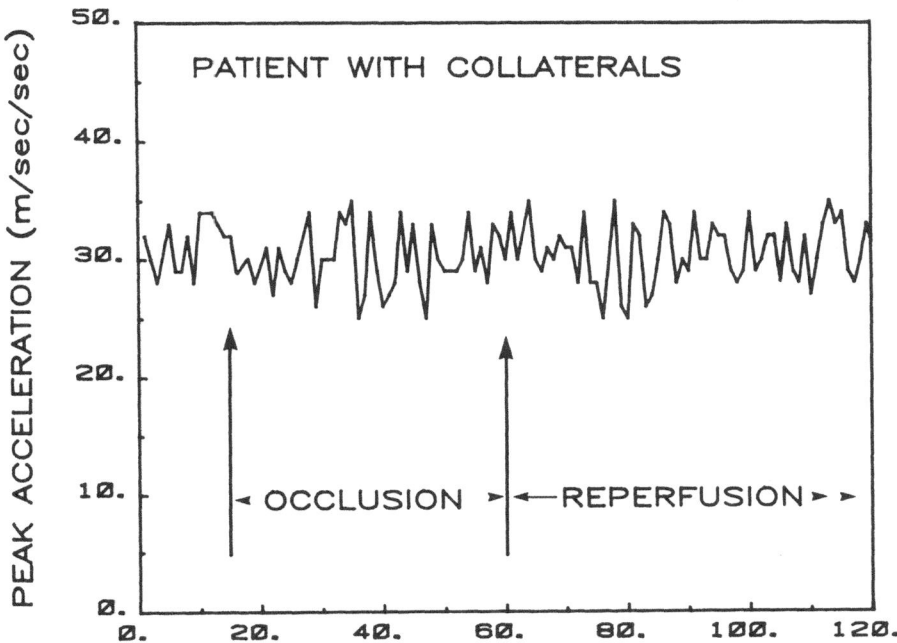

Figure 5. Time course of change of peak acceleration during coronary occlusion and reperfusion in a patient with collaterals supplying the coronary artery undergoing angioplasty. Note unchanged level of peak acceleration during coronary occlusion and reperfusion relative to preocclusion level. (Reproduced from Khaja *et al.*, Ref. [8], with permission).

[10]. In a study of 16 patients undergoing PTCA, collateral filling to the vessel undergoing angioplasty increased by one grade in 8 patients, by 2 grades in 5 patients, by 3 grades in two patients and remained unchanged relative to baseline in only one patient.

The observed depression of global left ventricular performance during brief periods of coronary occlusion in the absence of collateral vessels is consistent with observations by others [5,6,11–14]. Studies with 2-dimensional and M-mode echocardiography demonstrated regional left ventricular wall motion abnormalities during coronary occlusion in patients undergoing PTCA [5,6,11]. Under similar circumstances, others demonstrated a reduction of the peak rate of change of pressure (dP/dt) during coronary occlusion [13]. In a larger group of patients, Serruys *et al.* showed a gradual reduction of both peak dP/dt and left ventricular ejection fraction 20 to 50 seconds after occlusion of a coronary artery with the angioplasty balloon [12].

The data presented in this chapter are compatible with previous findings in laboratory animals; namely Doppler ejection indices of global left ventricular performance are sensitive to the presence of regional myocardial ischemia [4]. In applying these indices as adjuncts to the detection of coronary artery disease in patients, as with treadmill exercise testing, the user must be aware of two factors that can have a profound effect on the outcome of such measurements. First, preexisting collateral vessels and the potential recruitment of collaterals under conditions which increase myocardial oxygen demands may minimize the severity of ischemia and lead to no change of Doppler ejection indices even though coronary artery disease may be present. Second, if coronary disease promotes ischemia to a relatively small region, appropriate compensation by the residual normal myocardium will act to minimize global depression of left ventricular function [4].

References

1. Theroux, P, Franklin D, Ross J, Jr, Kemper WS. Regional myocardial function during coronary artery occlusion and its modification by pharmacologic agents in the dog. Circ Res 1974; 35:396–908.
2. Sabbah HN, Stein PD. Relation of intramyocardial and intracavitary pressure to regional myocardial asynergy in the canine left ventricle. Am Heart J 1983; 105:380–386.
3. Goldstein S, de Jong JW. Changes in left ventricular wall dimensions during regional myocardial ischemia. Am J Cardiol 1974; 34:56–62.
4. Sabbah HN, Przybylski J, Albert D, Stein PD. Peak aortic blood acceleration reflects the extent of left ventricular ischemic mass at risk. Am Heart J 1987; 113:885–890.
5. Alam M, Khaja F, Brymer J, Marzilli M, Goldstein S. Echocardiographic evaluation of left ventricular function during coronary angioplasty. Am J Cardiol 1986; 57:20–25.
6. Wohlgelernter D, Cleman M, Highman HA, Fetterman RC, Duncan JS, Zaret BL, Jaffe CC. Regional myocardial dysfunction during coronary angioplasty: Evaluation by two dimensional echocardiography and 12 lead electrocardiography. J Am Coll Cardiol 1986; 7:1245–1254.
7. Serruys PW, Wijns W, van den Brand M, Slager C, Schuurbiers JCH, Hugenholtz PG, Brower RW. Left ventricular function during transluminal angioplasty: a hemodynamic and angiographic study. Acta Med Scand 1984; 694:197–206.
8. Khaja F, Sabbah HN, Brymer JF, Stein PD. Influence of coronary collaterals on left ventricular function in patients undergoing coronary angioplasty. Am Heart J 1988; 116:1174–1180.
9. Sabbah HN, Khaja F, Brymer JF, McFarland TM, Albert DE, Snyder JE, Goldstein S, Stein PD. Noninvasive evaluation of left ventricular performance based on peak aortic blood acceleration measured with a continuous-wave Doppler velocity meter. Circulation 1986; 74:323–329.
10. Rentrop KP, Cohen M, Blanke H, Phillips RA. Changes in collateral channel filling immediately after controlled coronary occlusion by an angioplasty balloon in human subjects. J Am Coll Cardiol 1985; 5:587–592.
11. Hauser AM, Gangadharan V, Ramos RG, Gordon S, Timmins GC, Dudlets P. Sequence of mechanical, electrocardiographic and clinical effects of repeated coronary artery occlusion in human beings: Echocardiographic observations during coronary angioplasty. J Am Coll Cardiol 1985; 5:193–197.
12. Serruys PW, Wijns W, van den Brand M, Slager C, Schuurbiers JCH, Hugenholtz PG, Brower RW. Left ventricular performance, regional blood flow, wall motion, and lactate metabolism during transluminal angioplasty. Circulation 1984; 70:25–36.
13. Rothman MT, Baim DS, Simpson JB, Harrison DC. Coronary hemodynamics during percutaneous transluminal coronary angioplasty. Am J Cardiol 1982; 49:1615–1622.
14. Voyles WF, Anderson JL, Teague SM, Prasad R, Olson E, Schechter E, Thadani U. Abrupt coronary occlusion and left ventricular ejection during coronary angioplasty. Am J Noninvas Cardiol 1989; 3:125–130.

15. Doppler ultrasound assessment of left ventricular function – Risk stratification in acute myocardial infarction

NAWZER MEHTA and DAVID BENNETT

Department of Medicine 1, St. George's Hospital Medical School, London, England

15.1 Summary

Velocity ejection variables derived from Doppler ultrasonic interrogation of the ascending aorta were obtained in 92 acute myocardial infarction (AMI) patients and 73 age-matched normal subjects. As a means of stratifying for further risk assessment the AMI patients were divided into clinically defined Forrester subsets, and into survivors and non-survivors of the acute infarction period.

AMI patients had a 32% lower peak velocity, a 37% lower maximum acceleration ($p \leq 0.001$), a 49% lower systolic velocity integral ($p \leq 0.001$), and a 13% higher heart rate than the age-matched normal subjects ($p \leq 0.01$). Systolic velocity integral, peak velocity and maximum acceleration all showed a systematic significant decrease through the Forrester subsets ($p \leq 0.001$, $p \leq 0.001$ and $p \leq 0.001$ respectively), and were also significantly different between the survivor and non-survivor groups ($p \leq 0.01$, $p \leq 0.05$ and $p \leq 0.05$ respectively).

Thus, the non-invasive measurement of ascending aortic blood velocity and acceleration allows rapid assessment of left ventricular function, and provides indices closely related to the patients' clinical status, and subsequent risk of mortality: These observations underline the potential of the Doppler technique in the prognosis and subsequent management of myocardial infarction patients.

15.2 Introduction

Classically the diagnosis of acute myocardial infarction (AMI) and its subsequent progression has been by monitoring of clinical signs, such as the presence of hypotension, tachycardia, confusion, cyanosis, oliguria and abnormal electrocardiograms and chest X-rays. More recently, Forrester *et al.* (1977) [1], have used pulmonary arterial balloon catheter systems [2] to make objective haemodynamic measurements such as pulmonary artery pressure and cardiac output, and have correlated these with the more subjective bedside evaluations which still remain the cornerstone of clinical care. Forrester *et al.* (1977) [1] showed that the classification of AMI patients into recognizable subsets based on haemodynamic cardiac

Steve M. Teague (ed.) Stress Doppler Echocardiography, 191–203.

performance presents an acutely sensitive way of assessing patients at higher risk of subsequent mortality.

The measurement of velocity based indices of LV function to assess the dynamic contractile properties of the heart in ischemic heart disease (IHD) and particularly during AMI, has been assessed by several workers using the invasive electromagnetic catheter tip velocity probe both in dogs and in humans [3–6].

The invasiveness of both pulmonary arterial floatation catheters and electromagnetic catheter-tip velocity probes, and their inherent risks represent an obvious deterrent to their application to large numbers of AMI patients. The use of a non-invasive technique providing LV functional indices as sensitive as those described by Forrester et al. (1977) [1] would, therefore, provide a much more eloquent form of assessing these patients. Despite the obvious advantages of Doppler ultrasound to this application, very few studies have assessed Doppler velocity ejection measurements in the setting of AMI. Light and co-workers, during the initial evaluation of 'transcutaneous aortovelography', anecdotally documented aortic velocity (PV and SVI) information in groups of subjects (never numbering greater than 20 patients) suffering from myocardial infarction [7–8]. However, no systematic documentation of velocity measurements were presented in these earlier studies. Indeed no systematic study evaluating Doppler velocity indices in AMI existed in the literature prior to the initial publication of the data collection presented in this chapter [9].

15.3 Aims

The present study was undertaken to establish the normal range for the variables maximum acceleration peak velocity and systolic velocity integral. In particular, our aim was to determine whether Doppler velocity ejection indices could distinguish patients with AMI from age-matched normal subjects. In addition, we hoped to assess the usefulness of our Doppler velocity ejection indices in the setting of AMI, by relating velocity indices to clinical variables, and ascertaining the relative ability of the Doppler technique to detect patients at higher risk of mortality.

15.4 Materials and methods

A) Equipment

We have used a continuous-wave, bi-directional Doppler blood velocity meter (Bach-Simpson BVM 202, London, Ontario), transmitting ultrasound at a frequency of 2.2 MHz and receiving back-scattered frequencies from a distance of 6–14 cm from the transducer head. We have previously tested and documented the frequency response of this unit [10].

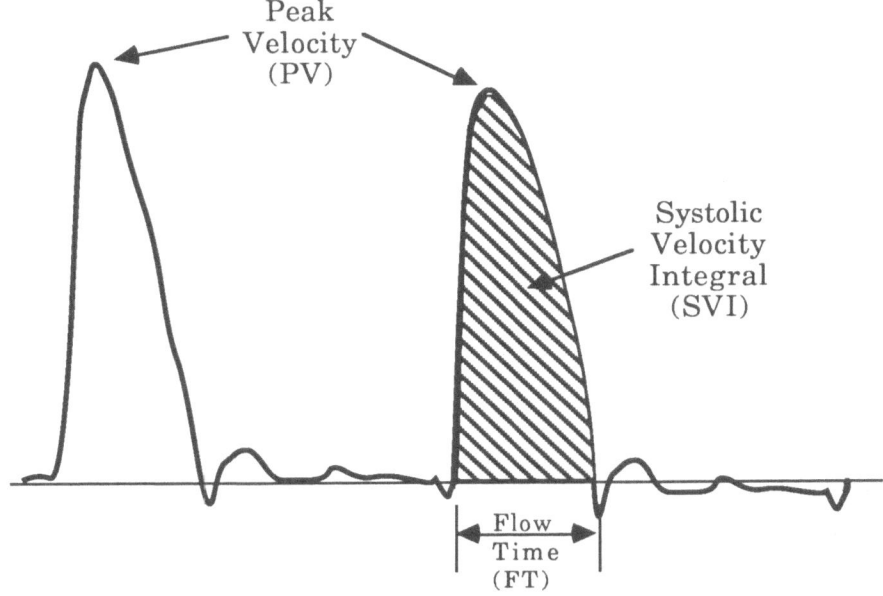

Figure 1. Diagrammatic representation of a typical ascending aortic velocity signal, showing derivation of Doppler ejection variables.

B) Signal analysis and derivation of Doppler ejection variables

The analogue voltage velocity signal (Figure 1) from the Bach-Simpson velocity meter is 'fed' to an analogue to digital converter under processor control (Signetics 2650 processor) which samples the signal at 250 Hz. The microprocessor is programmed to present 6 velocity ejection parameters; – peak velocity (PV), flow time (FT), maximum acceleration (MA), systolic velocity integral (SVI), mean (time-averaged) velocity (MV) and heart rate (HR), as a beat-by-beat digital display on a visual display unit, and to print these results as an average of every 10 beats. To account for any respiratory variation on the velocity parameters, which is particularly important in patients, the results presented here are an average of 50 consecutive beats. The detailed specifications of this equipment are described by Mehta N (1987) [11]. The peak velocity measured in $cm.s^{-1}$ represents the highest velocity achieved during systole. Maximum acceleration (1st differential of velocity) represents the greatest rate of rise of the velocity signal during the initial 30–50 msecs of systole, and is measured in $m.s^2$. The systolic velocity integral (the integral of velocity) is the area under the systolic portion of the velocity signal (see Figure 1) and represents the forward distance travelled by the blood during any particular systolic phase, as such it is measured in units of distance – centimetres (cm). The flow time (FT) is measured in milliseconds (ms) and represents the time over which forward velocity is occurring. The mean or time-averaged velocity (MV) is the SVI represented per unit of time (second), and thus accounts for differences in heart rate. While the SVI is a Doppler correlate of ejected volume, the MV is a Doppler correlate of flow, as shown by the following two equations.

$$\text{Volume} \quad = \quad \text{SVI} \quad \times \quad \text{Aortic Root Area} \qquad (1)$$
$$(\text{cm}^3) \qquad\qquad (\text{cm}) \qquad\qquad (\text{cm}^2)$$

$$\text{Flow} \quad = \quad \text{MV} \quad \times \quad \text{Aortic Root Area} \qquad (2)$$
$$(\text{cm}^3.\text{s}) \qquad\qquad (\text{cm.s}) \qquad\qquad (\text{cm}^2)$$

C) Signal acquisition

The Doppler transducer was placed in the suprasternal notch to obtain signals from the ascending aorta, and positioned to gain optimal velocity signals as adjudged by a combination of acoustic and visual feedback (the analogue voltage output of the Doppler instrument being monitored on an oscilloscope). The operator aims at obtaining the highest peak velocity signal which is associated with the loudest and clearest audio signal, thus ensuring that the ultrasound beam is aligned to within 0–20° of the long axis of the aorta. This form of signal acquisition is consistent with previous methodology [10]. The process of signal acquisition takes approximately 1–5 minutes, however, once the signal is optimized it is relatively easy to maintain this position.

D) Study groups

(i) Normal subjects
In order to compare Doppler velocity ejection data collected in the AMI patient group to that obtained in normal subjects, we studied 73 'normal' subjects. These normal subjects consisted of 35 males and 38 females, with a mean age of 56 ± 10 years (range 40–75 years), which in terms of age distribution represented an age-matched normal control group comparable to the AMI patient population (see Table 1). The normal population was recruited from the waiting room of the Accident and Emergency (A&E) ward, and consisted of relatives of people attending the A&E ward. Thus our normal population consisted of subjects unused to the hospital environment and of a similar anxious state of mind as that found in the majority of our AMI patients. Doppler measurements were made in the same semi-supine position (10° upper body-tilt) as that found in AMI patients.

(ii) AMI patients
167 patients were studied between the period October 1981 and November 1983 in the Intensive Therapy Unit (ITU) of St. George's Hospital. Doppler velocity signals

were obtained in the supine or semi-supine (10–15° upper body tilt) positions. All measurements were performed by one observer, and obtained within 0–18 hours (mean 8 hours) after admission to the ITU. Good quality velocity signals were obtained in 97% of these patients. Routine clinical data (blood pressure, 12-lead ECG, cardiac enzymes, peripheral temperature, pulse rate, respiratory rate, previous history) were all noted at the time of Doppler measurements, with all data computerized to aid information storage and retrieval.

Table 1. Demographic and clinical details of total AMI group, and AMI subsets. Peak enzyme levels have units µmol.ml.

| | AMI Total | Forrester subsets | | | Mortality subsets | | Normals |
		I	II	IV	Survivors	Non-sur-vivors	
N	92	45	21	20	78	14	73
Age (±1 SD)	61 ± 9	58 ± 10	65 ± 8	64 ± 10	61 ± 10	61 ± 11	56 ± 10
Sex							
Male	75	40	19	15	63	12	35
Female	17	5	2	5	15	2	38
Infarct Site							
Anterior	48	21	10	15	38	10	–
Inferior	41	21	11	5	37	4	–
Lateral	2	2	–	–	2	–	–
Peak Enzyme Level							
AST	209	187	205	271	191	303	–
HBD	689	666	748	742	658	852	–

AST: Aspartate Transaminase (normal < 30 I.U./L).
HBD: Alpha Hydroxy Buteric Dehydrogenase (normal > 0–230 I.U.).

Only data obtained in patients with documented AMI were subsequently analysed. AMI was established by predefined criteria requiring the presence of 2 of the following: (a) history of angina-like pain lasting greater than 15 minutes and unrelieved by nitrates; (b) development of new ECG Q-waves, in conjunction with evolutionary ST-T wave changes; (c) elevation of both serum (AST) Aspartate Transaminase and (HBD) Alpha Hydroxy Buteric Dehydrogenase levels above the upper limits of normals. In addition, patients with clinical, radiological or echocardiographic signs of aortic valve abnormalities were excluded from the study. 92 of 167 patients satisfied the above criteria. Details of this 'total' patient population are summarized in Table 1. Whilst Table 2 shows the percentage distribution of the 5 main drug regimens (anti-arrhythmic, β-blockade, diuretic, inotropic & vasodilator) within the total population.

Table 2. Percentage distribution of the five main drug regimens within the total AMI group and subsets.

	Total AMI Group	Forrester subsets I	II	IV	Mortality subsets Survivors	Non-survivors
Antidys-rhythmic	26%	33%	14%	30%	23%	43%
β-blockade	13%	18%	10%	5%	13%	7%
Diuretics	20%	9%	29%	40%	13%	50%
Inotropes	23%	4%	24%	60%	18%	50%
Vasodilators	67%	58%	81%	75%	67%	71%

(iii) AMI subset classification

(a) Clinical subsets. Classification of patients into readily recognizable subsets is of major clinical usefulness, since it has diagnostic, prognostic and therapeutic relevance for the management of patients with AMI. Forrester *et al.* (1977) [1] identified four distinct subsets, the fundamental assumption of their classification being that depression of Starling function is the direct cause of clinical manifestations of heart failure in AMI [12], i.e., increased LV end-diastolic pressure (LVEDP) results in pulmonary congestion and depressed cardiac output causes clinical signs of peripheral hypoperfusion.

Clinical pulmonary congestion was considered to be present if patients demonstrated both radiographic and auscultatory pulmonary congestion. Clinical peripheral hypoperfusion was identified by the presence of at least two of the following conditions: (a) a skin temperature of less than 32°C (measured on the foot by a skin temperature probe), (b) arterial hypotension as defined by a systolic pressure of less than 100 mmHg, (c) sinus tachycardia as defined by a heart rate greater than 100 b.min^{-1}.

Accordingly, four clinical subsets were identified as follows:

Subset   I – no pulmonary congestion or peripheral hypoperfusion,
Subset   II – pulmonary congestion only,
Subset III – hypoperfusion only,
Subset IV – both pulmonary congestion & peripheral hypoperfusion.

Table 1 defines the details of the patients populations in each of these clinical subsets. Subsets were analysed only if numbers were high enough for statistical evaluation (8 or more). Subset III did not fulfil that criteria in our patient population and so this subset was excluded from further analysis.

Table 2 identifies the percentage distribution of the 5 main drug regimens within the Forrester subsets.

(b) Mortality subsets. We identified two further subsets in our AMI patient population, based on mortality during the acute in-hospital phase (10 days). Table 1 includes details of these two mortality subsets, and indicates that 14 patients died during this acute phase. Table 2 indicates the percentage distribution of the 5 main

drug regimens in the two mortality subsets.

E) Statistical analysis

Unpaired Student-t tests or analysis of variance with multiple comparisons using Fisher's PLSD test, were utilized to assess the differences between groups ($p \leq 0.05$ being considered statistically significant). Chi-square analysis was used to determine significant differences in number distributions between subsets.

15.5 Results

Table 1 shows the clinical and demographic details of the total AMI population and its subsets. Although Forrester subset I had a lower mean age than either subsets II or IV, this was not significant, the age distributions being similar in all three subsets. The proportion of males was always greater than females in all subsets.

Analysis of infarction site indicated that there was an equal distribution of anterior and inferior infarctions in the total group. Forrester subsets I and II also had an equal distribution of anterior and inferior infarctions, however, subset IV had significantly greater anterior than inferior infarctions ($p \leq 0.05$). Similarly, non-survivors had significantly greater anterior infarctions than inferior ($p \leq 0.05$).

Analysis of the peak enzyme levels showed a systematic increase in enzyme levels from subset I to IV, with the difference in AST between subset I and IV, and that between survivors and non-survivors being statistically significant ($p \leq 0.05$). HBD levels were also higher in the non-surviving group, but this difference was not significant. Table 2 shows the percentage distribution of the 5 main drug regimens used in the treatment of AMI. Vasodilators were used in almost 70% of the patients, and the distribution among all the subsets was equal. Two further points emerge, namely that diuretics and inotropic agents were used in a greater proportion of subset IV patients and similarly, in a greater proportion of non-surviving patients.

Table 3. Doppler velocity data (mean ±SEM) in age-matched normal subjects and AMI patients. Statistical significance denotes differences between the two groups.

	Normals	AMI	Significance
PV (cm.s^{-1})	52.1 ± 1.0	35.3 ± 0.8	$p \leq 0.001$
MA (m.s^{-2})	19.1 ± 0.4	12.0 ± 0.3	$p \leq 0.001$
SVI (cm)	9.0 ± 0.2	4.6 ± 0.2	$p \leq 0.001$
MV (cm.s^{-1})	10.3 ± 0.3	6.0 ± 0.2	$p \leq 0.001$
FT (ms)	333 ± 5.5	243 ± 6.2	$p \leq 0.001$
HR (b.min^{-1})	73.2 ± 1.7	82.3 ± 2.3	$p \leq 0.01$

Table 4. Doppler velocity data and mortality rate in Forrester subsets. Mean values (±SEM) and statistical significance (NS=not significant).

	Forrester subsets			Significance		
	I	II	IV	IvsII	IvsIV	IIvsIV
PV (cm.s^{-1})	39.2 ± 1.1	33.9 ± 1.4	30.1 ± 1.7	p ≤ 0.01	p ≤ 0.001	NS
MA (m.s^{-2})	12.7 ± 0.3	11.7 ± 0.6	10.6 ± 0.4	NS	p ≤ 0.001	NS
SVI (cm)	5.4 ± 0.2	4.3 ± 0.3	3.2 ± 0.3	p ≤ 0.01	p ≤ 0.001	p ≤ 0.01
MV (cm.s^{-1})	6.6 ± 0.2	5.6 ± 0.3	5.1 ± 0.5	p ≤ 0.05	p ≤ 0.01	NS
FT (ms)	256 ± 8	235 ± 14	202 ± 8	NS	p ≤ 0.001	p ≤ 0.05
HR (b.min^{-1})	75.6 ± 2.5	80.0 ± 4.5	98.8 ± 5.7	NS	p ≤ 0.001	p ≤ 0.01
MAP (mmHg)	92.4 ± 1.9	93.9 ± 2.2	72.2 ± 3.4	NS	p ≤ 0.001	p ≤ 0.001
% Mortality	2%	0%	65%			
PV/HR	0.55 ± .03	0.45 ± .03	0.33 ± .03	p ≤ 0.05	p ≤ 0.001	p ≤ 0.05
MA/HR	0.18 ± .01	0.16 ± .01	0.12 ± .01	NS	p ≤ 0.001	p ≤ 0.05
SVI/HR	0.08 ± .01	0.06 ± .01	0.04 ± .004	p ≤ 0.05	p ≤ 0.001	p ≤ 0.05
FT/HR	3.7 ± 0.3	3.2 ± 0.3	2.3 ± 0.2	NS	p ≤ 0.01	p ≤ 0.05

Table 3 shows the results of Doppler velocity variables in the total AMI population compared to age-matched normal subjects, as mean values ±SEM. The statistical significance is also noted. All Doppler velocity ejection variables are significantly lower in the AMI population than in normal subjects, which is consistent with the impairment in LV function due to AMI. MA and SVI showed the greatest differences, with MA being 37% lower in AMI patients and SVI being 49% lower partially as a result of the 12% higher HR.

Table 4 shows the results of Doppler velocity variables in the Forrester subsets I, II and IV, as mean values ± SEM. The statistical significances between the groups are also indicated. Thus, all Doppler variables show a stepwise decrease through the Forrester subsets, indicating a fall in LV function despite a rising HR due to a compensatory increase in sympathetic drive [13]. Analysis of variance using multiple comparisons testing, indicated that all Doppler variables were significantly different between subsets I and IV, whilst SVI was significantly different between all the subsets. The poorer LV function in subset IV is confirmed by the higher level of mortality in this subset.

The significant differences in HR and MAP are not unexpected since Forrester's clinical separation uses HR and systolic BP as inherent variables in the classification. The differences in HR, particularly in subset IV are due to a reflex increase in sympathetic tone as the heart compensates for the fall in LV function due to myocardial infarction. To account for this reflex, we normalized the Doppler variables PV, MA, SVI and FT for the differences in HR by calculating the ratio (Doppler variable ÷ HR).

Clearly, if HR was higher in subset IV than in subset I or II, irrespective of a change in LV contractile state, then SVI and FT would be lower, since both these variables are negatively correlated with HR. Thus, when these two variables are normalized for HR, the marked differences are not as apparent, and a fall in significance levels is noted. However, HR is higher in subset IV because of a compensatory increase in sympathetic tone, this would clearly tend to increase MA and PV, because an increase in sympathetic state increases LV contractility. When these two Doppler variables are normalized for HR, they show more dramatic differences between the Forrester subsets. MA, for example, was 17% lower in subset IV when compared to subset I; however, when normalized for HR (MA/HR) it was 33% lower in subset IV when compared to subset I. In addition, whilst MA or PV could not statistically distinguish between subsets II and IV, the ratios MA/HR and PV/HR showed significant differences between the subsets. The percentage mortality data shown in Table 4 indicates that Forrester subset IV represents a high risk category, whilst subsets I and II represent low-risk categories.

Table 5. Doppler velocity data in mortality subsets. Mean values (±SEM) and statistical significance.

	Mortality subsets		Significance
	Survivors	Non-survivors	
PV (cm.s^{-1})	36.1 ± 0.9	31.0 ± 2.3	$p \leq 0.05$
MA (m.s^{-2})	12.2 ± 0.3	10.5 ± 0.4	$p \leq 0.05$
SVI (cm)	4.8 ± 0.2	3.5 ± 0.4	$p \leq 0.01$
MV (cm.s^{-1})	6.0 ± 0.2	5.7 ± 0.7	NS
FT (ms)	249 ± 7	213 ± 12	$p \leq 0.05$
HR (b.min^{-1})	78.8 ± 2.4	102.1 ± 4.3	$p \leq 0.001$
PV/HR	$0.50 \pm .02$	$0.31 \pm .02$	$p \leq 0.001$
MA/HR	$0.17 \pm .01$	$0.11 \pm .01$	$p \leq 0.001$
SVI/HR	$0.07 \pm .01$	$0.04 \pm .01$	$p \leq 0.01$
FT/HR	3.5 ± 0.2	2.2 ± 0.2	$p \leq 0.01$

Table 5 shows the results of Doppler velocity variables in the mortality subset (survivors and non-survivors), as means ± SEM. The statistical significances between the two groups are also indicated. Thus, all Doppler variables (except MV) are significantly lower in the non-surviving group. MV shows no significant difference, because HR is significantly higher due to augmented sympathetic tone. Normalizing the Doppler variables PV, MA, SVI and FT for the difference in HR, causes all Doppler variables to be even more significantly different between the two subsets.

Figures 2 and 3 summarize the data already presented by plotting the 3 Doppler variables which have provided the greatest discrimination between the subsets studied. Figure 2 clearly indicates the ability of the Doppler variables MA and SVI to gauge differing levels of LV dysfunction. Figure 3 takes the same format as that of Figure 2, but plots the data for PV against SVI.

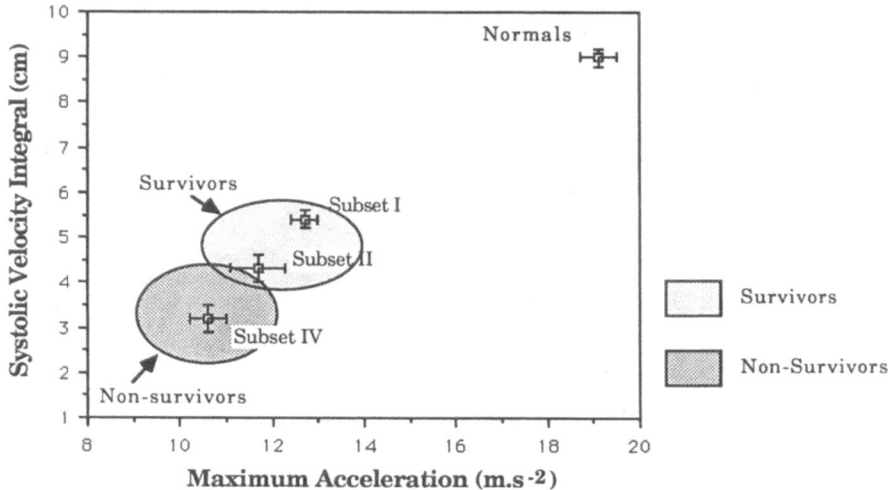

Figure 2. Scatterplot of MA vs SVI showing mean values ±SEM for normals and AMI Forrester subsets. Survivors and non-survivor data is superimposed as an area covering the mean value ±95% confidence intervals.

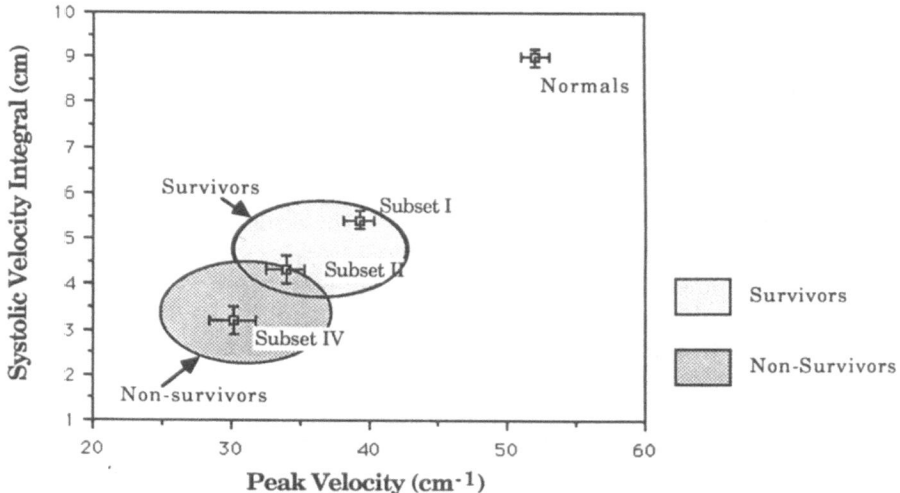

Figure 3. Scatterplot of PV vs SVI showing mean values ±SEM for normals and AMI Forrester subsets. Survivors and non-survivor data is superimposed as areas covering the mean value ±95% confidence intervals.

15.6 Discussion

A number of workers have shown that age is inversely related to the Doppler velocity variables MA and PV [14–15]. Thus, we age-matched our normal subjects, and established that there were no differences in age between the Forrester and mortality subsets (see Table 1).

Similarly, a number of workers have also shown that the Doppler variables MA and PV are significantly higher in males than in females [11, 14]. Although the distribution of males and females in the normal group was equal (35 vs 38), it was clearly not so in the AMI patient population. The differences between normals and AMI patients could then be partially attributed to this discrepancy in the distribution of the sexes. However, since more males are present in the AMI group, the mean values obtained in this group are higher than if the distribution were more equal. Clearly if similar gender distributions were maintained between these the normal and AMI groups, the differences in Doppler values of MA and PV would have been greater than the already highly significant differences shown in Table 3.

The Forrester classification was used in our study in order to determine the ability of the Doppler velocity variables to distinguish between patients with increasing levels of LV dysfunction. SVI represented the velocity variable with greatest discriminating power, being significantly different between all Forrester subsets. This is not surprising since SVI is dependent upon HR, and HR is an inherent factor in the Forrester classification. However, SVI reflects changes in both LV contractility and chronotropic influences. MA and PV (the two Doppler indices of contractility) showed a stepwise fall through the subsets, but only showed significant differences between subsets I and IV. It should be noted, however, that a greater percentage of subset II and IV patients were receiving inotropic support. This would tend to 'artificially' elevate MA and PV values in these subsets. It is clear, however, that despite the greater inotropic support and higher intrinsic level of sympathetic tone present in subset IV patients, these patients still have poorer LV function than their subset I counterparts, as indicated by the significantly lower Doppler values. Indeed the poorer LV function is reflected in the higher percentage mortality present in subset IV. This level of mortality is similar to that found by Forrester.

Finally it should be noted that the discriminating function of Doppler variables within the setting of clinical classification is best described in the situation where no concurrent drug therapy is administered, as was the case in Forrester's original work. The concurrent drug therapy in the AMI group would variously affect the Doppler variables [11, 16]. However, it is difficult to specify the relative effects of the drugs because there may be interaction between their influences on the Doppler variables. Some important influences should be noted, however:

(a) β-blockade would tend to reduce values of the Doppler variables MA and PV, whilst increasing SVI [11, 16]. However, only 13% of the total AMI group were beta-blocked and is therefore unlikely to affect the Doppler results within the various subsets;

(b) Similarly, diuretics and inotropes were present in only 20 and 23% of the total AMI group, respectively. Importantly however, a higher percentage of subset IV patients and non-survivors received inotropic support, which is in keeping with the therapeutic regime administered to these high-risk subsets with gross LV failure and cardiogenic shock [17]. This would tend to increase the mean values of the Doppler variables PV, MA and SVI [10–11] in these groups, above what would be expected in these patients without such pharmacological interventions;

(c) Vasodilators were by far the most commonly used therapeutic regime in the AMI group (67%). Vasodilatation in the setting of acute heart failure tends to increase stroke volume [18]. Thus SVI, our Doppler index of stroke volume, is higher in subset IV and non-surviving patients than would be expected if no vasodilator therapy were being used.

The significantly lower Doppler values in non-survivors of AMI found in our study is in keeping with previous literature. Jewitt *et al.* (1974) [6], studied 14 patients with myocardial infarction with an invasive electromagnetic catheter-tip system, and divided this group into survivors and non-survivors of the acute infarction period. They measured MA and PV and found these two variables to be significantly lower in the non-surviving group. Indeed they find very little overlap between the groups in terms of either PV or MA. They present no mean data on their mortality groups, but quote '...velocity measurements below 40 cm/s and maximum acceleration values below 7 m/s^2 were not associated with survival.' Although our data is not as distinct as that found by Jewitt *et al.* [6] in their limited study, the results are strikingly similar.

15.7 Conclusions

This study has established the usefulness of Doppler velocity measurements within the setting of AMI, by showing that a single non-invasive measure of ascending aortic blood velocity within 18 hours of admission can clearly differentiate those patients with AMI from age-matched normal subjects; and more importantly, that this one measure of velocity provides information related to both clinical status and subsequent prognosis.

References

1. Forrester JS, Diamond GA, Swan HJC. Correlative classification of clinical and haemodynamic function after acute myocardial infarction. Am J Cardiol 1977; 39:137–145.
2. Swan HJC, Ganz W, Forrester JS, Marcus H, Diamond G, Chonette D. Catheterization in the heart in man with use of flow directed balloon tipped catheter. N Engl J Med 1970; 283:447–451.
3. Bennett ED, Else W, Miller GHH, Sutton GC, Miller HC, Noble MIM. Maximum

acceleration of blood from the left ventricle in patients with ischaemic heart disease. Clin Sci 1974; 46:49–59.

4. Kezdi P, Stanley EL, Marshall WJ, Kordenat RK. Aortic flow velocity and acceleration as an index of ventricular performance during myocardial infarction. Am J Med Sci 1969; 257:61–71.

5. Kolettis M, Jenkins BS, Webb-Peploe MM. Assessment of left ventricular function derived from aortic flow velocity. Br Heart J 1976; 38:18–31.

6. Jewitt D, Gabe I, Mills CJ, Maurer B, Thomas M, Shillingford J. Aortic velocity and acceleration measurements in the assessment of coronary heart disease. Eur J Cardiol 1974; 1:299–305.

7. Light LH. Transcutaneous aortovelography. A new window on the circulation? Br Heart J 1976; 38:433–442.

8. Buchtal A, Hanson GC, Peisach AR. Transcutaneous aortovelography. Potentially useful technique in management of critically-ill patients. Br Heart J 1976; 38:451–456.

9. Mehta N, Bennett ED. Impaired LV function in acute myocardial infarction (AMI), assessed non-invasively by Doppler ultrasound. Clin Sci 1984; 67:6P (abstract).

10. Bennett ED, Barclay S, Davis AL, Mannering D, Mehta N. Ascending aortic blood velocity and acceleration using Doppler ultrasound in the assessment of left ventricular function. Cardiovascular Res 1984; 18:632–638.

11. Mehta N. The non-invasive assessment of left ventricular function by measurement of ascending aortic blood velocity and acceleration using Doppler ultrasound. PHD Thesis, Univ of London 1987; 88–100.

12. Swan HJC, Forrester JS, Diamond G, et al. Hemodynamic spectrum of myocardial infarction and cardiogenic shock: a conceptual model. Circulation 1972; 45:1097–1110.

13. Smith WW, Wikler NS, Fox AC. Haemodynamic studies of patients with myocardial infarction. Circulation 1954; 9:352–359.

14. Mowat DHR, Haites NE, Rawles JM. Aortic blood velocity measurement in healthy adults using a simple ultrasound technique. Cardiovasc Res 1983; 17:75–80.

15. Levy BI, Targett RC, Bardou A, McIlroy MB. Quantitative ascending aortic Doppler blood velocity in normal human subjects. Cardiovasc Res 1985; 19:383–393.

16. Harrison MR, Smith MD, Nissen SE, Grayburn PA, DeMaria AN. Use of exercise Doppler echocardiography to evaluate cardiac drugs: Effects of propranolol and verapamil on aortic blood flow velocity. J Am Coll Cardiol 1988; 19:383–393.

17. Goldberg LI, Dorney ER. Treatment of shock following myocardial infarction. Diverse action of drugs used. Postgrad Med 1965; 37:52–63.

18. Haq A, Rakowski H, Baigrie R, et al. Vasodilator therapy in refractory congestive heart failure: a comparative analysis of haemodynamic and non-invasive studies. Am J Cardiol 1980; 45:665–672.

16. Risk stratification following myocardial infarction using stress Doppler ultrasound

NAWZER MEHTA and DAVID BENNETT

Department of Medicine 1, St. George's Hospital Medical School, London, England

16.1 Summary

We assessed left ventricular (LV) function by Doppler ultrasound measurement of ascending aortic blood velocity and maximum acceleration in 165 patients (3–4 weeks after acute myocardial infarction) undergoing routine 12-lead electrocardiogram exercise stress testing, and in an age-matched group of 11 normal subjects. Patients were grouped into those with either positive or negative electrocardiograph stress tests as defined by ≥ 1mm ST segment depression in any lead. The Doppler velocity signal yields a number of variables of interest – the peak velocity, the maximum acceleration (an index of inotropic state), the systolic velocity integral (an index of stroke volume), and mean velocity (an index of cardiac output). All Doppler ejection variables were significantly lower at peak exercise in patients with a positive electrocardiograph stress test when compared to their negative test counterparts, with maximum acceleration showing most significance ($p \geq 0.001$). Coronary angiography was performed in 63 of the 67 positive test patients and patients were grouped into those with only 1&2 vessel coronary artery disease and those with 3 vessel disease. Peak velocity and maximum acceleration were significantly lower in the 3 vessel patients than in 1&2 vessel patients ($p \geq 0.01$, $p \geq 0.01$).

The ability to measure the LV functional response to exercise, rapidly and non-invasively using the Doppler technique, may provide a useful adjunct to routine exercise stress testing in identifying high mortality risk patients following myocardial infarction.

16.2 Introduction

Identification of non-invasive indices that reflect continuing myocardial ischaemia or marked impairment of left ventricular function has resulted in the development of strategies for assessment of patients following acute myocardial infarction. The principal aim of such strategies is to identify those patients at high risk of cardiac death and in whom myocardial revascularization (principally by coronary artery by-pass surgery) may be warranted. Measurement of ascending blood velocity using Doppler ultrasound has already been shown to be useful in assessing LV function at rest [1–3], but recently a number of workers have shown that it is also possible to apply this technique to the exercising patient [4–6].

Steve M. Teague (ed.) Stress Doppler Echocardiography, 205–218.

16.3 Aims

Our aims concentrated on identifying the value of Doppler velocity ejection variables within the setting of post myocardial infarction exercise stress testing. To that end, we compared Doppler velocity variables in patients with prior myocardial infarction (PMI) agains a comparable group of normal volunteers; secondly, we attempted to identify the relationship between Doppler indices of LV function and the more commonly associated variables obtained during stress testing, namely the presence of electrocardiographic ST segment depression and an inadequate blood pressure response; and lastly, we attempted to relate the changes in Doppler velocity variables to the severity of coronary artery disease.

16.4 Methods and materials

A total of 180 consecutive patients (mean age 59±24 years) were studied between the period November 1983 – July 1985 and enrolled into the myocardial infarction clinic at St. George's Hospital, London, England. All patients had a confirmed myocardial infarction as demonstrated by elevated cardiac enzymes and Q-wave ECG changes. The following exclusion criteria were used for this study:

− patients aged ≥ 70 years;
− patients with unstable angina;
− patients with previous CABG surgery;
− patients with valve replacements or primary valvular disease;
− patients with significant musculo-skeletal disorders (preventing exercise).

Of the 180 patients, 14 were excluded from the study on the basis of inferior or technically inadequate Doppler studies, representing a 8.3% rejection rate. Thus, the results from a total of 166 patients were analysed. Patient demographics are shown in Table 1.

A) Techniques

12-Lead Electrocardiogram (ECG). A conventional 12-lead configuration was used for recording the ECG with the exception of the limb leads which were attached to the four corners of the torso to reduce motion artefact produced by the moving limbs. An abnormal ECG response (positive exercise test) was defined by the presence of ≥ 1mm ST segment depression occurring 80ms after the J-point in any one of the 12 leads monitored (except leads already presenting Q-waves). The time taken to achieve significant ST segment depression (onset time) during the exercise protocol was noted to the nearest half minute.

Blood Pressure. Blood pressure was measured on the right arm using a standard cuff auscultation method. The increase in systolic blood pressure at peak exercise

Table 1. Patient details for the whole PMI group and ischaemic, functional and anatomical subdivisions.

	Total PMI group	Ischaemic division Negative exercise test	Positive exercise test	Functional division Good BP response	Poor BP response	Anatomical division Coronary vessel disease 1	2.	3
N	166 (144M, 22F)	98	68	109	57	21	11	32
MI Site								
Anterior	73	46	27	47	26	10	2	13
Inferior	70	41	32	45	25	9	7	14
Other	23	11	9	17	6	2	2	5
Drugs								
β-blockers	99/166 (60%)	58/98 (59%)	41/68 (60%)	65/109 (60%)	34/57 (59%)	17/21 (81%)	8/11 (73%)	16/32 (50%)
Nitrates	38/166 (23%)	21/98 (21%)	17/68 (25%)	19/109 (17%)	19/57 (33%)	5/21 (20%)	2/11 (18%)	7/32 (22%)
Ca antagonist	21/166 (13%)	10/98 (10%)	11/68 (16%)	9/109 (8%)	12/57 (21%)	2/21 (10%)	2/11 (18%)	5/32 (16%)
Exercise time (min)	5.6 ± 0.2	6.0 ± 0.2 **	5.0 ± 0.3	6.3 ± 0.2	*** 4.3 ± 0.2	6.2 ± 0.5 **	5.4 ± 0.5 **	4.4 ± 0.3
Onset time (min)	--	--	2.9 ± 0.2	--	--	5.3 ± 0.5 **	3.1 ± 0.5 * ***	1.8 ± 0.2
Recovery time (min)	--	--	6.5 ± 0.4	--	--	4.4 ± 0.6 ***	5.7 ± 1.1 ** ***	8.2 ± 0.5
Resting LVEF (%)	--	--	--	--	--	39 ± 3.3	36 ± 2.7	32 ± 2.5

Asterisks represent significant differences between groups.

* = p ≤ 0.05;
** = p ≤ 0.01;
*** = p ≤ 0.001.

was expressed as the percentage increase from the upright resting value. Patients who failed to increase their systolic blood pressure by ≥10% were considered to have a poor blood pressure response.

Doppler. Ascending aortic blood velocity was measured from the supra-sternal notch using a 2.2 MHz continuous-wave Doppler blood velocity meter (Bach-Simpson BVM 202), the characteristics of which we have previously documented [7]. The analogue velocity signal is 'fed' into an analogue to digital converter under microprocessor control (Signetics 2650) which samples the velocity signal at 250Hz (every 4 milliseconds). Dedicated software is then used to compute 6 velocity ejection parameters; peak velocity (PV) in cm.s, flow time (FT) in msecs, maximum acceleration (MA) in m/s^2, systolic velocity integral (SVI) in cm, mean (time-averaged) velocity (MV) in cm/s and heart rate (HR) in beats/min. These variables can be displayed on a beat-by-beat basis in 'real-time' on a video monitor, and are hard-copied to a thermal printer as the average of 10 beats. The Doppler transducer was placed in the supra-sternal notch to obtain signals from the ascending aorta, and positioned to gain optimal signals as judged by a combination of acoustic and visual feedback (Tektronix 7603 oscilloscope), such that the operator aims at obtaining the highest peak signal with the loudest and clearest audio signal. This process of signal acquisition takes approximately 1–5 minutes, but once the signal is optimised it is relatively easy to maintain this position. Blood velocity was monitored at rest and throughout exercise so that optimum position was always maintained, with only the last 40 beats of each exercise stage being analysed and averaged. Signals were obtained by the same observer in all patients. The percentage change from rest to peak exercise for each Doppler variable was calculated subsequently. Good quality Doppler velocity signals were obtainable throughout exercise in 166 out of 180 patients; thus 91% of patients were able to be studied adequately with this technique during exercise.

Exercise Stress Test Protocol. Exercise stress testing was performed as near as possible to three weeks after the acute event in patients who had been discharged from hospital. The stress tests were performed on a Quinton QT3000 (Quinton Instruments Co, Seattle, WA) system comprising an automatic motor driven treadmill, with a dedicated 12-lead ECG recording system. Exercise tests were performed using the symptom limited Bruce protocol [8]. All exercise tests were supervised by qualified medical personnel and full resuscitative equipment and drugs were available.

Following ECG electrode and lead attachment, the patient rested on a bed for about 5 minutes and the test procedure was explained. A 12-lead ECG, blood pressure and Doppler measurements were performed with the patient resting in the supine, and then in the upright position whilst standing astride the treadmill. The treadmill was then started and the patient stepped on in his own time. Timing of the protocol commenced when the patient started walking. Each stage was timed and the Bruce protocol advanced automatically. Three ECG channels were continuously monitored on the oscilloscope. 12-lead ECG, blood pressure and Doppler measurements were recorded at the end of each exercise stage and at peak exercise. Additionally a 12-lead ECG was recorded when evidence of ST segment depression was observed on the monitor.

Exercise was continued until one of the following end points was attained: 1) > 3mm ST segment depression 80ms after the J-point in any lead; 2) a fall in systolic blood pressure of > 10mm Hg below the upright resting value; 3) occurrence of chest pain, dyspnoea, fatigue or dizziness; 4) development of leg cramps. The development of chest pain and ventricular arrhythmias during exercise was noted.

Cardiac Catheterisation. Of the 67 patients who had a positive exercise stress test and/or a poor blood pressure response, 64 underwent subsequent coronary angiography. Multiple views of the coronary arteries were recorded for analysis by a radiologist (blinded to this study) for grading of the severity of coronary artery disease. For the purpose of this analysis each patient was considered to have three major coronary arteries: the left anterior descending (LAD), the left circumflex and the right coronary artery. A coronary artery stenosis of significance was defined by > 70% proximal luminal narrowing in any of the major coronary arteries. Thus patients were classified as having either single, double or triple vessel disease.

B) Patient subsetting

In order to fulfil the aims of this study, it was necessary to ascertain the result on Doppler variables in pre-determined patient subsets. Thus, to assess the effects of ischaemia on the Doppler variables, it was necessary to divide the patients into those without ST segment changes (negative (-ve) or normal test), and those with ST segment depression during exercise (positive (+ve) or abnormal test). The two groups formed by this division we have labeled the 'ischaemic' subsets.

The blood pressure (BP) response is commonly used in conventional stress testing to define a normal from abnormal exercise response. In order to determine the association between the BP response and Doppler velocity ejection variables, we have divided patients into those with a good BP response (> 10mm Hg increase in systolic blood pressure (SBP) from rest to peak exercise) and those patients with a poor BP response (≤ 10mm Hg increase in SBP from rest to peak exercise). The two groups formed by this division are labeled 'functional' subsets.

The relationship of Doppler velocity ejection variables to the severity of disease has been assessed by dividing the 63 patients in whom coronary angiography was performed into those with 1, 2 and 3 vessel disease. The three groups formed by this division we have labeled the 'anatomical' subsets. The details of patients within all the above subdivisions are presented in Table 1.

By way of comparison we have included the results of the 11 normal subjects, in whom we have collected similar exercise responses and who were also β-blocked (since the large majority of our patients were β-blocked (see Table 1)). The results of this normal group are compared against the total patient group.

Table 2. Doppler exercise response in the total PMI patient group and in 11 normal β-blocked subjects. Results are presented as means ±SEM. Asterisks represent significant differences between the groups (*=p ≤ 0.05, ¥=p ≤ 0.001).

	PV	MA	SVI	MV	FT	HR	N
PMI Pts							
Supine	43.9 ± 0.8	16.2 ± 0.3	6.7 ± 0.2	7.5 ± 0.2	297 ± 3.8	73 ± 1.4	166
Standing	40.8 ± 0.7	15.5 ± 0.2	5.9 ± 0.2	7.0 ± 0.2	278 ± 4.1	80 ± 1.5	166
Stage 1	44.4 ± 0.8	18.7 ± 0.3	5.7 ± 0.1	9.6 ± 0.2	258 ± 3.9	110 ± 1.7	166
Stage 2	46.4 ± 1.1	20.4 ± 0.4	5.7 ± 0.2	10.3 ± 0.3	248 ± 4.2	116 ± 2.2	99
Stage 3	49.1 ± 1.9	21.8 ± 0.7	5.8 ± 0.3	11.0 ± 0.6	246 ± 9.5	123 ± 3.3	35
Pk Ex	43.4 ± 0.8	19.5 ± 0.4	5.3 ± 0.1	9.7 ± 0.2	247 ± 3.9	119 ± 1.8	166
Normals							
Supine	56.7 ± 2.8¥	17.1 ± 1.4	9.3 ± 0.4¥	10.3 ± 0.2¥	268 ± 15.0	65 ± 3.2	11
Standing	52.9 ± 2.4¥	16.7 ± 1.2	8.6 ± 0.5¥	10.0 ± 0.4¥	255 ± 18.0	73 ± 3.7	11
Stage 1	65.2 ± 4.6¥	20.6 ± 1.5	9.5 ± 0.8¥	15.8 ± 1.1¥	279 ± 19.0	105 ± 3.7	11
Stage 2	67.5 ± 4.3¥	23.2 ± 2.1*	9.0 ± 0.6¥	16.0 ± 1.0¥	261 ± 16.0	113 ± 2.5	11
Stage 3	66.6 ± 4.3¥	25.4 ± 2.5*	8.4 ± 0.8¥	16.3 ± 1.2¥	256 ± 23.0	128 ± 3.6	11

C) Statistical analysis

Analysis of variance for repeated measures was performed for comparison of variables at the various stages of exercise in each group. The Fishers PLSD test was then applied to test for significance of differences. Independent t-tests were performed for comparison of variables between the different groups identified above.

16.5 Results

Table 2 shows the results of Doppler interrogation studies in the total group of 166 PMI patients during exercise testing 3 weeks post AMI. The mean results of 11 β-blocked normal subjects are included for comparison.

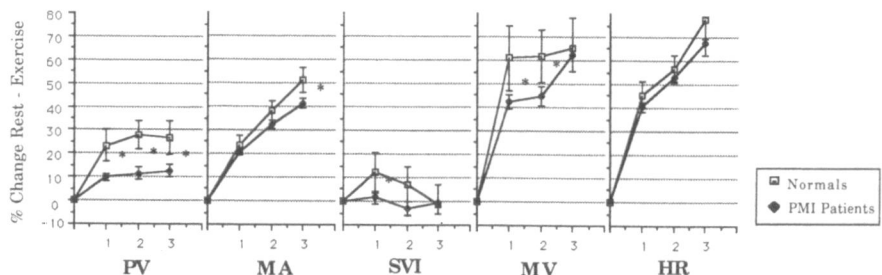

Figure 1. Exercise response of Doppler variables expressed as percentage change (mean ±SEM) from rest to each stage of exercise in normals subjects and PMI patients. Asterisk indicates significance of p ≤ 0.05.

Thus, it can be seen that the resting values for PV, SVI and MV in the PMI group, three weeks after AMI, are still significantly lower than in a group of β-blocked normal subjects. MA shows no significant difference at rest presumably because it is the one Doppler variable most affected by acute β-blockade [7, 9]. The higher values for SVI in the normal group are made up by a significantly higher PV and a slightly longer (but non-significant) ejection time. Although there are no significant differences in HR, the MV is significantly higher in normals due to the higher SVI. The results during exercise indicate again that PV, SVI and MV are significantly higher in normal β-blocked subjects than in PMI patients. MA, although not as significant as the other Doppler variables, is still significantly higher in normals. In order to show the exercise response we have plotted the % increase from upright rest to each stage of exercise for the Doppler variables PV, MA, SVI, MV and HR in both PMI patients and normal subjects. This data is shown in Figure 1 as mean values (±SEM). Clearly, the Doppler exercise response is significantly lower for PMI patients, with PV showing the most dramatic differences between the two groups. These Doppler differences are independent of HR, since there is no significant difference in the HR response in either group.

Table 3. Doppler data within 'ischaemic' subsets (-ve = negative stress tests, +ve = positive stress test (ST segment depression)). Results shown as mean values ±SEM. Asterisks represent significant differences between groups (* = $p \leq 0.05$, *** = $p \leq 0.001$).

		Supine	Standing	1	2	3	PkEx
N	-ve	98	98	98	65 (66%)	25 (26%)	98
	+ve	68	68	68	35 (51%)	10 (15%)	68
PV	-ve	44.1 ± 1.1	41.3 ± 1.0	45.7 ± 1.1	47.7 ± 1.4	49.2 ± 1.1	45.3 ± 1.1*
	+ve	43.6 ± 1.2	40.2 ± 0.9	42.6 ± 1.3	43.9 ± 1.9	48.9 ± 4.1	40.6 ± 1.6
MA	-ve	16.4 ± 0.3	15.7 ± 0.3	19.2 ± 0.4*	21.1 ± 0.5*	22.3 ± 0.7	20.6 ± 0.5***
	+ve	16.2 ± 0.5	15.3 ± 0.3	17.9 ± 0.5	18.9 ± 0.6	20.5 ± 1.3	17.8 ± 0.5
SVI	-ve	6.7 ± 0.3	6.1 ± 0.2	5.9 ± 0.2	5.9 ± 0.2	5.9 ± 0.4	5.6 ± 0.2*
	+ve	6.7 ± 0.2	5.6 ± 0.2	5.4 ± 0.2	5.3 ± 0.3	5.7 ± 0.5	5.0 ± 0.2
MV	-ve	7.5 ± 0.3	7.0 ± 0.2	9.8 ± 0.3	10.6 ± 0.4	11.0 ± 0.7	10.1 ± 0.3*
	+ve	7.6 ± 0.3	7.0 ± 0.2	9.4 ± 0.4	9.8 ± 0.5	11.0 ± 0.9	9.1 ± 0.3
FT	-ve	299 ± 5	280 ± 6	262 ± 5	251 ± 5	247 ± 5	249 ± 5
	+ve	295 ± 5	274 ± 6	252 ± 5	243 ± 6	242 ± 17	245 ± 6
HR	-ve	73 ± 1.9	79 ± 2.0	107 ± 2.2	115 ± 2.6	120 ± 3.6	117 ± 2.3
	+ve	73 ± 2.0	81 ± 2.3	113 ± 2.6	118 ± 3.9	129 ± 7.0	121 ± 2.7

Table 3 shows the Doppler data within the ischaemic subdivisions. Results are shown as mean values ± SEM, with asterisks representing significant differences between the two groups. Neither Doppler velocity ejection variables, nor HR, show any significant difference between the ischaemic subsets at supine or standing rest. However, during exercise, MA is significantly lower at each exercise stage (except at stage 3 where N values drop dramatically) in those patients with an abnormal

212

(+ve) exercise test. In addition, all Doppler variables (except FT) are significantly lower at peak exercise in the +ve test patients. Although this may be partly due to the fact that +ve test patients achieve less exercise (5.0 vs 6.0 mins, p ≤ 0.01), a more physiological explanation is that the exercise induced ischaemia occurring in +ve test patients results in deterioration of LV function, and this is reflected in the significantly lower Doppler values at peak exercise. It is also interesting to note that the decline in LV function is reflected in the significantly smaller number of +ve test patients able to complete exercise stage 3; so that whilst 26% of -ve test patients are able to complete exercise stage 3, only 15% of the +ve test patients are so able. Figure 2 shows the percentage changes from rest to peak exercise for all Doppler variables (except FT) in the ischaemic subsets. Clearly, patients with exercise induced ischaemia have significantly lower exercise responses at peak exercise.

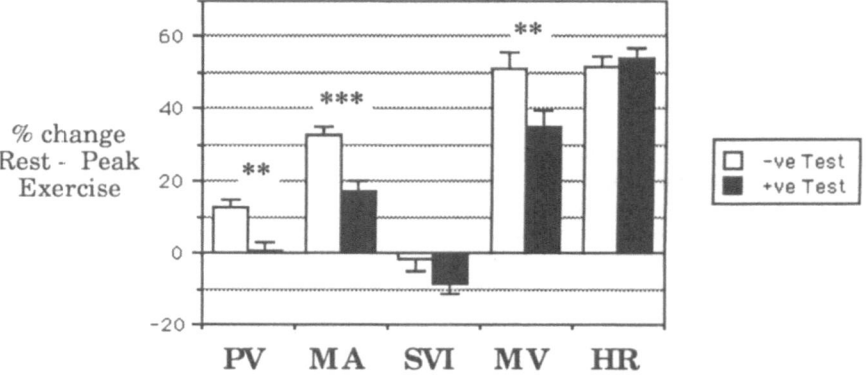

Figure 2. Exercise response of Doppler variable at peak exercise in the 'ischaemic' subsets. Results are shown as mean (≤ SEM) percentage changes between rest and peak exercise. Asterisks indicate the level of significance attained (**=p ≤ 0.01, ***=p ≤ 0.001).

Table 4 shows the results of Doppler studies within the 'functional' subsets, as defined by a good or poor BP response during exercise stress testing. There were no significant differences in Doppler velocity variables or HR at either supine or upright rest. However, during exercise all Doppler variables (except FT) were significantly lower at each stage of exercise in those subjects who exhibited a poor BP response. It should be noted that significant changes were not obtained at stage 3 due to the extremely small sample size in the poor BP group). The deterioration of LV function with each progressive exercise stage in the poor BP responders, is reflected in the extremely small numbers achieving stage 3; only 4% of poor BP responders achieved stage 3 of exercise, whilst almost 10 times more (30%) of the good BP responders achieved the same stage. As a result poor BP responders achieve a significantly lower exercise duration (6.0 vs 4.3 mins, p≤0.001). However, their HR is not significantly lower than their good BP counterparts, implying that poor BP responders in trying to sustain the fall in cardiac output

Table 4. Doppler data within 'functional' subsets. Results shown as mean values ± SEM. Asterisks represent significant differences between groups (* = p ≤ 0.05, **=p≤0.01).

		Supine	Standing	1	2	3	PkEx
N	Good	109	109	109	79 (72%)	33 (30%)	109
	Poor	57	57	57	20 (35%)	2 (4%)	68
PV	Good	44.3 ± 1.0	41.5 ± 0.9	46.0 ± 1.0**	47.5 ± 1.3*	49.5 ± 1.9	45.0 ± 1.0**
	Poor	43.1 ± 1.2	39.6 ± 1.2	41.3 ± 1.4	41.7 ± 2.0	43.9 ± 13.0	40.3 ± 1.3
MA	Good	16.1 ± 0.3	15.4 ± 0.3	19.2 ± 0.4*	20.8 ± 0.4*	21.7 ± 0.6	20.4 ± 0.4***
	Poor	16.7 ± 0.5	15.8 ± 0.5	17.7 ± 0.6	18.7 ± 1.1	23.3 ± 6.4	17.6 ± 0.6
SVI	Good	6.8 ± 0.2	5.9 ± 0.2	5.9 ± 0.2*	5.8 ± 0.2*	5.9 ± 0.3	5.5 ± 0.2
	Poor	6.5 ± 0.3	5.8 ± 0.3	5.3 ± 0.2	5.2 ± 0.3	5.3 ± 1.7	5.1 ± 0.2
MV	Good	7.6 ± 0.2	7.0 ± 0.2	10.1 ± 0.3**	10.6 ± 0.4*	11.0 ± 0.6	10.3 ± 0.3**
	Poor	7.5 ± 0.4	6.9 ± 0.3	8.8 ± 0.3	9.0 ± 0.5	10.7 ± 0.9	8.7 ± 0.3
FT	Good	302 ± 5	279 ± 5	261 ± 5	247 ± 5	241 ± 5	246 ± 5
	Poor	288 ± 6	275 ± 7	252 ± 7	251 ± 8	288 ± 46	250 ± 7
HR	Good	73 ± 1.7	80 ± 1.9	109 ± 2.0	117 ± 2.4	121 ± 3.1	121 ± 2.1
	Poor	73 ± 2.4	81 ± 2.5	110 ± 3.1	112 ± 5.1	145 ± 28.0	114 ± 3.1

Table 5. Doppler data within 'anatomical' subsets, defined as 1, 2 and 3 vessels diseased (VD). Results shown as mean values ±SEM. Asterisks represent significant differences between groups 1 and 3 (* = p ≤ 0.05).

		Supine	Standing	1	2	3	PkEx
N	1 VD	21	21	21	13(62%)	8 (38%)	21
	2 VD	11	11	11	7 (64%)	1 (9%)	11
	3 VD	32	32	32	13 (41%)	3 (9%)	32
PV	1 VD	48.2 ± 1.9	44.9 ± 1.8	48.7 ± 2.7	48.7 ± 3.8	53.4 ± 4.3	46.6 ± 2.8
	2 VD	44.1 ± 2.1	42.9 ± 2.8	44.9 ± 3.9	45.2 ± 3.7	46.4 ± --	43.6 ± 3.4
	3 VD	44.1 ± 1.9	39.9 ± 1.4	41.0 ± 1.7*	42.5 ± 2.8	49.3 ± 5.9	40.3 ± 1.3*
MA	1 VD	17.1 ± 0.7	15.7 ± 0.7	19.2 ± 0.7	20.5 ± 0.8	21.6 ± 1.5	19.7 ± 0.9
	2 VD	16.8 ± 0.7	15.6 ± 0.5	19.0 ± 1.5	19.9 ± 1.7	20.1 ± --	19.9 ± 1.4
	3 VD	16.5 ± 0.8	15.4 ± 0.6	17.1 ± 0.7*	18.9 ± 1.3	22.8 ± 4.0	17.0 ± 0.7*
SVI	1 VD	7.1 ± 0.4	6.0 ± 0.3	6.2 ± 0.4	5.6 ± 0.5	5.7 ± 1.4	5.5 ± 0.3
	2 VD	7.0 ± 0.5	6.3 ± 0.6	5.8 ± 0.5	6.0 ± 0.7	7.5 ± --	5.4 ± 0.5
	3 VD	6.5 ± 0.3	5.5 ± 0.3	5.2 ± 0.3	5.0 ± 0.3	5.4 ± 0.5	4.8 ± 0.3
MV	1 VD	7.6 ± 0.5	6.8 ± 0.4	10.1 ± 0.6	10.2 ± 0.8	11.6 ± 0.7	10.2 ± 0.6
	2 VD	7.2 ± 0.5	7.4 ± 0.8	10.2 ± 0.2	11.6 ± 1.8	15.3 ± --	10.0 ± 1.3
	3 VD	7.8 ± 0.5	7.0 ± 0.3	9.2 ± 0.5	9.1 ± 0.7	11.7 ± 1.1	8.9 ± 0.5
FT	1 VD	300 ± 10	277 ± 9	262 ± 10	238 ± 9	235 ± 13	246 ± 9
	2 VD	303 ± 14	283 ± 17	257 ± 13	269 ± 14	258 ± --	253 ± 15
	3 VD	284 ± 6	271 ± 9	248 ± 6	244 ± 12	268 ± 10	246 ± 10
HR	1 VD	68 ± 4	74 ± 4	105 ± 5	115 ± 8	128 ± 8	118 ± 6
	2 VD	65 ± 4	76 ± 6	111 ± 8	118 ± 10	114 ± --	122 ± 7
	3 VD	77 ± 3	83 ± 3	115 ± 4	117 ± 5	138 ± 11	120 ± 4

(associated with deteriorating LV function) increase their HR above values expected for the level of exercise they achieve. Clearly, the significantly lower MV at peak exercise in the poor BP responders would be lower still, if it were not for the fact that HR was being sustained at a higher level. The results in Table 4 reveal that the significantly lower value for MV in the poor responders at peak exercise is the result of a significantly attenuated contractile response as shown by the Doppler variables PV and MA. Figure 3 shows these changes in Doppler variables by plotting the percentage change from rest to peak exercise in the two functional subsets.

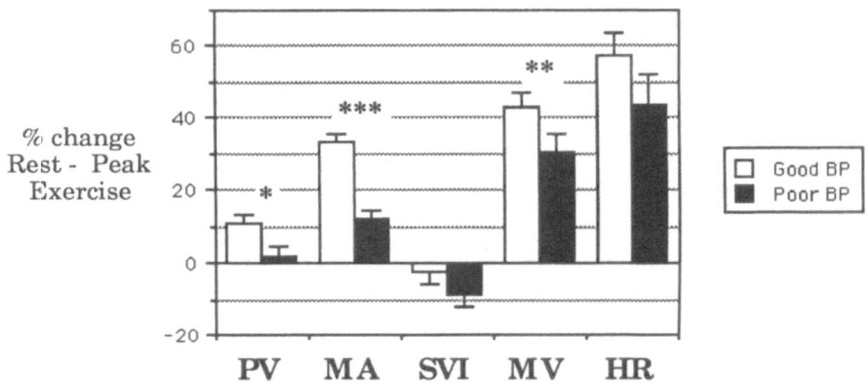

Figure 3. Exercise response of Doppler variable at peak exercise in the 'functional' subsets. Results are shown as mean (±SEM) percentage changes between rest and peak exercise. Asterisks indicate the level of significance attained (**=p ≤ 0.01, ***=p ≤ 0.001).

Table 5 documents the results of Doppler velocity variables within the 3 anatomical subsets defined by the severity of coronary artery disease. There was no association between severity of disease and Doppler velocity variables at either supine or upright rest. This was confirmed by the fact that LVEF (obtained at rest during coronary angiography) also failed to show any association (see Table 1). During exercise, only PV and MA show any statistical differences between the three groups, being significantly higher in 1 vessel disease patients than in patients with 3 vessel disease. Although SVI and MV showed no differences, it was striking to note that both 1 and 2 vessel disease patients appeared to have similar mean values for these two variables, whilst 3 vessel disease patients had lower values, though these differences were non-significant.

With the premise that 3 vessel disease patients presented a high risk subset and 1&2 vessel disease patients were a low risk subset, we re-analysed the data by combining 1&2 vessel disease patients into single group and compared their data to the 3 vessel disease patients. This re-analysis reveals SVI (6.1 vs 5.2 cm, p ≤ 0.05) and MV (10.2 vs 9.2 cm/s, p ≤ 0.05) to be significantly higher at stage 1 of exercise in those patients with less severe disease. This trend in SVI and MV was also apparent at peak exercise, where SVI was 5.5 vs 4.8 cm (p ≤ 0.05) and MV was 10.2

vs 8.9 cm/s (p ≤ 0.05). PV and MA were also significantly different at peak exercise. These changes are more readily seen in Figure 4, where we have plotted the percentage changes from rest to peak exercise in the combined 1&2 vessel subset against the 3 vessel subset. As can be seen the HR response between the two subsets is not significantly different, although 1&2 vessel disease patients achieve a slightly higher HR due to the fact that they achieve significantly more exercise (5.9 vs 4.5 mins, p ≤ 0.01). PV showed hardly any change at peak exercise and this was reflected in the falls in SVI. MA, however, showed a significantly better response in those patients with less severe disease, presumably reflecting the greater degree of LV function in these patients. This is corroborated by the significantly better MV response in the 1&2 vessel disease patients, indicating that these patients are better able to augment cardiac output during exercise than their counterparts with more severe disease.

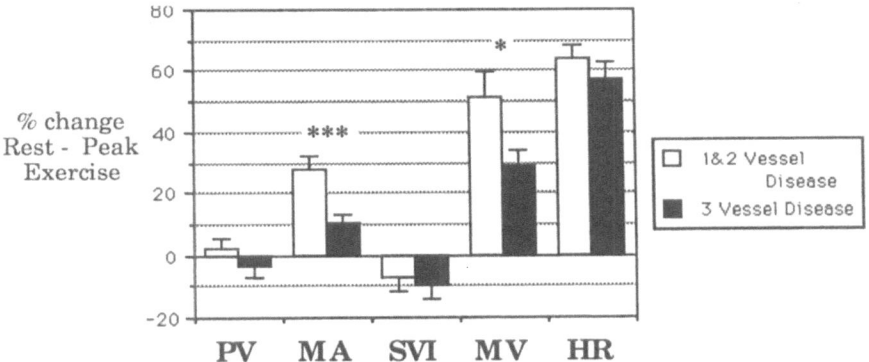

Figure 4. Exercise response of Doppler variable at peak exercise in the newly defined 'anatomical' subsets (1&2 vessel disease and 3 vessel disease). Results are shown as mean (±SEM) percentage changes between rest and peak exercise. Asterisks indicate the level of significance attained (**=p ≤ 0.01, ***=p ≤ 0.001).

As with the ischaemic and functional subsets, the anatomical subsets achieved varying levels of exercise (see Table 1), and this again is reflected in the disparity in numbers of each group reaching stage 2 and 3 of exercise. Thus, whilst 62% and 64% of 1 and 2 vessel disease patients achieve stage 2, only 41% of 3 vessel disease patients do similarly. This disparity is continued and becomes more apparent at stage 3 of exercise.

16.6 Discussion

This study shows that the LV functional response to exercise can be assessed with ease, rapidity and great accuracy in the majority of patients (91%) undergoing treadmill exercise stress testing 3 weeks after acute myocardial infarction, using a simple, non-invasive Doppler ultrasonic technique.

The evaluation of global left ventricular function during exercise is a useful technique to assist in distinguishing normal subjects from patients with CAD. To that end we have described Doppler velocity variables both at rest and during exercise in normal subjects and patients 3 weeks after acute MI, and shown that there was a significant difference in all Doppler variables between these two groups. These differences were independent of HR, since HR was similar between the two groups. Similar findings have also been documented by other workers using Doppler ultrasound [4, 10–11]. Thus, the findings of our study and those of other workers using Doppler are in agreement with the more recognized literature using radionuclide ventriculography [12–14], who also show significant differences in exercise LVEF between normal subjects and patients with CAD.

The finding that Doppler velocity variables were significantly different between patients with and without ST segment depression, has not been previously documented by other workers. The fact that most of the Doppler variables were only significantly different at peak exercise could be partially attributed to the differences in exercise time between these two subsets. However, MA was significantly lower in positive test patients at exercise stages I and II, implying that ventricular contractility is impaired in the ischaemic ventricle. Recently, Sabbah *et al.* (1987) have shown in an experimental dog preparation that peak velocity and acceleration are severely compromised by the induction of acute regional ischaemia, as long as the ischaemic mass was greater than 20% of the total LV mass [15]. These same workers have also shown that peak velocity and particularly maximum acceleration were severely reduced during the acute coronary occlusion induced during the course of percutaneous coronary angioplasty in patients [16]. Thus, Doppler velocity variables present an invaluable tool in the investigation of patients prone to exercise induced ischaemia.

The finding that Doppler velocity variables were significantly lower in patients who exhibited a poor BP response during exercise was not altogether unexpected, since an unchanged or frankly hypotensive response during exercise has long been used to indicate an impairment in LV function [17]. Importantly, however, we have shown an association between the BP response and Doppler velocity variables during exercise, and have been able to document LV functional impairment in more quantitative terms using Doppler velocity variables.

Within the protocol of the Infarction Clinic at St. George's Hospital, only patients with a positive exercise test underwent catheterisation, and as such our anatomical subset consisted of only 39% of the overall study group (64/166). Within this subset, we have shown that patients with 1 and 2 vessel disease have a significantly better haemodynamic response at peak exercise than their 3 vessel disease counterparts. This is in keeping with literature using radionuclide angiography to assess LV haemodynamics during exercise [13–14]. Nicod *et al.* (1983) observed that in 16 patients with single vessel disease LVEF increased by 2%, whilst 26 patients with multi-vessel disease decreased LVEF by 6%, this being a statistically significant difference [14].

Mehdirad *et al.* (1987) have used Doppler ultrasound to study 14 subjects with

CAD, and extrapolation from their raw data shows that patients with 1 vessel disease had a better % rest-to-exercise response than their counterparts with multivessel disease, though again lack of sample size prevents any statistical observations [11]. Bryg *et al.* (1986) used the same Doppler equipment as that described by Mehdirad *et al.* (1987), but were unable to obtain high quality signals during exercise. They do, however, document the percent change from rest to immediately post-exercise and show that the response of eight 1 vessel disease patients is markedly different from that obtained in nine multi-vessel disease patients [10]. Both groups of workers were, however, unable to measure acceleration from their 'spectrally' derived velocity signal.

There were certain logistic and technical limitations in the study described here. Firstly, we made no attempt to account for the effect of β-blockade. However, analysis of the percentage of patients receiving β-blockade therapy (see Table 1) indicate a similar distribution within each of the subsets described in this study. Thus whilst β-blockade undoubtedly affects the resting HR and therefore SVI, this effect is likely to exist in all the subsets with equal degree.

A second limitation was the difficulty of obtaining velocity signals during treadmill exercising. Ascending aortic velocity signals are undoubtedly harder to obtain during treadmill exercise, since motion artefacts become more prominent during exercise. Thus, the number of patients in whom adequate velocity signals are obtained throughout exercise falls (9% of patients were lost due to this factor). More importantly, motion artefacts cause collection of muted, low-amplitude signals which could result in false-positive responses. Although signals with poor signal to noise ratio and marked beat-to-beat variation can be excluded from the on-line analysis by software algorithms, it must be stressed that operator experience is essential in judging the quality of the obtained data. Indeed the reproducibility of the Doppler technique during exercise has been addressed by both Gardin *et al.* (1988) and Mehta *et al.* (1988), who both show excellent reproducibility in the hands of trained operators [6, 18].

16.7 Conclusions

In conclusion, the Doppler technique is readily applied to the exercising situation, since it allows a rapid non-invasive assessment of LV function. The ease and reproducibility with which Doppler studies are performed allows monitoring of patients over an extended time period and through medical and surgical interventions. Further studies are required to establish the usefulness of Doppler ultrasound within the setting of exercise stress testing, especially in comparison to other techniques such as radionuclide ventriculography and exercise echocardiography.

References

1. Bennett ED, Barclay S, Davis A, Mannering L, Mehta N. Ascending aortic blood

218

velocity and acceleration using Doppler ultrasound in the assessment of left ventricular function. Cardiovasc Res 1984; 18:632–638.

2. Light LH. The transcutaneous aortovelograph in the assessment of left ventricular function – an effective alternative to cardiac output measurements. In: Jageneau AHM (ed.). Non-invasive methods on cardiovascular haemodynamics. Amsterdam, Elsevier/North Holland Biomedical Press 1981; 497–501.

3. Elkayam U, Gardin J, Berkley R, Hughes C, Henry WL. The use of Doppler flow velocity measurement to assess the haemodynamic response to vasodilators in patients with heart failure. Circulation 1982; 67:377–382.

4. Teague SM, Corn C, Sharma M, et al. A comparison of Doppler and radionuclide ejection dynamics during ischemic exercise. Am J Card Imaging 1987; 1:145–151.

5. Mehta N, Bennett ED, Mannering D, Dawkins K, Ward DE. Usefulness of noninvasive Doppler measurement of ascending aortic blood velocity and acceleration in detecting impairment of the left ventricular functional response to exercise three weeks after acute myocardial infarction. Am J Cardiol, 1986; 58:879–884.

6. Gardin JM, Kozlowski J, Dabestani A, et al. Studies of Doppler aortic flow velocity during bicycle exercise. Am J Cardiol 1986; 57:327–332.

7. Mehta N. The non-invasive assessment of left ventricular function by measurement of ascending aortic blood velocity and acceleration using Doppler ultrasound. PHD Thesis, Univ of London 1987; 88–100.

8. Bruce RA, Blackmon JR, Jones JW, et al. Exercise testing in adult normal subjects and cardiac patients. Paediatrics 1963; 32:742–748.

9. Harrison MR, Smith MD, Nissen SE, Grayburn PA, DeMaria AN. Use of exercise Doppler echocardiography to evaluate cardiac drugs: Effects of propranolol and verapamil on aortic blood flow velocity and acceleration. J Am Coll Cardiol 1988; 11:1002–1009.

10. Bryg RJ, Labovitz AJ, Mehdirad AA, Williams GA, Chaitman BR. Effect of coronary artery disease on Doppler derived parameters of aortic flow during upright exercise. Am J Cardiol 1986; 58:14–19.

11. Mehdirad AA, Williams GA, Labovitz AJ, Bryg RJ, Chaitman BR. Evaluation of left ventricular function during upright exercise: correlation of exercise Doppler with post exercise two-dimensional echocardiographic results. Circulation 1983;75:413–419.

12. Osbakken MD, Bocher CA, Okada RD, Bingham JD, Strauss W, Pohost GM. Spectrum of global left ventricular responses to supine exercise. Am J Cardiol 1983; 51:28–35.

13. Manyari DE, Kostuk WJ. Left and right ventricular function at rest and during bicycle exercise in the supine and sitting positions in normal subjects and patients with coronary artery disease. Assessment by radionuclide ventriculography. Am J Cardiol 1983; 15:36–42.

14. Nicod P, Corbett JR, Firth BG, et al. Prognostic value of resting and submaximal exercise radionuclide ventriculography after acute myocardial infarction in high-risk patients with single and multi-vessel disease. Am J Cardiol 1983; 52:30–36.

15. Sabbah HN, Przybylski J, Albert DE, Stein PD. Peak aortic blood acceleration reflects the extent of left ventricular mass at risk. Am Heart J 1987; 113:885–890.

16. Khaja F, Sabbah HN, Brymer JF, Stein PD. Influence of coronary collaterals on left ventricular function in patients undergoing coronary angioplasty. Am Heart J 1988; 116:1174–1180.

17. Jennings K, Reid DS, Hawkins T, Julian DJ. Role of exercise testing early after myocardial infarction in identifying candidates for coronary surgery. Br Med J 1984; 288:185–187.

18. Mehta N, Boyle G, Bennett ED, et al. Hemodynamic response to treadmill exercise in normal volunteers – An assessment by Doppler ultrasonic measurement of ascending aortic blood velocity and acceleration. Am Heart J 1988; 116:1298–1307.

17. Evaluation of exercise performance in mitral stenosis using Doppler echocardiography

KIRAN B. SAGAR and L. SAMUEL WANN

Cardiology Division, Milwaukee County Medical Complex, 8700 West Wisconsin Avenue, Milwaukee, Wisconsin 53226, U.S.A.

Patients with significant heart disease may have normal resting hemodynamics during cardiac catheterization. Since most cardiac symptoms are precipitated by exertion, it is important that hemodynamic performance be assessed both at rest and during some form of stress, such as muscular exercise, pharmacologic intervention or artificially induced tachycardia. This kind of evaluation enables one to assess both the severity of hemodynamic impairment and the level of cardiovascular reserve. Physiological information thus obtained is helpful in reaching a diagnosis, prescribing treatment, selecting patients for surgery and predicting prognosis. Since the stress of muscular exercise closely resembles the life situation in which the patient with heart disease may become symptomatic, exercise is commonly used in the evaluation of patients with heart disease.

17.1 Static versus dynamic exercise

Cardiovascular responses to dynamic and static exercise are different. Dynamic or isometric exercise causes an increase in heart rate, systemic arterial blood pressure and cardiac output with a fall in peripheral arterial resistance. Static or isometric exercise results in a predominant increase in systemic arterial pressure, a minor increase in heart rate and cardiac output [1–5]. Due to the differences in cardiovascular responses, dynamic exercise is particularly useful in the assessment of valvular heart disease and may also be employed to assess the integrated physiological response of the cardiovascular system to stress. These differences in cardiovascular responses have resulted in the use of dynamic exercise in the evaluation of valvular disease. Isometric exercise has been employed to assess left ventricular function.

17.2 Exercise and mitral stenosis

Hemodynamic effects of dynamic exercise are integrated effects of tachycardia, catacholamine stimulation and Frank-Starling mechanism. In patients with mitral stenosis, filling of the left ventricle and consequently cardiac output is dependent on the diastolic filling period, hence tachycardia impinges on left ventricular filling

Steve M. Teague (ed.) Stress Doppler Echocardiography, 219–225.
© 1990 *Kluwer Academic Publishers.*

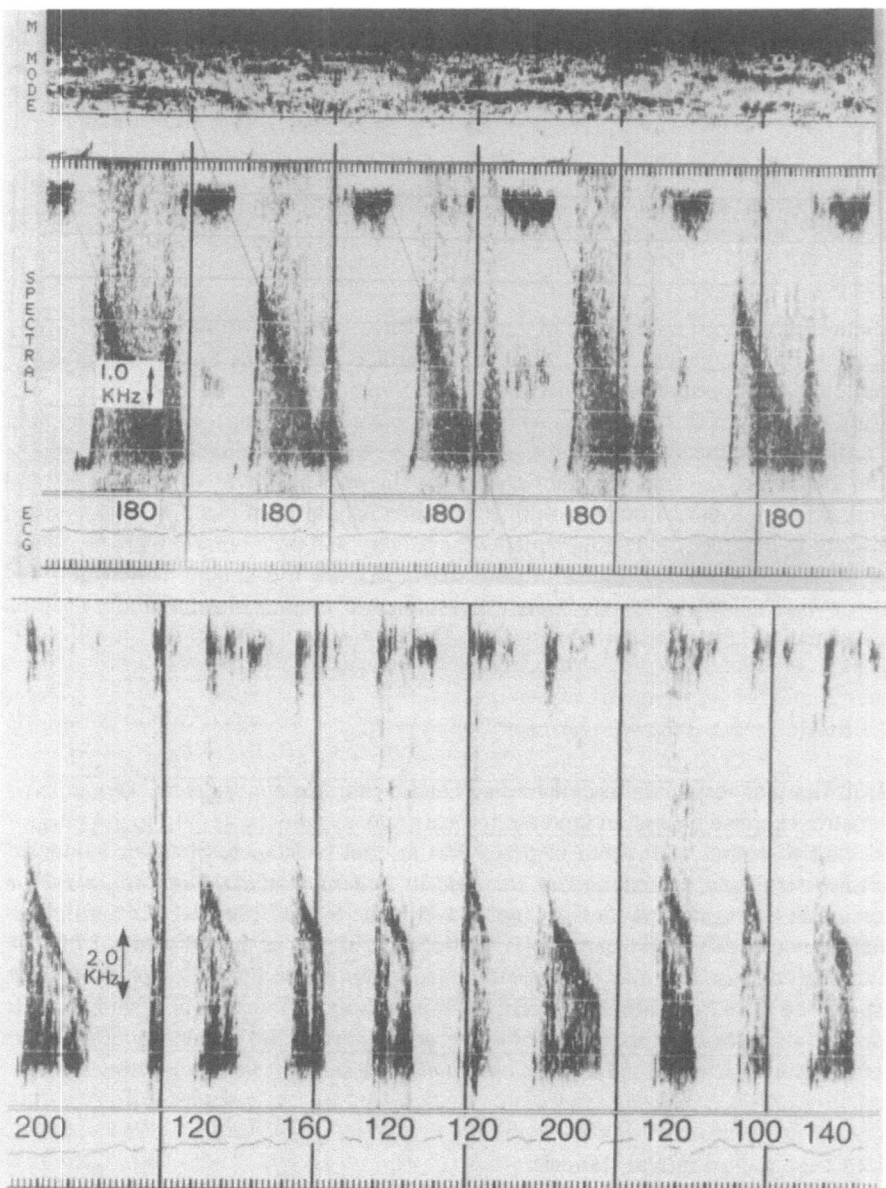

Figure 1. Representative examples of Doppler recording of mitral flow at rest (A:left) and during exercise (B:right). Heart rate increased from 60 bpm at rest to 95 bpm during exercise. Mitral pressure half-time decreased from 120 ms at rest to 124 ms during exercise.

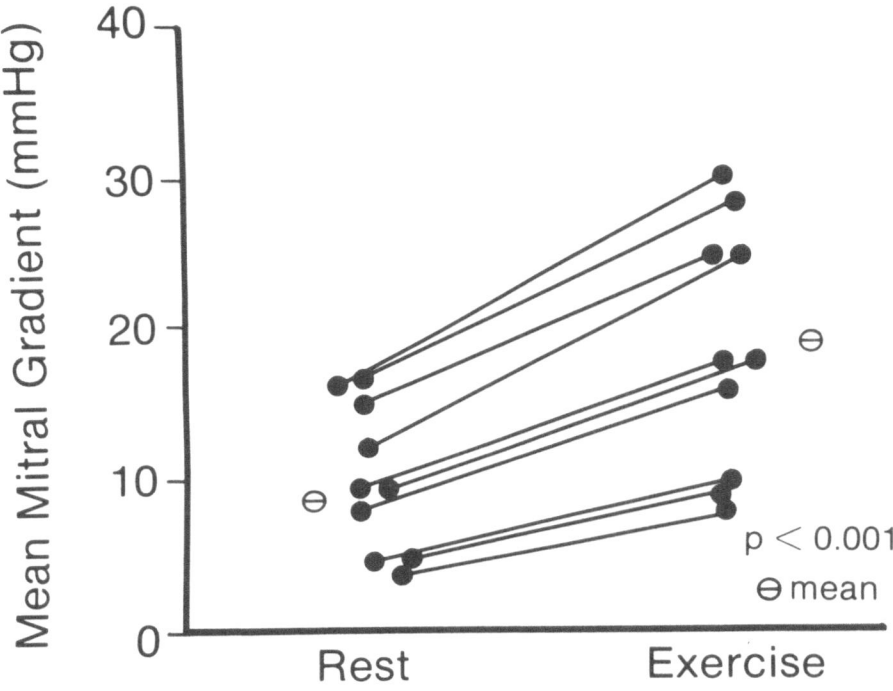

Figure 2. Mean mitral valve gradient at rest and during peak exercise.

by decreasing this interval leading to an increase in valve gradient. In addition, increase in mitral flow due to the inotropic effect of catacholeamine stimulation in the presence of a relatively fixed mitral valve orifice can increase valve gradient. Therefore, evaluation of hemodynamics during exercise for patients with mitral stenosis has been in practice for several decades. Gorlin & Gorlin in 1951 demonstrated a significant increase in mitral valve gradient (MVG), heart rate and cardiac output, and a fall in diastolic filling period without any change in mitral valve area (MVA), during dynamic supine exercise [6]. Since then several studies have confirmed their findings [7–9]. Ilesons & Ryan [7] studied cardiovascular responses to isometric exercise in patients with mitral stenosis. MVG increased from 11.5 mmHg at rest to 16.7 mmHg (P = 0.002) during exercise whereas MVA did not change. There was no significant change in left ventricular end diastolic pressure. Huikuri & associates [10] studied the value of isometric exercise testing during cardiac catheterization and used it to predict outcome of surgery. They demonstrated a positive correlation between the change in mean MVG during isometric exercise and changes in measures of left ventricular function. The patients who increased MVG > 4 mmHg, left ventricular ejection fraction remained unchanged and whose peak systolic pressure/end systolic volume ratio increased

222

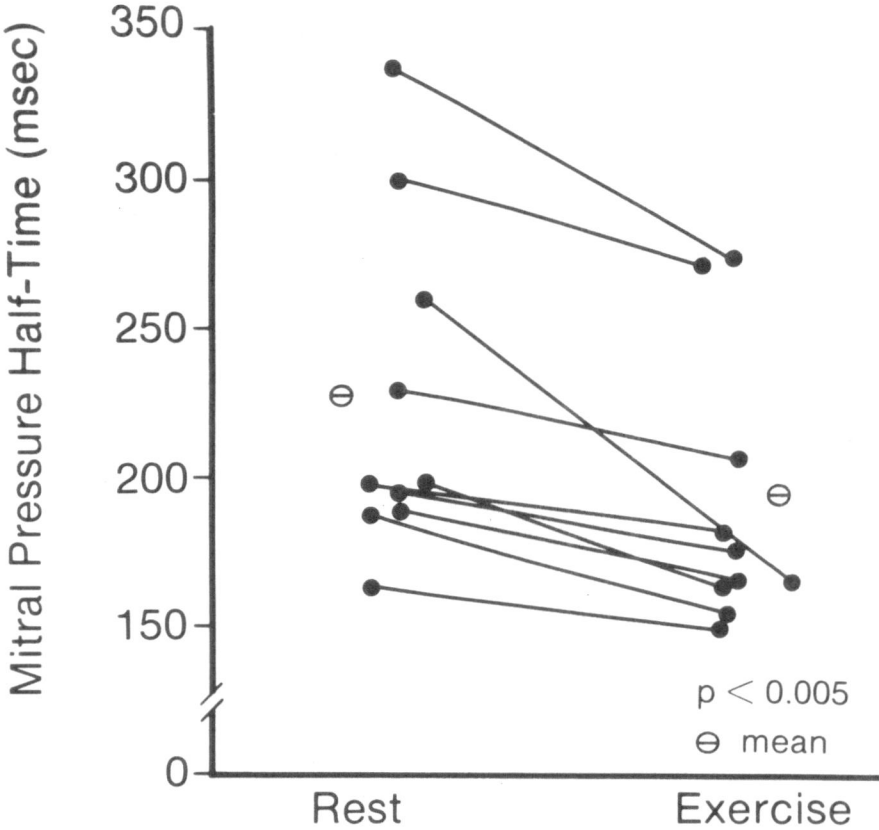

Figure 3. Mitral pressure half-time at rest and during peak exercise.

during isometric exercise had a significant improvement in symptoms following surgery.

Until 1984, most hemodynamics evaluations of mitral stenosis during exercise had been performed during cardiac catheterization. Introduction and validation of Doppler echocardiography for estimation of MVG and MVA provided a noninvasive technique to evaluate the response of mitral stenosis during exercise [11]. To date, only a few studies have used Doppler echocardiography for evaluation of mitral stenosis during exercise. Theoretically, exercise Doppler echocardiography offers an opportunity to evaluate not only severity of mitral stenosis, but also to assess left ventricular function.

17.3 Stress Doppler protocol for mitral stenosis

A symptom-limited exercise test using a supine bicycle ergometer (Engineering Dynamic Corp Model 2420, Echostat Table Picker Corp) was used in the study by Sagar *et al.* [12]. Exercise was performed under basal conditions, initiated at a load of 20 Watts and was increased by 20 W until symptoms occurred. Heart rate and blood pressure were recorded every minute during exercise and recovery period. Patients were examined in the left lateral decubitus position with the head elevated at 30 degrees. An apical four chamber view was used for interrogation of mitral inflow velocities with the sample volume positioned below the tip of the mitral valve. The orientation of Doppler beam parallel to suspected flow was verified with simultaneous real time imaging and monitoring of audiocardiac output to ensure highest velocities throughout the study. Mean mitral valve gradient was estimated by modified Bernoulli's equation and mitral pressure half time was measured by the method of Hatle *et al.* [11].

Hatle & associates [12] reported a moderate decrease in mitral pressure half time from a mean of 190 ml at rest to 160 ml (P < 0.001) during supine bicycle exercise in 37 patients with mitral stenosis. There was a more pronounced simultaneous increase in mitral valve gradient (7.6 to 16 mmHg).

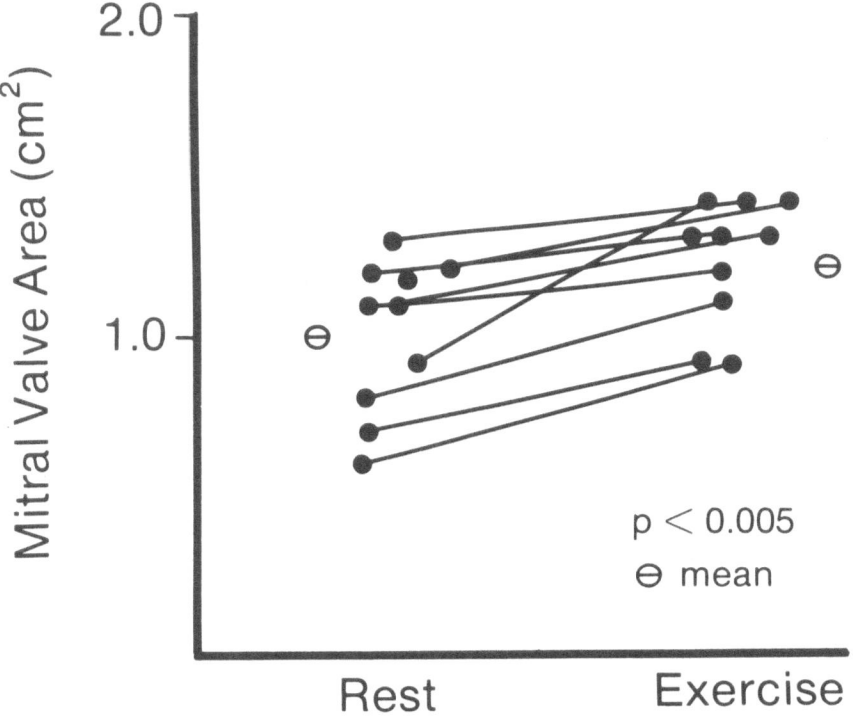

Figure 4. Estimated mitral valve area at rest and during exercise.

Sagar *et al.* [13] performed Doppler echocardiography at rest and during exercise in ten patients with mitral stenosis. Figure 1A and 1B show a representative example of mitral flow velocity at rest and during exercise. This patient developed transient atrial fibrillation during exercise which resolved spontaneously after exercise. During exercise the heart rate increased from 74 ± 14 beats/min (mean ± SD) at rest to 110 ± 8 beats/min (P < 0.001) during exercise. The mean MVG (Figure 2) increased from 9 ± 5 mmHg at rest to 18 ± 7 mmHg (P < 0.01) during exercise. The mitral pressure half-time decreased from 225 ± 62 ms at rest to 190 ± 92 ms during peak exercise (P < 0.005) (Figure 3). The estimated mitral valve area increased from 1.0 ± 0.4 cm^2 at rest to 1.2 ± 0.3 cm^2 at peak exercise (P < 0.005) (Figure 4). In the same study the authors showed excellent correlation between the Doppler derived and catheterization derived MVG at rest and during exercise. Correlation for mitral valve area was excellent at rest, however during exercise the correlation coefficient dropped.

Both of the preceding studies indicate that an increase in flow may lead to decrease in pressure half-time causing an increase in estimated mitral valve area. Stewart *et al.* [14] in an experimental study observed a flow related increase in orifice size of normal mitral valves. It is likely that other factors such as diastolic filling period, and left atrial and left ventricular compliance may also influence mitral pressure half-time.

Measurements of peak velocity and acceleration of Doppler derived ascending aortic and pulmonary artery flow velocity can provide assessment of left and right ventricular function respectively [15–17].

In summary, exercise Doppler echocardiography can be performed for assessment of severity of mitral stenosis and assessment of left and right ventricular function. In the future, exercise Doppler echo may also aid in evaluation of prosthetic mitral valves.

References

1. Dexter L. Effects of exercise on circulatory dynamics of normal individuals. J Applied Physiol 1951; 3:439.
2. Donald KW, Bishop TM, Cumming G, Wade BL. The effect of exercise on the cardiac output and cirucatory dynamics of normal subjects. Cln Sci 1955; 14:37.
3. Sonnenblick EH, Braunwald E, Williams JF, Erlick G. Effects of exercise on myocardial force-velocity relations in intact unanethetized man. Relative rate of changes in heart rate, sympathetic activity and ventricular dimensions. J Clin Invest 1958; 44:205.
4. Donald KW, *et al.* Cardiovascular responses to static contraction. Circ Res 1987; 20(Suppl 1):15.
5. Helfant RH, de Ville MA, Meister SG. Effect of sustained isometric handgrip exercise on left ventricular performance. Circulation 1971; 44:982.
6. Gorlin R, Gorgin SG. Hydraulic formula for calucation of the area of the stenotic mitral valve, other cardiac values and central circulatory shunts. Am Heart J 1951; 41:1.
7. Flessas AP, Ryan T. Cardiovascular responses to isometric exercise in patients with mitral stenosis. Arch Int Med 1982; 142:1629.
8. Nakhjavan FR, Katz MR, Maranhao V, Goldberg H. Analysis of influence of

catacholeamines and tachycardia during supine exeriçse in patients with mitral stenosis and sinus rhythm. Brit Heart J 1989; 31:753.

9. Rudolph FKW. Symptoms exercise capacity and exercise hemodynamics: Interrelationships and their role in quantification of valvular lesion. Herz 1987; 9:187.

10. Hiukuri VH, Takkunen JT. Value of isometric exercise testing during cardiac catheterization in mitral stenosis. Am J Cardiol 1983; 22:540.

11. Hatle L, Augelsen BA, Techn DR, Tramedie A. A noninvasive assessment of atrioventricular pressure half-time by Doppler ultrasound. Circulation 1979; 60:1096.

12. Hatle L, Andersen B. Doppler ultrasound in cardiology: Physical principles and clinical applications. Philadelphia: Lee & Febiges page 110, 1985.

13. Sagar KB, Wann LS, Paulsen WJH, Levin S. Role of exercise Doppler echocardiography in isolated mitral stenosis. Chest 1987; 92:27.

14. Stewart WJ, Jiang L, Mich R, Pandian W, Guerrero JL, Weyman AE. Variable effects of changes in flow rate through the aortic, pulmonary and mitral valves on valve area and flow velocity: Impact on quantitative Doppler flow calculations. J Am Coll Cardiol 1985; 6:653.

15. Daley PJ, Sagar KB, Wann LS. Supine versus upright exeriçse: Doppler echocardiographic measurement of ascending aortic flow velocity. Br Heart J 1985; 54:562–567.

16. Vaska KJ, Sagar KB, Wann LS. Effect of heart rate on Doppler indices of right ventricular function. Clin Res 1988; 36(3):325A.

17. Vaska KJ, Sagar KB, Wann LS. Can Doppler ultrasonic recordings of pulmonary arterial blood flow be used to track pulmonary arterial pressure? Clin Res 1988; 36(3):326A.

18. Left ventricular ejection force and impulse: Noninvasive assessment using Doppler ultrasound*

KARL ISAAZ

Service de Cardiologie A, CHU de Nancy-Brabois, Université de Nancy, 54511 Vandoeuvre-les-Nancy, France

18.1 Introduction

The importance of the mass-acceleration concept for the evaluation of cardiac function has been emphasized many years ago [1–6] and re-emphasized more recently [7–9]. In 1964, Rushmer [7] concluded that the left ventricle acts as an impulse generator and that the 'initial ventricular impulse' represents a reliable index of myocardial performance. Based on this concept, Rushmer suggested the use of measurement of peak aortic blood velocity and acceleration as indices of LV function [7]. Noble et al. [8] have suggested from a series of animal experiments that the maximal aortic blood acceleration is closely related to the maximum force exerted by the left ventricle in early systole and directed towards overcoming inertia. The force is a well established physical term defined as the product of mass and acceleration according to Newton's second law of motion:

$$\text{Force} = \text{mass} \times \text{acceleration}$$

The ability of Doppler echocardiography to measure aortic blood flow velocity and acceleration has led to the use of this ultrasound technique in the noninvasive assessment of left ventricular (LV) performance [10–14]. Since Doppler echocardiography has been shown to be a reliable method for the measurement of stroke volume [15–17], it provides a potential method to measure the mass of blood which flows through the cross-section of aorta during a given time interval. Recently, we reported preliminary results using Doppler echocardiography to determine the mean ejection force imparted to the aortic blood over the time from the onset of ejection to the attainment of peak flow. In a small number of patients, we showed that the ejection force was capable of differentiating normal subjects from patients with dilated cardiomyopathy [18]. In a larger series of patients, we have shown recently that the mean ejection force calculated over the acceleration time relates closely to the left ventricular performance as assessed by angiographic ejection

* Supported by an International Research Fellowship (1 F05 TW04099) from the Fogarty International Center, National Institutes of Health, Bethesda, Maryland, and supported in part by the Simone del Duca Foundation, Paris, France.

fraction [19]. The impulse is another physical term defined as the product of force and time. In a recent report [20], we have shown that Doppler echocardiography may be used for the noninvasive assessment of left ventricular ventricular impulse during the acceleration time.

The object of this paper is to analyze the utility of Doppler echocardiography in the noninvasive assessment of left ventricular performance based on the mass-acceleration concept. Different mathematical models of force and impulse calculation are reviewed. Finally, in view of the relationship between ejection force and left ventricular load, the significance of aortic blood flow velocity and acceleration as well as their potential role in the left ventricular load are discussed.

18.2 Theory: Simplified approach derived from the system formulation

In the system formulation, we 'isolate in the mind's eye' a bolus of fluid and follow his motion. Newton's second law states that the sum of all external forces acting on a body in motion relative to a fixed coordinate system is equal to the product of the mass and the acceleration of the body, that is $F = m \times a$ where m is the mass, a the acceleration, and F the resultant of forces acting on the body. For aortic blood flow, Newton's second law applies to the mass of a bolus of blood which flows through the cross-section of aorta during a given time interval. Accordingly, the basic principle of estimating a force consists in calculating the mass of blood which is ejected over a given time interval and multiplying this mass by its acceleration. This mathematical approach of calculation of force which acts to accelerate a given mass of blood has been used previously in ballistocardiography theory [1–6]. The mass of blood which flows through the aortic cross-sectional area during a time interval is proportional to the flow area, to the spatial average velocity and to the duration of the time interval. Consequently, different mathematical models of force can be studied depending on the mass of blood which is arbitrarily considered and depending on the time interval over which the force is averaged [1–6, 19].

The mass of blood (m) which crosses through the aortic cross-sectional area (CSA) over a time interval Δt is calculated as

$$m = \rho \times CSA \times V \times \Delta t \tag{1.1}$$

where ρ is the mass density of blood (1.06 gm/cm^3), V is the spatial mean velocity (in cm/sec). During the same time interval the blood undergoes an average acceleration γ as

$$\gamma = \Delta V / \Delta t \tag{1.2}$$

where ΔV represents the velocity increment over the time interval Δt. Let us consider the initial part of the aorta over a short distance as a circular cylindrical tube, thus the velocity varies only with time due to the unsteady state of flow (local or transient acceleration). If Δt represents the acceleration time (AT) which is the time from the onset of ejection to the attainment of peak flow, thus Equation (1.1) is rewritten

$$m_{at} = \rho \times CSA \times V_{at} \times AT \tag{1.3}$$

where V_{at} is the mean velocity calculated over AT, and m_{at} is the mass of blood which flows over the acceleration time, and the average acceleration γ is written

$$\gamma = PkV/AT \tag{1.4}$$

where PkV is the peak aortic blood velocity. According to the second law of motion (force = mass × acceleration), we obtained from the Equations (1.3) and (1.4)

$$MFAT = \rho \times CSA \times V_{at} \times PkV \tag{1.5}$$

where MFAT is called the *mean force over the acceleration time*. From multiplication of MFAT by AT (impulse = force × time) we obtain:

$$MIAT = MFAT \times AT = \rho \times CSA \times V_{at} \times PkV \times AT \tag{1.6}$$

where MIAT is called the *mean impulse over acceleration time*. Multiplying the mass of blood m_{at} as calculated from Equation (1.3) by the peak instantaneous acceleration (PA) gives

$$PFAT = \rho \times CSA \times V_{at} \times AT \times PA \tag{1.7}$$

where PFAT is called the *peak instantaneous force over acceleration time*.

The mass of blood which flows through the aortic cross-sectional area over the ejection time (ET) or stroke volume mass is given by Equation (1.1) by substituting ET for Δt

$$m_{et} = \rho \times CSA \times V_{et} \times ET \tag{1.8}$$

where V_{et} is the mean velocity calculated over ET.

Multiplying m_{et} by the peak acceleration we obtain the *peak instantaneous force over ejection time*

$$PFET = \rho \times CSA \times V_{et} \times ET \times PA \tag{1.9}$$

Multiplying m_{et} by the mean acceleration γ as calculated from Equation (1.4) we obtain the *mean force over ejection time*

$$MFET = \rho \times CSA \times V_{et} \times ET \times PkV/AT \tag{1.10}$$

The product of MFET by ET gives the *mean impulse over ejection time* (MIET):

$$MIET = \rho \times CSA \times V_{et} \times PkV/AT \times ET^2 \tag{1.11}$$

Consider now Δt in Equation (1.1) approaching zero (Δt->0), thus ΔV also approaches zero. The Equation (1.1) can be rewritten

$$dm = \rho \times CSA \times V(t) \times dt \tag{1.12}$$

where dm is an element of mass which flows through the cross-section of the aorta during an infinitesimal time interval, and the ratio $\Delta V/\Delta t$ assumes a finite value called the instantaneous acceleration γ_i as

$$\gamma_i = \lim_{\Delta t \to 0} \Delta V/\Delta t = dV/dt \tag{1.13}$$

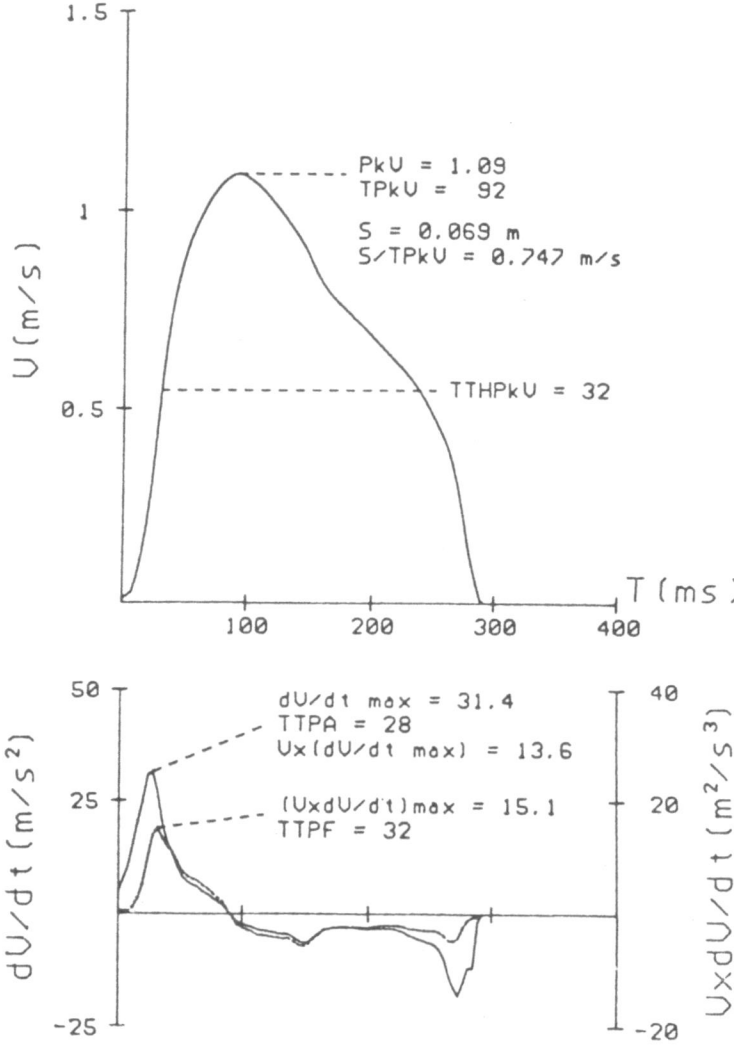

Figure 1a. Example of digitized tracing recorded from a normal subject. *Top*, digitized aortic blood flow velocity tracing. *Bottom*, instantaneous acceleration graph (solid line) and graph of the instantaneous product velocity × acceleration (broken line). The instantaneous rate of change of ejection force is obtained from the product of [V × dV/dt] with the blood mass density and the aortic cross-sectional area. PkV = peak velocity; V = velocity; S = velocity time integral over the acceleration time. TPkV = time to peak velocity (acceleration time); TTHPkV = time to half-peak velocity; TTPA = time to peak acceleration; TTPF = time to peak rate of change of ejection force.

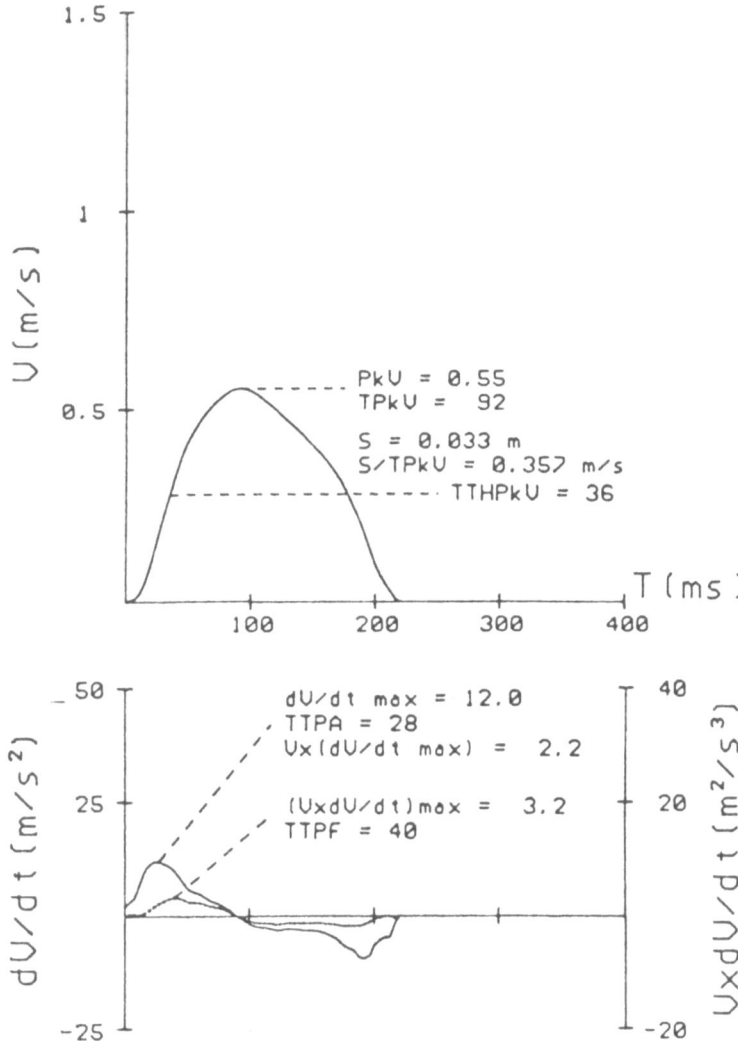

Figure 1b. Example of digitized tracing obtained from a patient with depressed left ventricular function.

From the product of the Equations (1.12) and (1.13) we obtain

$$dF = dm \times \gamma_i$$

$$= \rho \times CSA \times V(t) \times dV \tag{1.14}$$

where dF is an element of force. From Equation (1.14) we obtain

$$dF/dt = \rho \times CSA \times V(t) \times dV/dt \tag{1.15}$$

where dF/dt is called the *rate of change of ejection force* [21]. The *rate of change of ejection force at the time of peak acceleration* (dF/dt at PA) is expressed as:

$$dF/dt \text{ at } PA = \rho \times CSA \times V(t) \times PA \tag{1.16}$$

The *peak rate of change of ejection force* (peak dF/dt) [21] is calculated as the maximum value of [$\rho \times CSA \times V(t) \times dV/dt$]. Figure 1a shows a typical example of digitized aortic blood flow velocity and acceleration tracings and the graph of the product $V(t) \times dV/dt$ obtained from a normal subject. An example of recording obtained in a patient with LV dysfunction is shown in Figure 1b. Multiplying the value of $V(t) \times dV/dt$ max by $\rho \times CSA$, we obtain the rate of change of ejection force at the time of peak acceleration (dF/dt at PA) according to the Equation (1.16). Multiplying the maximum value of $V(t) \times dV/dt$ by $\rho \times CSA$, we obtain the peak rate of change of ejection force (peak dF/dt) [21].

18.3 Theory: Approach derived from the generalized linear momentum equation applied to the left ventricular/aortic coupling

As mentioned previously [19] the models of calculation the ejection force based on the product of a given mass ejected into the aorta with its acceleration take into account only a fraction of the force involved in the ejection of blood. In fact, at any instant, the sum of all the forces exerted by the ventricle to accelerate the blood is equal to the sum of the force which acts to accelerate the blood into the aorta plus the force that acts to move the blood within the ventricle. Thus a more complete approach would include the calculation of the force involved in the acceleration of the ventricular blood mass. Because the mass of blood in the ventricle is changing continuously with time during ejection it is more convenient to use another method of description to apply the basic laws of motion which is the control-volume formulation. A control volume refers to a region in space and is useful in the analysis of situations where flow occurs into and out of the space. The boundary of a control volume is its control surface. The control-volume concept is related to the system in terms of a general property of the system. The major task in going from the system to the control volume formulation of the basic laws is to express the rate of change of the arbitrary extensive property for a system in terms of time variations of this property associated with a control volume.

The general equation which relates the rate of change of any arbitrary extensive property, **N**, of the system to the time variations of this property associated with the control volume is expressed as:

$$dN/dt \big|_{system} = \partial/\partial t \iiint_{cv} n\rho \, dV + \iint_{cs} n\rho v \, dS,$$

where cv = control volume, cs = control surface, n = the amount of property N per unit of mass, dV = element of volume, ρ = blood mass density, v = velocity, dS = area element. The term $dN/dt \big|_{system}$ is the total rate of change of the extensive property N. The term $\iiint_{cv} n\rho \, dV$ is the total amount of the extensive property N which is contained within the control volume. The term $\partial/\partial t \iiint_{cv} n\partial \, dV$ is the time rate of change of the extensive property N within the control volume. The term $\iint_{cs} n\rho v \, dS$ is the net rate of efflux of the extensive property, N, through the control surface. $\rho v \, dS$ is the rate of mass efflux through the area element dS per unit time. To derive the control volume formulation of Newton's second law of motion, we set:

$$N = mv \text{ (momentum)}$$

Thus, Newton's second law is expressed as:

$$\Sigma F = d(mv)/dt = \partial/\partial t \iiint_{cv} v\rho \, dV + \iint_{cs} \rho vv \, dS \tag{2.1}$$

which is called the linear momentum equation in its integral form. In words, the resultant force acting on a control volume is equal to the time rate of increase of linear momentum within the control volume plus the net efflux of linear momentum from the control volume. The application of this equation to the left ventricle implies that the force exerted by the contracting myocardium which acts to cause ejection is equal to the sum of the net rate of momentum efflux into the aorta plus the rate of exchange of momentum of blood in the ventricle [22]. According to the second right side term of the Equation (2.1) and assuming that the velocity profile at the aortic orifice is flat, the momentum efflux (F1) into the aorta is calculated as:

$$F1 = \rho \, CSA \, v_a^2,$$

where v_a is the aortic blood velocity. The net inward flux of momentum provided by the motion of the ventricular wall can be neglected when compared to $\rho CSA \, v_a^2$. The momentum of the blood in the ventricle is equal to the mass of blood in the ventricle times the velocity of ejection times a scaling factor k. Thus, the rate of change of momentum in the ventricle (F2) is written as:

$$F2 = d(kv_a\rho V)/dt,$$

where V is the instantaneous ventricular volume.

Thus, the total force which acts to cause ejection is given by:

$$\Sigma F = F1 + F2 =$$
$$= \rho S_a v_a^2 + d(kv_a \, \rho V)/dt \tag{2.2}$$

The factor k is a dimensionless number which would be constant if the ventricle remains geometrically similar during contraction. Assuming the fluid motion within the left ventricle as irrotational, we can calculate the factor k by solving the Laplace equation using the Legendre polynomials. In the physiological range the calculation can be greatly simplified and k can be derived from the square of the aortic/LV radius ratio (Isaaz K et al., unpublished data). We showed recently that the variation in its value in time from the onset of flow to the peak flow is slow (Isaaz et al., unpublished data). Thus it is reasonable to assume k as a constant specifically if we consider the early systole. Thus, considering at a first approximation k as a constant during early systole, we obtain from Equation (2.2):

$$\Sigma\,F = \rho\,CSA\,v_a^2 + k\rho[v_a dV/dt + dv_a/dt\,V] \qquad (2.3)$$

The rate of change of left ventricular volume (dV/dt) is equal to the volumetric flow rate into the aorta in the absence of mitral insufficiency and considering that the systolic flow into the coronary arteries is negligible:

$$dV/dt = -\,CSA \times v_a \qquad (2.4)$$

From Equations (2.3) and (2.4), we obtain:

$$\Sigma\,F = (1-k)\rho CSA\,v_a^2 + k\rho V\,dv_a/dt \qquad (2.5)$$

The instantaneous left ventricular volume V can be derived from the equation:

$$V = LVEDV - CSA \int v_a dt \qquad (2.6)$$

where LVEDV is the left ventricular end-diastolic volume.

Substituting the right side term of Equation (2.6) in the Equation (2.5) we obtain:

$$\Sigma\,F = (1-k)\,\rho CSA\,v_a^2 + k\rho[LVEDV-CSA \int v_a\,dt]\,.\,dv_a/dt \qquad (2.7)$$

The Equation (2.7) shows that at the time of peak velocity (Pkv), the total force can be written as:

$$\Sigma\,F = (1-k)\,\rho CSA\,v_a^2 \;(\text{since } dv_a/dt = 0) \qquad (2.8)$$

From Equation (2.4) and (2.7), we can derive the rate of change of ejection force dF/dt as:

$$dF/dt = \rho CSA\,v_a\,dv_a/dt\,(2-3k) + \rho kVd^2v_a/dt^2 \qquad (2.9)$$

At the time of peak acceleration PA ($d^2v_a/dt^2 = 0$), Equation (2.9) reduces to:

$$dF/dt = \rho\,CSA\,v_a\,PA\,(2-3k) \qquad (2.10)$$

We see that dF/dt at the time of peak acceleration as derived from the linear momentum equation is close to dF/dt as calculated by Equation (1.16). Both expressions differ only by the term $(2-3k)$. In a recent study (Isaaz K et al., unpublished data) we showed that the factor $(2-3k)$ ranged from 1.60 to 1.80 in a population consisting in 9 normal subjects and 10 patients with dilated cardiomyopathy. Therefore, dF/dt at the time of peak acceleration can be calculated from Equation (1.16) since $2-3k$ remains almost constant from an individual to another one.

From Equation (2.7), it is possible to calculate the impulse I of the force over a given time interval. By definition, the linear impulse I of the resultant force $\Sigma\,F$ is the integral of $\Sigma\,F$ over the time interval $[t_1, t_2]$ during which the force F acts:

$$I = {}_{t_1}\!\int^{t_2} F \, dt$$

Thus, the linear impulse of the left ventricular ejection force applied between the onset of flow and peak flow can be expressed as:

$$I_{at} = {}_0\!\int^t \{(1-k)\, \rho \, CSA \, v_a^2 + k\rho \, V \, dv_a/dt\} \, dt \qquad (2.11)$$

where t = acceleration time

Using integration by parts and the Equation (2.4), Equation (2.11) becomes:

$$I_{at} = [\rho CSA \, {}_0\!\int^t v_a^2 \, dt] + [k\rho \bullet (LVEDV) \bullet PkV] -$$
$$[k\rho \, CSA \bullet \{{}_0\!\int^t v_a \, dt\} \bullet PkV]$$

$$(2.12)$$

Table 1. Doppler indexes derived from the mass acceleration concept.

Doppler indexes	Study population			
	Normals (n = 11)	LVEF > 60% (n = 17)	60% ≤ LVEF>40% (n = 9)	LVEF ≤ 40% (n = 10)
MIAT	27.3 ± 8	28.7 ± 8	23.5 ± 4.1	12.8 ± 4.9[AB]
PFAT	78.8 ± 23	73.7 ± 22	46 ± 10.5[B]	22.7 ± 6[AB]
PFET	261 ± 42.3	241 ± 63.2	141.5 ± 30.7[B]	51.8 ± 19.9[BD]
MFET	101 ± 26.2	97 ± 28.8	68 ± 8.5[C]	27.5 ± 12.4[BD]
MIET	90.7 ± 12.2	91.5 ± 18.4	72 ± 8.1[CD]	32 ± 16.4[BD]
dF/dt at PA	457 ± 103	400 ± 112.6	244 ± 78.8[AB]	114.3 ± 57.5[AB]
Peak dF/dt	542.6 ± 143	509 ± 169	328.5 ± 82.6[AB]	159 ± 56.8[AB]

dF/dt at PA = rate of change of ejection force at the time of peak acceleration (in Kdyn/sec); MFET = mean force over ejection time (in Kdyn); MIAT = mean impulse over acceleration time
(in dyn × sec × 10^2); MIET = mean impulse over ejection time (in dyn × sec × 10^2); peak dF/dt = peak rate of change of ejection force (in Kdyn/sec); PFAT = peak instantaneous force over acceleration time (in Kdyn); PFET = peak instantaneous ejection force over ejection time (in Kdyn).
[A] $p<0.01$ vs 60%≤ LVEF > 40%;
[B] $p < 0.001$ vs normals and LVEF > 60%;
[C] $p < 0.01$ vs normals and LVEF > 60%;
[D] $p < 0.001$ vs 60% ≤ LVEF > 40%.
All values are expressed as mean ± SD.

18.4 Results: Doppler indexes derived from the method based on the system formulation

We have shown recently [19] that the mean left ventricular ejection force over the acceleration time (MFAT) as calculated from Equation (1.5) using Doppler echocardiography relates closely to the left ventricular performance as assessed by angiographic ejection fraction. In a series of 36 patients undergoing cardiac catheterization, we found a linear correlation coefficient of 0.86 between MFAT

236

and angiographic LVEF. When the data were fitted to a power curve, the correlation coefficient improved to 0.91. Peak aortic blood velocity and mean acceleration showed less good correlations with LVEF ($r = 0.73$ and $r = 0.64$ respectively; power fit, $r = 0.76$ and $r = 0.72$ respectively). Moreover, no significant difference was found between normal subjects and patients with LVEF between 60% and 40% regarding peak aortic blood velocity and mean acceleration [19]. Table 1 shows the values for MIAT (Equation (1.6)), PFAT (Equation (1.7)), MFET (Equation (1.10)), PFET (Equation (1.9)), MIET (Equation (1.11)), dF/dt at the time of peak acceleration (Equation (1.16)) and peak dF/dt in 11 normal subjects and 36 patients subgrouped into three groups based on LVEF. The correlations between each of the indices and angiographic ejection fraction are shown in Figure 2 and Figure 3.

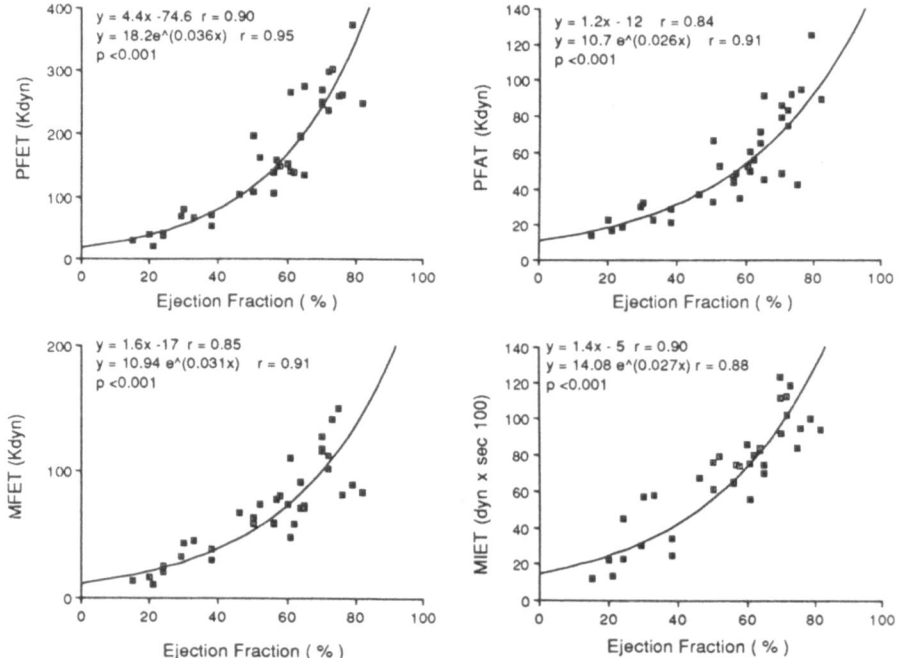

Figure 2. Relationship between angiographic ejection fraction and peak force over ejection time (PFET), peak force over acceleration time (PFAT), mean force over ejection time (MFET), and mean impulse over ejection time (MIET).

18.5 Results: Doppler calculations based on the generalized linear momentum equation

In a recent study (Isaaz K et al., unpublished data) we assessed noninvasively the time course of the instantaneous LV ejection force in 10 patients with dilated

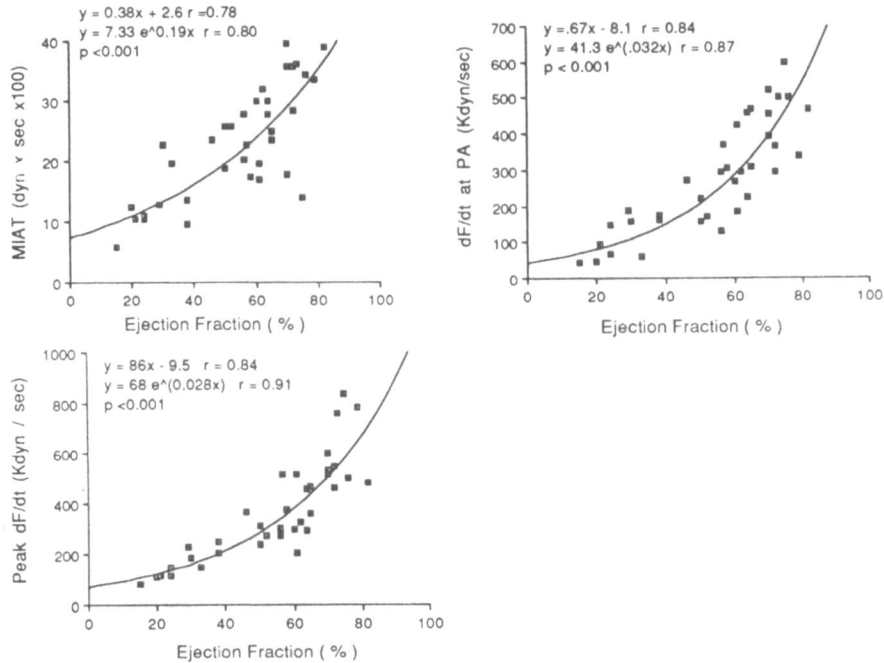

Figure 3. Relationship between angiographic ejection fraction and mean impulse over acceleration time (MIAT), rate of change of ejection force at the time of peak acceleration (dF/dt at PA), and peak rate of change of ejection force (peak dF/dt).

cardiomyopathy using Doppler echocardiography and applying Equation (2.7). We found a significant decrease in the maximum value of ejection force in patients with cardiomyopathy when compared to normal subjects ($p = 0.0001$). In both groups, the maximum value of ejection force was attained early in ejection at the time of peak acceleration, and was mostly accounted for by local acceleration effects. We found a significant linear correlation between peak acceleration and maximum LV ejection force ($r = 0.91$). We found that, at the time of peak aortic velocity, the LV ejection force had fallen to 84% of its maximum value in normals whereas it had fallen to 64% in patients with cardiomyopathy ($p < 0.01$). The maximum LV ejection force resulted into a pressure gradient between the LV and the aorta ($\Sigma F_{max}/CSA$) of 9.8 mmhg in normals and 6 mmhg in dilated cardiomyopathy ($p = 0.0001$). The values of the pressure gradient in our normal subjects calculated noninvasively was in close agreement with the results reported by Murgo et al. [23] who published multisensor catheter measurements.

18.6 Discussion

The present study shows that Doppler echocardiography, a noninvasive technique, may be used for the assessment of left ventricular performance based on measurements of indexes derived from the mass-acceleration concept.

The acceleration of blood, a term of the force, has been proposed many years ago as an index of left ventricular performance. Rudewald in 1962 speculated about the possible correlation between the acceleration of the ascending aortic blood flow and the mechanical properties of the left ventricular myocardium [24]. In 1964, Rushmer [7] suggested that the left ventricle acts as an impulse generator and that the 'initial ventricular impulse' appears to be an appropriately descriptive term for the dynamic properties of ventricular ejection. The potential use of the impulse impressed by the heart on the blood as a quantitative criterion of ventricular ejection was already suggested by Masini et al. in 1953 [4]. Then, Noble et al. [8] suggested from a series of animal experiments that the peak acceleration is closely related to the maximum force exerted by the heart in early systole.

However, acceleration is only one of the two terms of the force, the second term being the accelerated mass. Thus, for a complete assessment of left ventricular ejection dynamics, the two terms should be considered according to the basic concept of mass-acceleration. A first attempt of constructing the cardiovascular forces in man from the product of the mass of blood ejected with its acceleration has been made many years ago [1-6] and the potential utility of the mass-acceleration concept applied to the heart has been emphasized more recently by Rushmer [7,9]. However, at this time, the application of the concept was limited by the technology. In particular, the flow ejection curve, upon which were based the calculments, was derived from animal ejection curves [1] or derived from the pressure pulse contour [3] with arbitrarily assigned coordinates [1,3]. When related to ballistocardiography, the predicted cardiovascular ejection forces [1,3] were found to be greater than those reconstructed from the ballistocardiogram [3]. Ballistocardiography is also a technique derived from the application of Newton's second law of motion, and has been proposed to estimate the cardiac force from the movements of the body imparted by the moving blood mass [1-6]. However, this latter technique, although valid in its basic concept, presented limitations related to the instrumentation and to the numerous assumptions which were required. This partially explains why the forces involved in ejecting blood were recorded with an unknown degree of diminution in the ballistocardiogram [3]. By contrast, Doppler echocardiography has been validated for the measurement of aortic blood flow characteristics [25]. Thus, this technique offers the possibility of direct calculation of mass flow rate and acceleration, and therefore provides an accurate method for the estimation of the ejection force. We have shown that the mean LV ejection force as calculated from Equation (1.5) relates better to global left ventricular performance as assessed by angiographic ejection fraction than the mean acceleration alone does [18, 19]. It is reasonable to state that a greater mass of blood requires a greater force than a smaller mass to undergo the same acceleration, implying a higher level of cardiac performance. Our previous data [19] have shown that peak aortic blood velocity and mean acceleration do not achieve any significant difference between normals and patients with mild to moderate LV dysfunction. This suggests that conventional Doppler indexes, namely peak aortic velocity and mean acceleration, are not significantly decreased as long as a severe alteration of LV function does not occur, and that other indexes should be used for the diagnosis of mild to moderate LV dysfunction at rest. Although a high correlation with ejection fraction was found for PFET and MFET, we don't state that these indexes represent an appropriate physical model of calculation of the force but rather a semi-empirical model.

Multiplying at any instant the all stroke volume mass by the local acceleration measured at the aortic orifice level implies that the stroke volume moves as a unit and that the convective component of acceleration is neglected. That is obviously difficult to support. Due to the flow area reduction from the left ventricle to the aortic anulus, especially in patients with dilated left ventricle, the local acceleration at the level of aortic anulus is not equal at any instant to the local acceleration at any point of the centerline within the ventricle. The difference, at any instant, between the local acceleration at a given position within the ventricle and the local acceleration at the aortic anulus, is dependent on the ratio of aortic orifice to ventricular flow section areas. Similarly, if we consider the motion of the stroke volume as the motion of a unit within the aorta, we see that the length of that column of blood (stroke distance) may attain about 25 cm in a patient with normal cardiac index. Due to the changes in the geometry of the aorta over such a distance, it is obvious that we cannot apply the same local acceleration to any point within the space occupied by the stroke volume. Thus, the mathematical model of estimation the force from the product of instantaneous local acceleration measured at aortic level with the stroke volume mass, as suggested previously [1,5] appears to be an oversimplification of the problem. Therefore, PFET and MFET appear to be semi-empirical indexes that are not based on an appropriate physics model although closely related to cardiac function as assessed by ejection fraction. Furthermore, these indexes, that can be used for the noninvasive assessment of global LV performance at rest, must be obviously sensitive to acute changes of loading conditions since the stroke volume is included in their calculation.

The determination of the LV ejection force and its impulse, as indexes of left ventricular performance, from the product of acceleration with the mass ejected only during the acceleration time appears to be more valid for many reasons. First, it would seem more logical to multiply a positive acceleration (be it mean or peak) by a mass which undergoes acceleration during the same period that the acceleration is positive. Second, due to the small volume occupied at any instant by the mass ejected during the acceleration time, the instantaneous local acceleration can be approximated as being the same at any point of the space within the mass with minor error. Furthermore, it has been suggested from experimental studies [26–28] that the left ventricle is contributing little to the ejection in late systole. In late systole, after the positive acceleration is over and maximum velocity has been attained, the blood would then continue to flow under its own momentum until resistance stops it [26–28]. More importantly, it has been shown that changes in stroke volume due to variations in preload resulted essentially from a change in late systolic flow, and that during early systole, inertiance dominates the opposition to left ventricular ejection while resistance and compliance are less important [26–28]. Thus, the ejection force and impulse estimated over the early systole, namely the acceleration time (as MFAT, MITA and PFAT) appear to be conceptually more appropriate than those indexes calculated over the ejection time (as MFET, MIET and PFET) to assess the left ventricular function.

The calculation of the LV ejection force and impulse from the linear momentum equation applied to the LV/aortic coupling provides a more complete approach since the events within the LV are involved in the calculation. However, although all the factors involved in Equations (2.7) and (2.12) can be determined noninvasively, the calculations remain more complex than those involved in the simplified models derived from the system formulation. Using the linear momentum equation in a recent study (Isaaz K et al., unpublished data), we confirmed the hypothesis of Noble et al. [8] who suggested that peak aortic blood flow acceleration is closely related to the maximum LV ejection force. Moreover, we found that the fall in the instantaneous LV ejection force from the onset of ejection to the time of peak flow was greater in patients with dilated cardiomyopathy (36%) than in normals (16%, p < 0.01) (Isaaz K et al., unpublished data).

It is known that in normal subjects, the LV wall stress declines rapidly once its maximum value is attained soon after the aortic valve opening [29]. In a study performed recently at the Cardiovascular Research Institute of San Francisco, University of California, we have shown that the afterload attains its peak value at the time of peak aortic flow acceleration (unpublished data). Thus, in normal subjects, once the aortic blood flow acceleration is attained, the afterload declines rapidly and consequently the negative feedback between the afterload and the velocity of fiber shortening is less operative at the time of peak aortic flow. Conversely, in patients with dilated cardiomyopathy the afterload remains elevated during the entire ejection period [29] and the negative feedback is fully operative throughout the ejection.

Assuming the left ventricle as an ellipsoid of revolution, we can show that the aortic blood flow velocity is proportional to the velocity of circumferential fiber shortening; the aortic blood flow acceleration is proportional to the sum of the square of velocity of circumferential fiber shortening and the acceleration of fiber shortening. Given the force-velocity relationships of the myocardium, the time course of the shortening load and the time course of the instantaneous ejection force, we suggested in a recent study that decreased peak aortic blood acceleration and velocity in cardiomyopathy result from adjustments of feedback loading functions in addition to alteration in contractile state (Isaaz K et al., unpublished data). The hypothesis of a negative feedback loop through which the aortic blood acceleration and velocity allow the contracting myocardium to regulate partially its own load has been suggested previously [30, 32]. The calculation of the LV ejection force according to the Equation (2.7) provides a noninvasive method for the analysis of the intrinsic component of the load (inertial effect) on the myocardium which must be considered in the assessment of the total systolic load, especially in case of vigorous ejection as during exercise. During exercise, the inertial effects related to peak acceleration and velocity become relatively important [23,32] and consideration of only the extrinsic component (aortic blood pressure) of the total systolic load could be misleading in the assessment of cardiac mechanics [32].

References

1. Starr I, Rawson AJ, Schroeder HA, Joseph NR. Studies on the estimation of cardiac output in man, and of abnormalities of cardiac function, from heart recoil and the blood impacts. The ballistocardiogram. Am J Physiol 1939; 127:1.
2. Starr I, Rawson AJ. The vertical ballistocardiograph; experiments on the changes in the circulation on arising with a further study of ballistic theory. Am J Physiol 1941; 134:403–425.
3. Hamilton WF, Dow P, Remington JW. The relation between the cardiac ejection curve and the ballistocardiographic forces. Am J Physiol 1945; 14:557–570.
4. Masini V, Rossi P. A new index for quantitative ballistocardiography: The velocity of body displacement. Circulation 1953; 8:276–281.
5. Wolf-Wito von Wittern. Ballistocardiography with elimination of the influence of the vibration properties of the body. Amer Heart J 1953; 46:705–714.
6. Starr I, Noordergraaf A. Evaluation of the ballistocardiogram using mathematical models. In Ballistocardiography in cardiovascular research; physical aspects of the circulation in health and disease. Philadelphia, 1967, JB Lippincott, p44.
7. Rushmer RF. Initial ventricular impulse. A potential key to cardiac evaluation. Circulation 1964; 29:268–283.
8. Noble MIM, Trenchard D, Guz A. Left ventricular ejection in conscious dogs. 1. Measurement and significance of the maximum acceleration of blood from the left ventricle. Circ Res 1966; 19:139–147.
9. Rushmer RF. Hemodynamic measurements. In: Rushmer (ed.). Organ physiology – Structure and function of the cardiovascular system (ed. 2), Philadelphia, 1976, W.B. Saunders, p. 37.
10. Bennett ED, Barclay SA, Davis AL, Mannering D, Mehta N. Ascending aortic blood velocity and acceleration using Doppler ultrasound in the assessment of left ventricular function. Cardiovasc Res 1984; 18:632–638.
11. Gardin JM, Iseri LT, Elkayam U, Tobis J, Childs W, Burth CS, Henry WL. Evaluation of dilated cardiomyopathy by pulsed Doppler echocardiography. Am Heart J 1987; 106:1057–1067.
12. Elkayam U, Gardin JM, Berkley R, Hugues CA, Henry WL. The use of Doppler flow velocity measurement to assess the hemodynamic response to vasodilators in patients with heart failure. Circulation 1983; 67:377–383.
13. Sabbah HN, Khaya F, Brymer JF, Mc Farland TM, Albert DE, Snyder JE, Goldstein S, Stein PD. Noninvasive evaluation of left ventricular performance based on peak aortic blood acceleration measured with a continuous-wave Doppler velocity meter. Circulation 1986; 74:323–329.
14. Teague SM, Corn C, Sharma M, Prasad R, Burow R, Voyles WF, Thadani U. Comparison of Doppler and radionucleide ejection dynamics during ischemic exercise. Am J Cardiac Imaging 1987; I–2:145–151.
15. Huntsman LL, Stewart DK, Barnes SR, Franklin SB, Colocousis JS, Hessel EA. Noninvasive Doppler determination of cardiac output in man. Clinical validation. Circulation 1983; 67:593–602.
16. Lewis JF, Kuo LC, Nelson JG, Limacher MC, Quinones MA. Pulsed Doppler echocardiographic determination of stroke volume and cardiac output: clinical validation of two new methods using the apical window. Circulation 1984; 70:425–431.

242

17. Ihlen H, Amlie JP, Dale J, Forfang K, Nitter-Hange S, Otterstad JE, Simonsen S, Myhre E. Determination of cardiac output by Doppler echocardiography. Br Heart J 1984; 51:54.
18. Isaaz K, Cloez JL, Thompson A, Pernot C. Assessment of ventricular ejection dynamics by Doppler using a new method in congestive cardiomyopathy. Circulation 1986; 74 (supp II): II–13.
19. Isaaz K, Ethevenot G, Admant P, Brembilla B, Pernot C. A new Doppler method of assessing left ventricular ejection force in congestive heart failure. Am J Cardiol 1989; 64: 81–89.
20. Isaaz K, Cloez JL, Thompson A, Pernot C. Noninvasive-assessment of left ventricular performance based on initial ventricular impulse measured by Doppler echo-cardiography. J Am Coll Cardiol 1987; 9:18A.
21. Isaaz K, Ethevenot G, Cherrier F, Pernot C. The peak rate of change of ejection force: A new Doppler index of left ventricular performance. Circulation 1987; 76(supp IV):IV–528.
22. Caro CG, Pedley TJ, Schroter RC, Seed WA. The heart. In Caro CG, Pedley TJ, Schroter RC, Seed WA editors: The mechanic of the circulation, Oxford, 1978, Oxford University Press, p. 236.
23. Murgo JP, Dorethy JF, Alter BR, McGranahan GM, Jr. Aortic valve gradients in normal man during exercise and isoproterenol infusion. Relationship to pulsatile flow. Circulation 1978; 57–58 (suppII–30).
24. Rudewald B. Hemodynamics of the human ascending aorta as studied by means of a differential pressure technique. Acta Physiol Scandinav 1963; (supp) 187:55–61.
25. Mehta N, Noble M, Mills C, Pugh S, Drake-Holland A, Bennett D. Doppler measured ascending aortic blood velocity and acceleration. Validation against an electromagnetic catheter-tip system in humans (abst.). Circulation 1987; 76:(supp IV) 94.
26. Noble MIM. The contribution of blood momentum to left ventricular ejection in the dog. Circ Res 1968; 28:663–670.
27. Noble MIM, Trenchard D, Guz A. Left ventricular ejection in conscious dogs. II. Determinants of stroke volume. Circ Res 1966; 19:148–152.
28. Spencer M, Greiss FC. Dynamics of ventricular ejection. Circ Res 1962; 10:274–279.
29. Gault JH, Ross J Jr, Braunwald E. Contractile state of the left ventricle in man. Instantaneous tension-velocity-length relations in patients with and without disease of the left ventricular myocardium. Circ Res 1968; 22:451.
30. Hoadley SD, Pasipoularides A. Are ejection phase Doppler/echo indices sensitive markers of contractile dysfunction in cardiomyopathy: role of afterload mismatch. Circulation 1987; 76:(supp IV) 404.
31. Milnor WR. Arterial impedance as ventricular afterload. Circ Res 1975; 36:565.
32. Pasipoularides A, Murgo JP, Miller JW, Craig WE. Noninvasive left ventricular ejection pressure gradients in man. Circ Res 1987; 61:220.

19. Theoretical analysis of the left ventricular ejection pulse

STEVE M. TEAGUE

University of Oklahoma Health Sciences Center, Oklahoma City, Oklahoma 73190, U.S.A.

19.1 Introduction

The preceding chapters have discussed analysis of the Doppler ejection pulse based upon descriptive time domain measurements. Maximal acceleration, peak velocity, stroke integral, and the systolic time intervals all key upon features of the flow profile easily measured in hard copy records. Clinical evaluations have been restricted to correlative studies evaluating pulse timing, rate of rise, and peak deflection with commonly accepted invasive and noninvasive reference standards of ventricular performance; dP/dt, ejection fraction, Vcf, and power of left ventricular ejection. Ischemic mass, extent of coronary disease, exercise tolerance, and thallium perfusion defects have also been referenced. No prior study has addressed the genesis of the flow pulse in the ascending aorta.

The earliest clinical studies of Doppler aortovelography correlated the contour of the Doppler ejection pulse with patient clinical status [1–7]. Low, rounded pulses were associated with congestive heart failure or cardiogenic shock, while high amplitude pulses peaking early in systole were observed in septic shock or other high output states. However, these analyses were completely descriptive, offering no quantitative means by which diseases could be categorized.

It is the purpose of this chapter to quantiate the contour, or shape of the velocity-time curve in the ascending aorta utilizing frequency domain analysis. Pragmatically, mathematical techniques and computational hardware are available to implement this approach for existing Doppler instrumentation. The hypothesis of the following mathematical exercise is that the shape of the ventricular ejection pulse is quantitatively related to ventricular performance.

19.2 Mass balance considerations

The following will develop a mathematical model that couples left ventricular size, rate, and contractility to flow pulse contour in the ascending aorta. These ends are accomplished by implementing the law of mass conservation. We begin by realizing that blood is incompressible under physiologic conditions. Thus, if ventricular septal defect and significant mitral regurgitation are absent, blood displaced from the ventricle during systolic contraction must appear in the ascending aorta.

Steve M. Teague (ed.) Stress Doppler Echocardiography, 243–253.

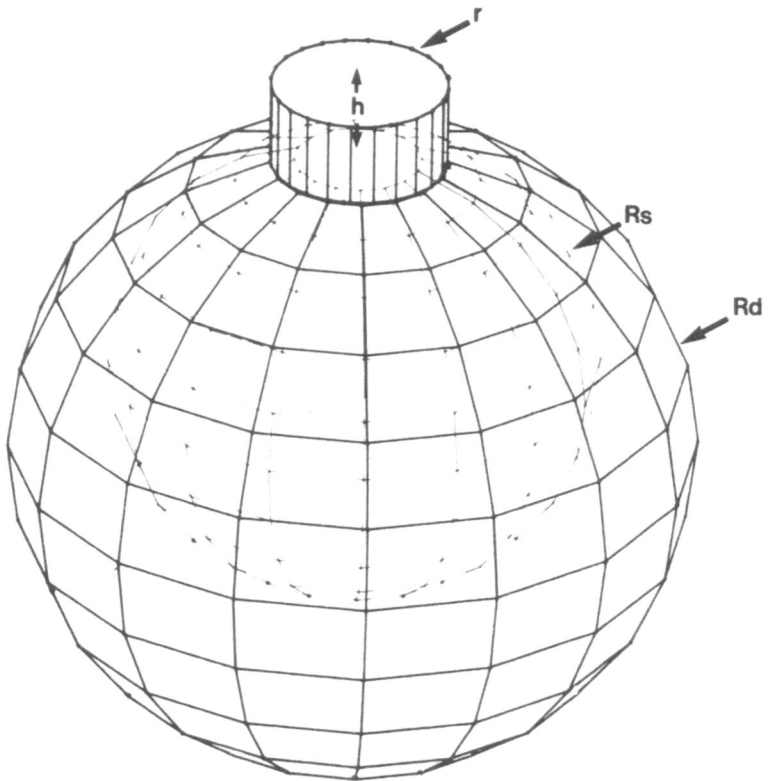

Figure 1. The ejecting ventricle is modeled as a sphere with radius [R(t)] varying between diastolic (Rd) and systolic (Rs) limits. The aorta is modeled as a cylinder of radius r and height h. For discussion, see text.

For mathematical simplicity (and with surprising physiologic accuracy), we will assume the aorta to be an indistensible cylinder and the ventricle to be a sphere of varying radius:

$$4/3 \ \pi R^3 \quad \text{(Volume of sphere)} \tag{1}$$
$$\pi r^2 h \quad \text{(Volume of cylinder)} \tag{2}$$

As shown in Figure 1, the sphere radius varies from an end-diastolic radius (Rd) to an end-systolic radius (Rs) during systole. The aortic radius is r. Over a brief time interval, Δt, the ventricular radius changes by a small amount, ΔR, while the height ·of the blood column in the aorta changes by similar small amount, Δh. Following conservation of mass, volume lost must equal volume gained:

$$\pi r^2 \Delta h = 4\pi R^2 \Delta R \tag{3}$$

If we take the limit as Δt, Δh, and ΔR approach 0, a differential equation is produced that describes dh/dt in terms of dR/dt and associated geometrical radii.

Note that dh/dt at any instant represents the velocity of flow into the ascending aorta. This differential equation describes the systolic aortic velocity-time curve. For simple application of this model, we must assume that there is no mitral regurgitation or ventricular septal defect, no systolic expansion of the aorta, and that the ventricular contractile pattern is precisely symmetrical in three dimensions. The velocity profile in the aortic inlet is assumed to be blunt. Although actual biologic conditions violate many of these assumptions, this model generated surprisingly physiologic pulses.

19.3 Ventricular contractile patterns

We must make additional assumptions regarding the time course of ventricular radius during systole. The radius must decrease from a maximum (Rd) to a minimum (Rs) over systole. At both Rd and Rs, the rate of radius change is zero. Between these endpoints, the rate of radius change accelerates, reaches a maximum and then decelerates. It is reasonable to approximate the timecourse of systolic radius change [r(t)] as sinusoidal between Rd and Rs:

$$R(t) = 1/2(Rd + Rs) + 1/2 (Rd–Rs)COS \ \Omega t \tag{4}$$

Clinical evidence supports sinusoidal-type variation described in the above equation. Radionuclear left ventricular time-activity curves and digitized high resolution M-mode echocardiograms (Figure 2) disclose this quasi-sinusoidal systolic ventricular diameter variation. Diastolic radius changes are complex, and not adequately described by a simple sinusoid. The above model is only required to address systolic function, however.

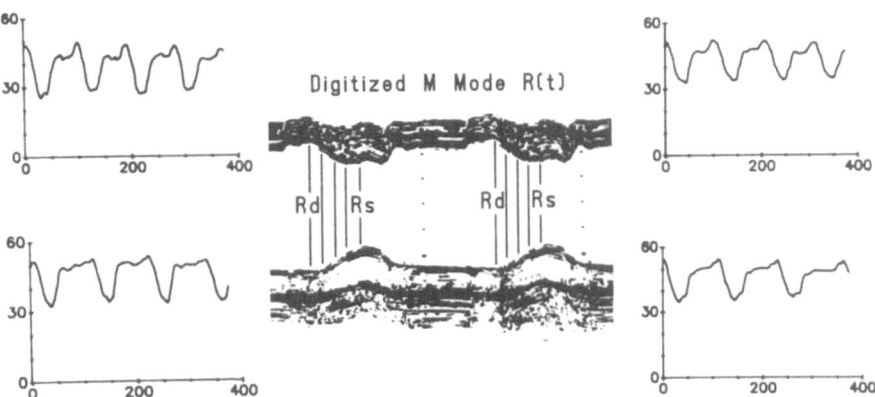

Figure 2. The validity of sinusoidal variation in ventricular chamber radius between diastolic (Rd) and systolic (Rs) endpoints can be evaluated by high resolution digitization of endocardial borders in M-mode echocardiograms. The data of four normals are plotted over four seconds. The units of the y axis are millimeters while the units of the x axis are centiseconds.

The amplitude of the sinewave is determined by Rd and Rs, while the radial frequency (Ω) of the sinusoidal variation is determined by left ventricular ejection time. It can be shown that left ventricular ejection time is equal to the time of the systolic half cycles shown in Figure 2:

$$\Omega = \pi/\text{LVET} \tag{4.5}$$

An additional reason for assuming R(t) to be sinusoidal with time is that sine function first and second time derivatives are relatively simple compared to more complex R(t) functions:

$$\dot{R}(t) = -\Omega/2(\text{Rd–Rs})\text{SIN } \Omega t \tag{5}$$

$$\ddot{R}(t) = \Omega^2/2(\text{Rd–Rs}) \text{ COS } \Omega t \tag{6}$$

These first (5) and second (6) time derivatives of the input function R(t) will be required in the generation of velocity and acceleration Equations (7) and (8).

19.4 Pulse equations

We can now write equations for velocity and acceleration as functions of time based upon Equations (3) through (6). Velocity depends upon the squared radius of the aorta, diastolic and systolic radii of the ventricle, and left ventricular ejection time. Rearranging Equation (3):

$$V(t): \quad 4/r^2(R^2\dot{R}) \tag{7}$$

Acceleration is the first time derivative of velocity, with similar dependence on the above variables:

$$A(t): \quad 4/r^2(\ddot{R} R^2 + 2R\dot{R}^2) \tag{8}$$

where R(t), R, and R are described in Equations (4), (5), and (6).

Relatively simple expressions for V(t) and A(t) may be written after appropriate substitution for R(t) and its first and second time derivatives, trigonometric simplification, and algebraic reduction:

$$V(t) = MV [KV_1\text{COS } \Omega t + KV_2\text{COS } 2\Omega t + KV_3 \text{ COS } 3\Omega t] \tag{9}$$

$$A(t) = MA [KA_1\text{SIN } \Omega t + KA_2\text{SIN } 2\Omega t + KA_3\text{SIN } 3\Omega t] \tag{10}$$

Notice that equations for velocity and acceleration are described by three harmonically related sine or cosine functions preceded by a common multiplier. The following table discloses the composition of the multiplier (Mx) and the sine or cosine amplitude terms (Kx_1, Kx_2, Kx_3) for velocity and acceleration:

	Mx	Kx_1	Kx_2	Kx_3	
V(t):	$4B\Omega/r^2$	A^2	2AB	$1/3B^2$	(11)
A(t):	$4B\Omega^2/r^2$	$A^2+1/4B^2$	2AB	$3/4B^2$	(12)

where:
$$A = 1/2(Rd + Rs), \quad \text{and} \quad B = 1/2(Rd - Rs) \tag{13}$$

Notice that V(t) and A(t) are (mathematically speaking) Fourier expansions of the input function, R(t). Amplitudes of the Fourier components, Kx_1, Kx_2, and Kx_3, are solely determined by diastolic and systolic radii of the ventricle through A and B. In the multiplier reside terms describing ventricular shortening (Rd – Rs), aortic radius (r), and the heart rate dependent contractile frequency of the ventricle (Ω).

An interpretation of these equations would include the strong dependence of aortic flow velocity and acceleration upon heart rate (Ω), aortic radius (r), and ventricular size (Rd) as well as systolic shortening performance (Rd–Rs). Implicit to the multiplier is the Doppler angle cosine Θ.

The shape of V(t) is defined by the harmonically related cosine amplitudes, while overall pulse amplitude is determined by the multiplier. If the goal of ejection pulse analysis is to elucidate systolic ventricular performance, attention must focus upon the Fourier amplitude components Kx_1, Kx_2, and Kx_3, for they are determined solely by the sum and differences of diastolic and systolic ventricular radii. Ratios of these Fourier amplitudes would thus contain ventricular dimensional measurements, but be independent of the traditional Doppler limitations carried in the multiplier; angle, aortic size, and heart rate. The following ratios are defined:

$$\begin{aligned} K_1 &= KV_1/KV_2, \\ K_2 &= KV_2/KV_2, \\ K_3 &= KV_1/KV_3 \end{aligned} \tag{14}$$

The following section presents both theoretical and clinical experience with this mathematical approach to ejection pulse shape analysis.

19.5 Clinical studies

We first sought to elucidate the performance of the above detailed model with physiologic input variables:

$$\begin{aligned} &\text{Rd: 1 cm to 4 cm by 0.2 cm} \\ &\text{Rs: 0.8 cm to (Rd – 0.2) cm by 0.2 cm} \\ &\text{r: 1.2cm} \\ &\text{LVET: 0.1 to 0.34 sec by 0.02 sec} \end{aligned} \tag{15}$$

These input variables were allowed to vary singularly while the others were held constant, so that all permutations and combinations could be evaluated. This large data set simulated the range of ejection pulses observable in small and large ventricles under the various conditions of heart rate and contractile performance that might be experienced during Doppler stress testing.

To illustrate the theoretical superiority of shape analysis over the traditional time domain descriptors of maximal acceleration and peak velocity, three pulses were selected from this data set and plotted in Figure 3. For all pulses, the left ventricular ejection time is 0.3, the aortic radius is 1.2 cm, and ventricular diastolic and systolic radii are variable and recorded in the figure legend. All pulses were selected for maximal accelerations of 16 m/s/s, while peak ejection velocities are quite similar, ranging between 98 and 120 cm/s.

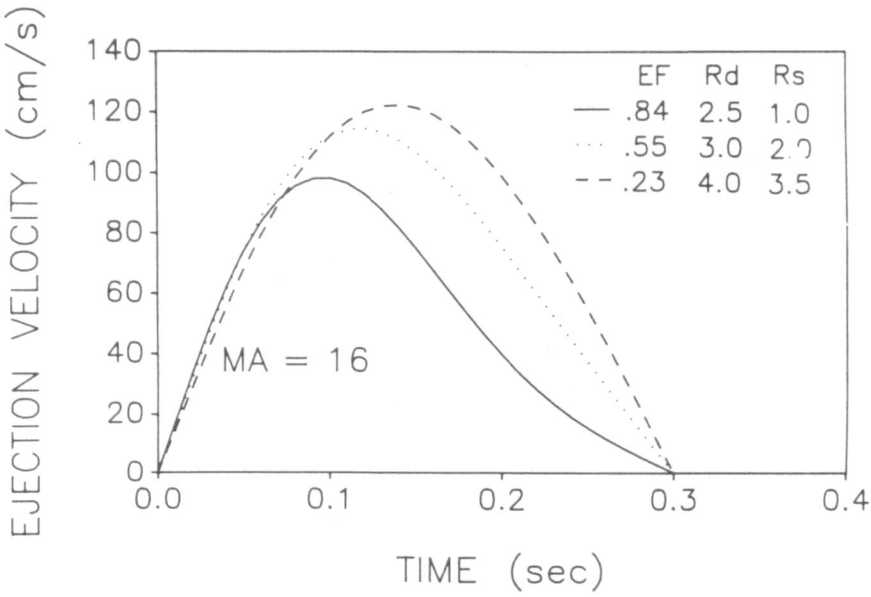

Figure 3. Selected ejection pulses with equivalent maximal accelerations and similar peak velocities generated from spherical model ventricles. Ejection fractions (EF) range from 0.84 to 0.23. The diastolic and systolic radii of spheres generating these pulses are indicated. Note that the shapes of the pulses are dramatically different.

Interestingly, ejection fractions of spherical model ventricles generating these pulses were between 0.84 and 0.23. Even though maximal accelerations were equivalent, shapes of the pulses varied significantly. The high performance ventricle (0.84) achieved peak ejection velocity in the first third of systole, and the deceleration phase of the pulse was concave. The impaired ventricle (0.23) achieved peak ejection velocity in the middle of systole and had a convex downslope. The normally performing ventricle (0.55) had curve contour between these two extremes. The surprising finding of this analysis is that the downslope of the ejection pulse, rather than the upstroke, appears to contain the information disclosing ventricular performance.

We can observe the Fourier frequency mix responsible for these pulse contours by plotting the Fourier sine wave components in Figure 4. The ejection pulse of the high performance ventricle has frequency components rich in second and third order harmonics, while the fundamental frequency is attenuated. On the other hand, the ejection pulse of the impaired ventricle is dominated by first order fre-

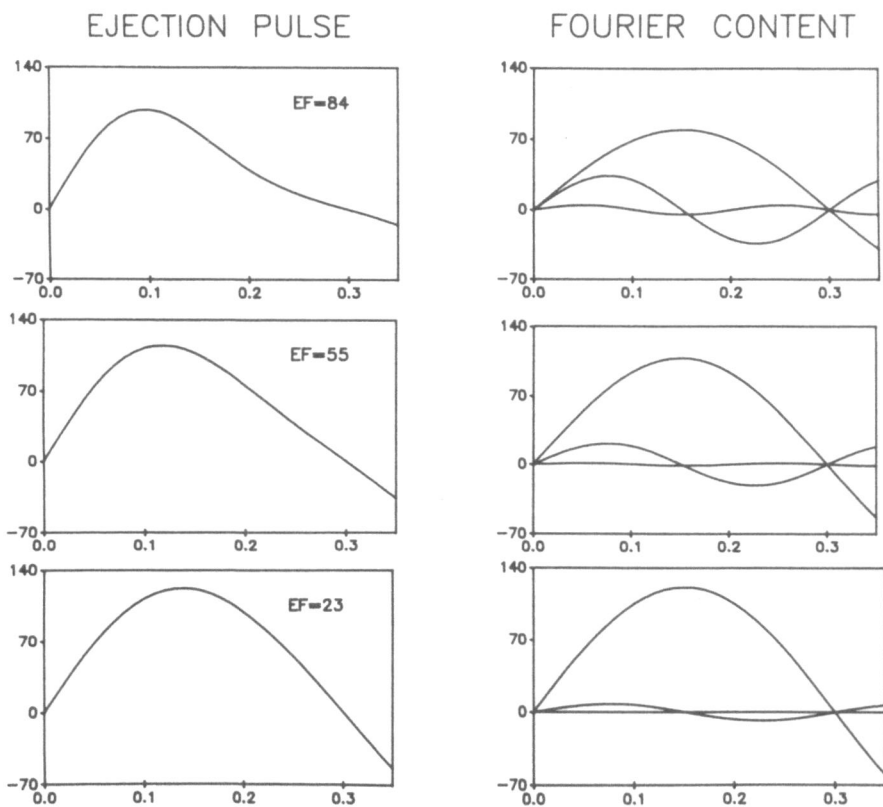

Figure 4. Fourier analysis of ejection pulse shapes depicted in Figure 3. The Fourier content of the EF = 0.84 pulse is dominated by second and third order harmonics, while the frequency content of the EF = 0.23 pulse is dominated by the fundamental frequency. For further discussion, see text. Y axis: velocity in cm/s; X axis: time in seconds.

quencies, with severely attenuated second and third order harmonics. The dependence of the Fourier harmonic amplitudes upon ventricular contractile performance is also illustrated in Figure 5. Notice that decreasing ventricular performance is accompanied by increasing fundamental frequency content in the ejection pulse, while increasing ventricular performance is indicated by increasing second and third order harmonic content.

We then became interested in evaluating the clinical merit of these ejection pulse contour observations. We collected ascending aortic Doppler flow profiles in ten patients with clinical heart failure undergoing resting radionuclear blood pool scanning, and in ten patients with coronary artery disease but no clinical evidence of ventricular dysfunction. Ejection pulses from representative patients appear in

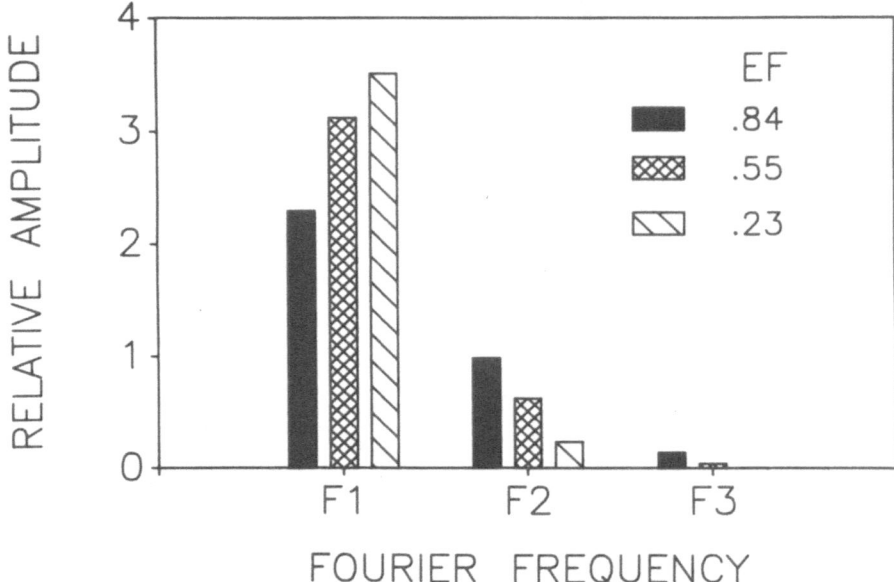

Figure 5. Sine wave amplitudes of Fourier components depicted in Figure 4 are plotted as a function of the Fourier harmonic frequency, F1 to F3. Notice the inverse dependence of fundamental frequency with EF, and direct dependence of EF upon second and third order harmonics.

Figure 6. The first patient has heart failure and a fractional shortening (FS) of 6, but a peak ejection velocity of 1.1 m/s. Notice that the ejection pulse peaks in mid-systole, and the deceleration phase is convex. In contrast, a patient with high normal ventricular performance marked by fractional shortening of 51% and peak velocity of 1.5 m/s has an ejection pulse peak in early systole and a concave deceleration phase. Since time domain observations suggested the validity of our model, we traced pulse envelopes of all 20 patients and proceeded to Fourier shape analysis.

High quality pulses were ensemble averaged over thirty-five cycles using a proprietary AT computer-based signal acquisition system. 1024 point fast Fourier transforms were performed using MATLAB or ILS-PC software [8, 9]. Based upon heart rate dependent omega, the fundamental frequency and its harmonics were identified in the frequency domain. Fourier amplitude ratios as defined in Equation (14) were calculated and plotted in Figure 7. Patients with radionuclear ejection fractions between 19 and 26% are indicated by solid bars, while patients with ejection fractions in the normal range from 45 to 66% are shown by crosshatched bars. All Fourier ratios successfully discriminated patients with abnormal and normal ventricular performance. The hypothesis that poor ventricular function results in ejection pulse contours dominated by the fundamental Fourier frequency (Ω) was supported.

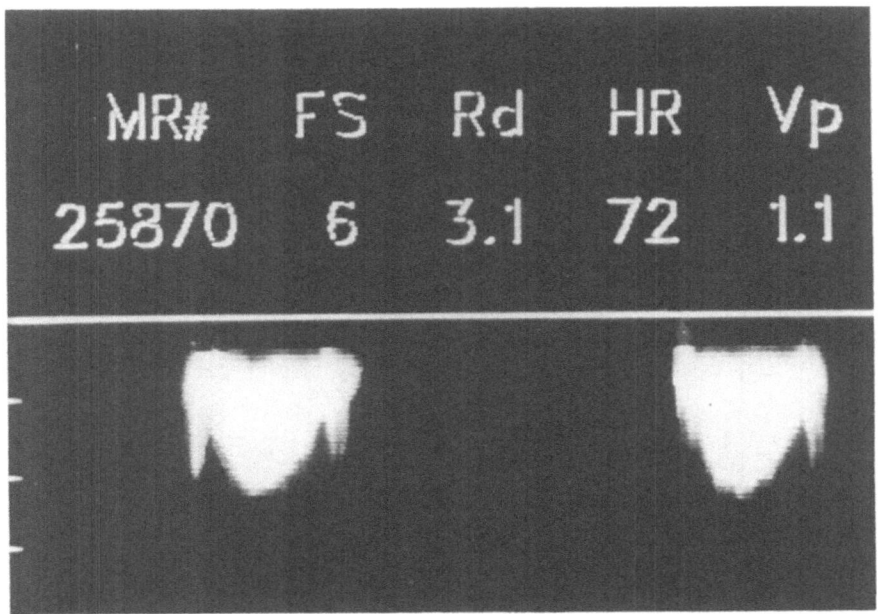

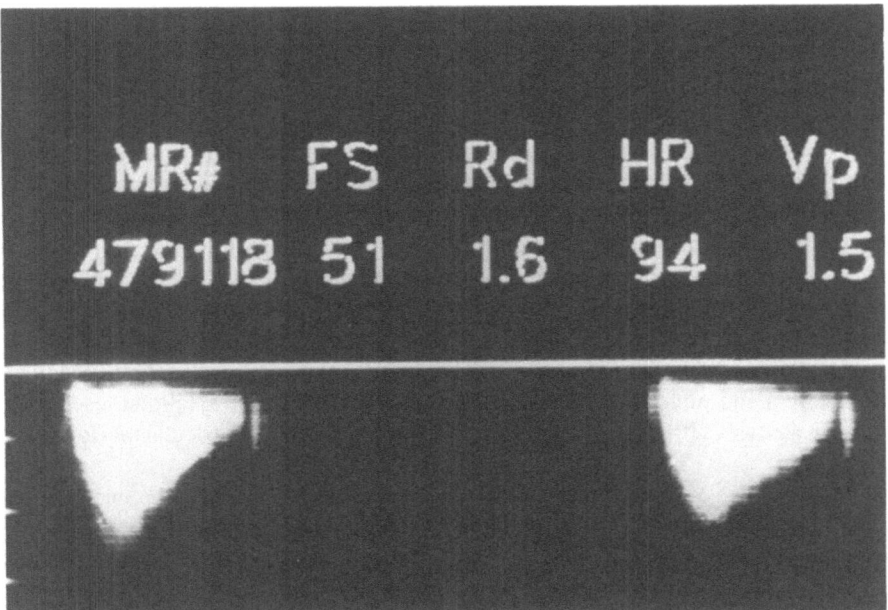

Figure 6. Representative Doppler ejection profiles acquired from the ventricular apex in patients with cardiomyopathy (Panel A) and high normal ventricular performance (Panel B). Medical record numbers (MR), fractional shortening (FS), diastolic radii (Rd), heart rates (HR), and peak ejection velocity values (Vp,M/s) are indicated. Note that pulse shapes of patients with excellent and poor ventricular performance are similar to model pulses depicted in Figure 3.

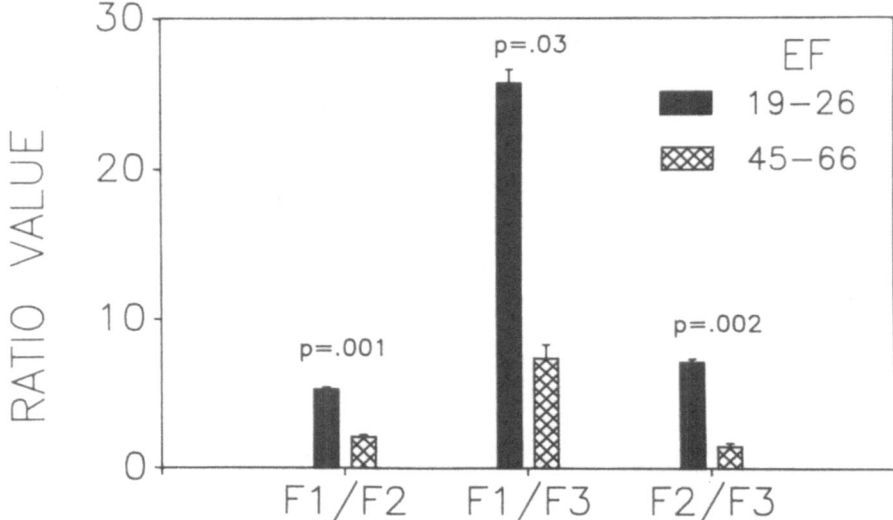

Figure 7. Comparison of Fourier amplitude ratios F1, F2, and F3 (x axis) for patients with poor ventricular performance (EF = 19 to 26: solid bars) versus patients with normal function (EF = 45 to 66: cross-hatched bars). All ratios were statistically successful in discrimination of the two groups. See text discussion.

19. 6 Discussion

The above analyses illustrate the limitations of traditional time domain measurements applied to Doppler ejection pulses. Maximal acceleration and peak velocity are heavily dependent upon heart rate, the size of the aorta, and the size and contractile performance of the ejecting ventricle. Doppler angle scales pulse amplitude in an unknown fashion during each and every clinical study. Successful correlations of peak velocity and acceleration against ejection fraction, Vcf, and dP/dt have unbewittingly relied upon similarities in the approach angles, heart rates, aortic sizes, and ventricular dimensions of patient or animal groups under study. Maximal acceleration and peak velocity evaluate only two points on the ejection pulse, while contour analysis shows that each and every point carries ventricular performance information.

The analyses and data presented here suggest that patients will be encountered who have compensated for contractile impairment by appropriately increasing ventricular size or elevating heart rate, achieving normal maximal acceleration and peak velocity despite low resting ejection fractions. This is, in fact, the case. It is extremely unusual to encounter a clinical echocardiographic study where resting ejection velocity is not between 0.8 and 1.3 m/s (if the aortic valve is normal), even in the most impaired ventricle.

The shape of the Doppler ejection pulse quantified by Fourier analysis is independent of many pitfalls inherent to time domain analysis. Since the scaling multiplier carries the heart rate, Doppler angle, and aortic diameter, the Fourier amplitude components of harmonically related sine waves synthesizing the pulse depend upon diastolic and systolic ventricular dimensions alone. Our preliminary clinical studies do suggest that shape analysis discloses ventricular performance status. Certainly, limitations exist in this first approach to this complex problem.

Assumptions of our model do not consider patients with very compliant aortas, severe aortic valve narrowing with resulting flow turbulence, or regional ventricular wall motion abnormalities. Further studies will be required to validate the shape analysis concept in many types of disease categories under many sets of loading conditions. Moreover, all existing clinical Doppler instrumentation has been developed for time domain measurements, so that new algorithms and processing techniques for shape analysis will require derivation and implementation. The Doppler flow signal is stochastic, and frequently resembles noise. It will be challenging to develop methods for reliable shape analysis considering the quality of signals obtained during the majority of clinical studies. Nonetheless, this theoretical analysis lends credence to the earliest clinical Doppler studies of ascending aortic flow, illustrating the importance of ejection pulse contour in the evaluation of ventricular performance.

References

1. Light LH, Cross G. Cardiovascular data by transcutaneous aortovelography. In: Roberts C (ed.). Blood Flow Measurement. London: Sector Publishing, 1972:60–63.
2. Light LH. Transcutaneous aortovelography. A new window on the circulation. Br Heart J 1976; 38:433–442.
3. Buchtal A, Hanson GC, Peisach AR. Transcutaneous aortovelography, potentially useful technique in management of critically ill patients. Br Heart J 1976; 38:451–456.
4. Sequeira RF, Light LH, Cross G, Raftery EB. Transcutaneous aortovelography. A quantitative evaluation. Br Heart J 1976; 38:443–450.
5. Bilton AH, Brotherhood J, Cross G, Hanson GC, Light LH, Sequeira RF. Transcutaneous aortovelography as a measure of central blood flow. J Physiol 1987; 281:4–5.
6. Light LH, Sequeira RF, Cross G, Bilton A, Hanson GC. Flow-orientated circulatory patient assessment and management using transcutaneous aortovelography, a noninvasive Doppler technique. J Nucl Med All Sci 1979; 23:137–144.
7. Light LH, Cross G. Convenient monitoring of cardiac output and global left ventricular function by transcutaneous aortovelography – an effective alternative to cardiac output measurements. In: Spencer M (ed.). Cardiac Doppler Diagnosis. Boston: Martinus Nijhoff, 1983:69–80.
8. Rabiner LR, Gold B. Theory and Application of Digital Signal Processing. Englewood Cliffs NJ, Prentice-Hall, 1975.
9. Brodersen RW, Hewes CR, Buss DD. A 500 stage CCD transversal filter for spectral analysis. IEEE Trans Electron Dev 1976; ED-23:143–152.

20. The use of color Doppler ultrasound in exercise testing

JOHN W. COOPER and NAVIN C. NANDA
University of Alabama at Birmingham, Birmingham, Alabama, U.S.A.

Vigorous exercise of the large skeletal muscles produces an increase in myocyte oxygen demand which must be satisfied by an increase in cardiac output of up to, or even exceeding, 500% in normal individuals. Since this is accomplished by a combination of increased heart rate and contractile force, myocardial oxygen demand also rises, and this demand, in turn, is satisfied by an increase in blood flow in the coronary arteries. In patients with ischemic heart disease, this increased flow produces a pressure drop distal to any narrowed coronary arterial segment. If this pressure drop is high enough, transient myocardial ischemia will result. Such ischemia causes changes in both electrical and functional properties of the heart muscle, and since these changes may be detected non-invasively in various ways, exercise stress testing has been useful in the detection and assessment of ischemic heart disease since 1931 [1].

Although a fairly wide variety of exercise modes have been employed, the two which are currently the most popular are the upright treadmill and the bicycle ergometer (usually with the patient supine). Each of these methods has its own set of advantages and limitations. With upright treadmill exercise, the oxygen demand is greater because more muscle groups are employed than with the bicycle, and ventilation is improved as well. Also, high work rates can be obtained with less active patient cooperation. This is a more important consideration in America than in other countries where bicycles are a common primary transportation source. On the other hand, the walking patient inherently has more movement artifact than the supine bicycling patient, and venous return is not quite as good, and the exercise induced increase in stroke volume may not be as prominent. In general, while upright treadmill exercise stresses the patient more and is therefore more likely to induce myocardial ischemia, movement artefact precludes intraexercise assessment of many parameters.

With the introduction of imaging ultrasound in the late 1960's came indices of cardiac performance which were of potential use in an exercise setting, although this was limited by the poor anatomic orientation of M-mode echocardiography. With the advent of two-dimensional echocardiography, the use of ultrasound in conjunction with stress electrocardiography began in earnest, and the use of stress echocardiography was demonstrated to improve the rather low sensitivity of stress electrocardiography without interfering with its generally high specificity. Recently, Doppler analysis of blood flow during exercise has been used to supple-

Steve M. Teague (ed.) Stress Doppler Echocardiography, 255–261.

ment the stress ECG and/or echocardiographic findings, and more recently a few studies have been done in this setting using the new modality, color Doppler or Doppler color flow mapping.

20.1 Color Doppler

This is essentially a pulsed Doppler system, but shifts in phase rather than frequency of the reflected sound are considered, and auto-correlation rather than fast Fourier transform analysis is used to manage the phase shift data [2, 3]. This allows a large number of very small sample regions to be sampled, on the order of 256 for each scan line position. Thus, phase shift signals from moving blood cells can be displayed directly on the two-dimensional sector image. These signals are color coded for transducer-relative flow direction, blue representing flow away from and red, flow toward the probe.

A variety of other parameters are displayed along with the basic colors, and these alter flow display appearance in certain predictable ways under certain circumstances. The lighter the color, for example, the higher velocity below the Nyquist limit. Any region of a flow exceeding the Nyquist limit will be seen to alias, as in conventional pulsed Doppler, but this phenomenon appears as a reversal of color in the region exceeding the Nyquist limit. The amplitude, or intensity, of the signals is influenced by the number of reflectors (cells) passing through a sampling region and determines the brightness of the color signal. In most systems the color green is added in proportion to the 'variance' in the flow, which is essentially the same parameter as the degree of 'spectral broadening' in a conventional spectral trace Doppler display.

These elements combine to allow a virtually instantaneous appreciation of blood flow, its direction, its character (whether smooth and normal or disturbed), and within certain limits its velocity, as it moves around within the chambers and vessels of the cardiovascular system.

This aspect of color Doppler allows the potential variation and error in flow pattern sampling mentioned by several authors [4, 5] studying exercise conventional Doppler to be reduced by aiding in confident placement and then maintenance of a conventional Doppler sample volume in a discrete and well defined portion of the flow within a vessel (for example, the region of highest velocity near the center of the lumen in the ascending aorta), guaranteeing that all sampling done will be as consistent and as uniform as possible.

20.2. Exercise induced mitral regurgitation

In addition to providing improved beam steering capability, color Doppler also allows flow parameters other than ejection acceleration and velocity to be used in an exercise setting. Color Doppler is an ideal means for both detecting and assessing the severity of the mitral regurgitation which can occur in the presence of acute myocardial ischemia. This was examined by our group in 1987 [6]. The mode of exercise chosen for this study was supine bicycle ergonometry using a specially designed bicycle table which could be tilted so that the subjects were effectively in 45 degree left decubitus position. Thirty-nine subjects (seventeen normal volunteers and twenty-two patients with angiographically demonstrated coronary disease, none of whom had mitral regurgitation at rest), were exercised to maximum tolerance through a series of increasing work stages. Prior to exercise, a complete cardiac ultrasound examination, including color Doppler, was done. Because of the relative stability of these patients due to the nature of the exercise, a two-dimensional structural and color Doppler examination from the apical position was possible throughout exercise and for three minutes after exercise in each subject, using alternating views of the apical 2 and 4 chamber planes.

Although there was no significant correspondence between the semi-quantitative degree of severity of any exercise induced mitral regurgitation and the severity of the subjects' coronary disease [7], the very occurrence of an exercise induced leak was seen to be a significant indicator of both the presence and the degree of severity of coronary artery disease (Figure 1). As an indication of the existence of disease, this parameter increased the sensitivity of the exercise test from 54% to 59% and the specificity from 88% to 100%. If the development of left ventricular wall motion abnormalities was also taken into consideration, the 100% specificity was retained and the sensitivity further improved to 82%. When the electrographic changes were used in combination with the color Doppler and echocardiographic criteria, the specificity declined to the original 88%, but the sensitivity increased to 91%. Thus, this combination of criteria not only resulted in very high sensitivity and specificity but also in near equality of those indices, an important consideration.

In addition, as mentioned, this study also suggested that the development of mitral regurgitation during exercise can aid in the assessment of disease severity as well. A mitral leak developed in 89% of subjects with 3 vessel disease, in 36% of those with 1 or 2 vessel disease, and in none of the normal subjects. Thus, just over 10% of those subjects with 2 vessel disease or less developed mitral regurgitation, while it was seen in nearly 90% of those with three vessel disease, and only those subjects with coronary artery disease developed it.

20.3 Carotid flow studies

Color Doppler has helped to add another potential sampling site for use in Doppler exercise testing. Occasionally, the suprasternal window is unavailable due to reasons such as patient body habitus or unusual heart position, so the flow in the ascending aorta is difficult or impossible to interrogate. A study done at this center indicates that the common carotid arteries may be used as an alternative when changes in the parameters of volume and velocity are being considered [8].

In this study, twenth-two subjects (ten normal volunteers and twelve patients with a previously established diagnosis of coronary artery disease) underwent

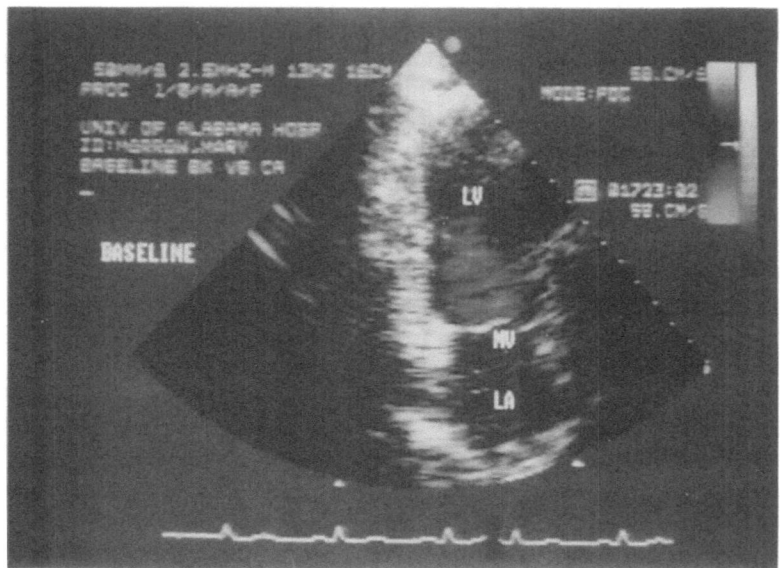

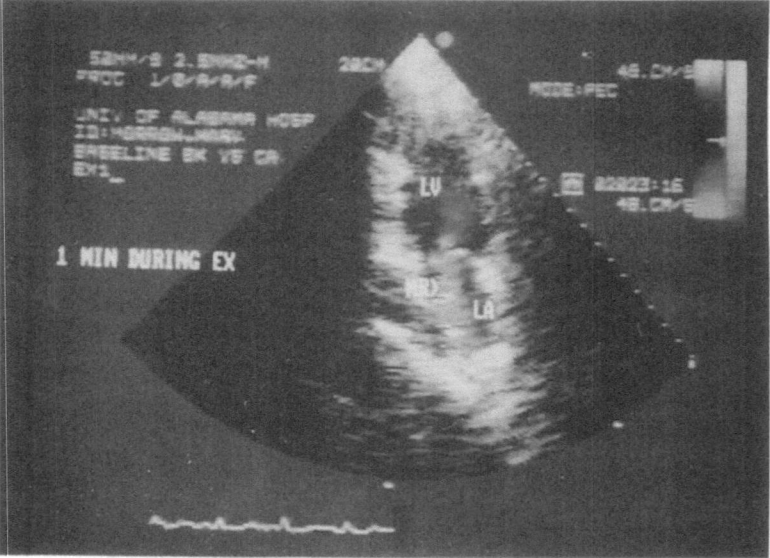

Figure 1. Color Doppler exercise echocardiography. A) The apical four chamber view in an elderly female patient shows no evidence of mitral regurgitation at baseline. B) One minute into the supine bicycle exercise, bluish green signals are visualized originating from the mitral valve (MV) and occupying a large area of the left atrium (LA) indicative of significant mitral regurgitation (MR) resulting from exercise induced myocardial ischemia. LV = left ventricle. Reproduced with permission from: Cooper J, Nanda NC. Exercise conventional, color and carotid Doppler echocardiography. In: Patient decision making in cardiac artery disease: present role and future prospectives of echocardiography. Kluwer Academic Publishers, Dordrecht, the Netherlands, 1989 (in press).

staged exercise during which color guided conventional pulsed Doppler was used to interrogate both the right common carotid artery and left ventricular outflow tract (from the apical position). The mode of exercise used was again supine bicycle ergometry because of the inherently increased patient stability and ease in maintaining transducer position. The ten normal volunteers exhibited a proportional increase in flow velocity and calculated flow volume in both channels. This exercise-induced percentage change in the left ventricular outflow tract velocity was found to be similar to changes in the carotid flow velocity, making it possible to use Doppler interrogation of the carotid artery to monitor changes in stroke volume produced by exercise. An increase in velocity and volume occurred in those patients with documented disease but no resting wall motion abnormalities, but not to the extent seen in the normal cohort. The patients with contractile abnormalities at rest showed a decrease in both parameters in both channels. Since the common carotid artery and its flow is nearly universally available to two-dimensional structural and color Doppler interrogation because of the relative immobility of the neck region during exercise, the proximity of the artery to the transducer, and lack of interposition of obstacles to ultrasound such as lung or bone, it appears to be a viable alternative sampling position when changes in velocity or calculated flow volume are to be considered.

20.4 Limitations to the use of color Doppler

There are two major limitations to the use of color Doppler as a part of an exercise examination. In the first place, the learning curve is long and considerable operator experience is required before the modality can be used reliably in any setting. The relationships of the color control settings to one another are more complex than in conventional Doppler equipment and until the effects of these relationships on the video display are fully understood, the examinations will not be of optimal quality and may be confusing and misleading. The second major limitation is the presence of 'ghosting', an artifact caused by the assignment of color values to moving structures. The resultant display appears as transient sheets or 'flashes' of color splashed across the screen, and although these bear no relation to chamber and vessel contours, they can cause confusion. This type of display is very common during exercise because the heart tends to be hyperdynamic. Adjusting filter, compression, frame rate and pulse repetition frequency settings can help, but experience and familiarity with the equipment and its display are the most important factor in circumventing this limitation.

20.5 Conclusion

The field of exercise color Doppler ultrasound is very new, and few studies have been done. These preliminary studies suggest that it can add important information to a conventional electrocardiographic stress test, and increase sensitivity and the ability to assess severity of coronary artery disease, although specificity may not be much improved. The parameters considered, primarily related to changes in ejection velocity and acceleration during exercise and to the development of mitral regurgitation, all appear useful. Changes in acceleration and the development of mitral regurgitation appear to add the most information. It is also worthy of note that the best results have been achieved using a combination of modalities, each supplementing the others. In the mitral regurgitation study by our group, high sensitivity and specificity were best achieved using a combination of electrocardiographic, echocardiographic and Doppler criteria. Ejection velocity and acceleration were not included in this study as parameters, so it is not known what affect consideration of these additional criteria might have had on overall sensitivity, specificity, and severity assessment. This might be a subject for future consideration.

The use of color Doppler appears to have the additional utility of allowing enhanced appreciation of these parameters by allowing visual guidance to flow interrogation using more conventional Doppler modalities. It also appears to allow quicker acquisition of potential sampling regions such as the left ventricular outflow tract, ascending aorta and the common carotid arteries, and time is an important consideration in an exercise examination.

The studies seem to indicate that while upright treadmill exercise produces the greater degree of work, both because of the larger amount of skeletal muscle involved and because of its increased familiarity (at least to Americans), supine bicycle exercise may also play an important role in the non-invasive evaluation of patients with suspected or proven coronary artery disease. This is not only because of the more stable transducer positions involved but because the use of the cycle allows employment of all of the ultrasound modalities throughout exercise, in addition to before and after. We have found that subjects respond well to encouragement as the work load increases, and are able to achieve and maintain a high degree of performance on the bicycle.

The studies which have been done suggest that color Doppler ultrasound can be a desirable addition to exercise testing in patients with ischemic heart disease.

References

1. Sheffield LT, Exercise stress testing. In: Braunwald E (ed.). Heart Disease: A textbook of cardiovascular medicine. Philadelphia, W.B. Saunders & Co., Harcourt, Brace-Jovanovich, Inc. 1988. pp. 223–242.
2. Nanda NC (ed.). Textbook of color Doppler echocardiography. Philadelphia, Lea & Febiger, 1989.
3. Nanda NC (ed.). Atlas of color Doppler echocardiography. Philadelphia, Lea & Febiger, 1989.
4. Fisher DC, Sahn DJ, Friedman MJ, et al. The effects of variations on pulsed Doppler sampling site on calculations of cardiac output: An experimental study in open-chested dogs. Circulation 1983; 67:370.
5. Louie EK, Maron BJ, Green KJ. Variations in flow-velocity waveforms obtained by pulsed Doppler echocardiography in the normal human aorta. Am J Cardiol 1986;

58:821–826.
6. Zachariah ZP, Hsiung MC, Nanda NC, Kan MN, Gatewood, Jr. RP. Color Doppler assessment of mitral regurgitation induced by supine exercise in ischemic heart disease. Am J Cardiol 1987; 59:1266–70.
7. Helmcke F, Nanda NC, Hsiung MC, Soto B, Adey C, Goyal RG, Gatewood R. Color Doppler assessment of mitral regurgitation with orthogonal planes. Circulation 1987; 75:175.
8. Moos S, Fan P, Chopra HK, Kapur KK, Shah VK, Helmeck F, Oberman A, Nanda NC, University of Alabama at Birmingham, AL. Exercise carotid artery Doppler: A new method to assess cardiac function in coronary artery disease. Clin Res 1989; 37:280A.

Index

Developments in Cardiovascular Medicine

Developments in Cardiovascular Medicine

23. J. Roeland (ed.): *The Practice of M-Mode and Two-dimensional Echocardiography.*
1983   ISBN 90–247–2745–6
24. J. Meyer, P. Schweizer and R. Erbel (eds.): *Advances in Noninvasive Cardiology.*
Ultrasound, Computed Tomography, Radioisotopes, Digital Angiography. 1983
ISBN 0–89838–576–8
25. J. Morganroth and E.N. Moore (eds.): *Sudden Cardiac Death and Congestive Heart
Failure.* Diagnosis and Treatment. Proceedings of the 3rd Symposium on New Drugs
and Devices, held in Philadelphia, Pa., U.S.A. (1982). 1983   ISBN 0–89838–580–6
26. H.M. Perry Jr. (ed.): *Lifelong Management of Hypertension.* 1983
ISBN 0–89838–582–2
27. E.A. Jaffe (ed.): *Biology of Endothelial Cells.* 1984   ISBN 0–89838–587–3
28. B. Surawicz, C.P. Reddy and E.N. Prystowsky (eds.): *Tachycardias.* 1984
ISBN 0–89838–588–1
29. M.P. Spencer (ed.): *Cardiac Doppler Diagnosis.* Proceedings of a Symposium, held in
Clearwater, Fla., U.S.A. (1983). 1983   ISBN 0–89838–591–1
30. H. Villarreal and M.P. Sambhi (eds.): *Topics in Pathophysiology of Hypertension.*
1984   ISBN 0–89838–595–4
31. F.H. Messerli (ed.): *Cardiovascular Disease in the Elderly.* 1984
Revised edition, 1988: see below under Volume 76
32. M.L. Simoons and J.H.C. Reiber (eds.): *Nuclear Imaging in Clinical Cardiology.*
1984   ISBN 0–89838–599–7
33. H.E.D.J. ter Keurs and J.J. Schipperheyn (eds.): *Cardiac Left Ventricular Hyper-
trophy.* 1983   ISBN 0–89838–612–8
34. N. Sperelakis (ed.): *Physiology and Pathology of the Heart.* 1984
Revised edition, 1988: see below under Volume 90
35. F.H. Messerli (ed.): *Kidney in Essential Hypertension.* Proceedings of a Course, held
in New Orleans, La., U.S.A. (1983). 1984   ISBN 0–89838–616–0
36. M.P. Sambhi (ed.): *Fundamental Fault in Hypertension.* 1984   ISBN 0–89838–638–1
37. C. Marchesi (ed.): *Ambulatory Monitoring.* Cardiovascular System and Allied
Applications. Proceedings of a Workshop, held in Pisa, Italy (1983). 1984
ISBN 0–89838–642–X
38. W. Kupper, R.N. MacAlpin and W. Bleifeld (eds.): *Coronary Tone in Ischemic Heart
Disease.* 1984   ISBN 0–89838–646–2
39. N. Sperelakis and J.B. Caulfield (eds.): *Calcium Antagonists.* Mechanism of Action
on Cardiac Muscle and Vascular Smooth Muscle. Proceedings of the 5th Annual
Meeting of the American Section of the I.S.H.R., held in Hilton Head, S.C., U.S.A.
(1983). 1984   ISBN 0–89838–655–1
40. Th. Godfraind, A.G. Herman and D. Wellens (eds.): *Calcium Entry Blockers in
Cardiovascular and Cerebral Dysfunctions.* 1984   ISBN 0–89838–658–6
41. J. Morganroth and E.N. Moore (eds.): *Interventions in the Acute Phase of Myocardial
Infarction.* Proceedings of the 4th Symposium on New Drugs and Devices, held in
Philadelphia, Pa., U.S.A. (1983). 1984   ISBN 0–89838–659–4
42. F.L. Abel and W.H. Newman (eds.): *Functional Aspects of the Normal, Hyper-
trophied and Failing Heart.* Proceedings of the 5th Annual Meeting of the American
Section of the I.S.H.R., held in Hilton Head, S.C., U.S.A. (1983). 1984
ISBN 0–89838–665–9

Developments in Cardiovascular Medicine

Developments in Cardiovascular Medicine

Developments in Cardiovascular Medicine

Developments in Cardiovascular Medicine